Consciousness and Self-Regulation

Advances in Research and Theory

VOLUME 2

Consciousness and Self-Regulation

Advances in Research and Theory

VOLUME 2

Edited by
GARY E. SCHWARTZ
Yale University

and
DAVID SHAPIRO
University of California, Los Angeles

PLENUM PRESS · NEW YORK AND LONDON

Library of Congress Cataloging in Publication Data

Main entry under title:

Consciousness and self-regulation.

Includes bibliographical references and index.
1. Consciousness. 2. Self-control. I. Schwartz, Gary E., 1944-
II. Shapiro, David, 1924-
BF311.C64   153   76-8907
ISBN 0-306-33602-2

© 1978 Plenum Press, New York
A Division of Plenum Publishing Corporation
227 West 17th Street, New York, N.Y. 10011

Printed in the United States of America

Dedication

This volume is dedicated to the memory of Professor A. R. Luria, a pioneer in the field of neuropsychology and its application to fundamental problems of human consciousness and self-regulation. Professor Luria combined the unique skills and gifts of a critical researcher, comprehensive theorist, and creative and caring clinician. His concern for patterning of neuropsychological processes and the dynamic, interactive nature of complex functional systems in the brain has provided an important model for linking mind, body, and behavior to the central nervous system. We believe that history will place Professor Luria among the small group of eminent, interdisciplinary biobehavioral scientists as exemplified by William James.

Contributors

GYÖRGY ÁDÁM, Department of Comparative Physiology, Eötvös Loránd University, Budapest, Hungary

BERNARD C. GLUECK, Research Department, Institute of Living, Hartford, Connecticut

RUBEN C. GUR, Department of Psychology, University of Pennsylvania, Philadelphia, Pennsylvania

A. R. LURIA, Late of the Department of Sociology, University of Moscow, Moscow, USSR

WESLEY C. LYNCH, John B. Pierce Foundation Laboratory, New Haven, Connecticut

F. J. McGUIGAN, Performance Research Laboratory, University of Louisville, Louisville, Kentucky

MARTIN T. ORNE, Unit for Experimental Psychiatry, The Institute of Pennsylvania Hospital and University of Pennsylvania, Philadelphia, Pennsylvania

KENNETH S. POPE, Department of Psychiatry, University of California, San Francisco, California

LARRY E. ROBERTS, Department of Psychology, McMaster University, Hamilton, Ontario, Canada

JUDITH RODIN, Department of Psychology, Yale University, New Haven, Connecticut

HAROLD A. SACKEIM, Department of Psychology, Columbia University, New York, New York

UWE SCHURI, Max-Planck-Institut für Psychiatrie, München, West Germany viii

JEROME L. SINGER, Department of Psychology, Yale University, New Haven, Connecticut

CHARLES F. STROEBEL, Research Department, Institute of Living, Hartford, Connecticut

STUART K. WILSON, Unit for Experimental Psychiatry, The Institute of Pennsylvania Hospital and University of Pennsylvania, Philadelphia, Pennsylvania

Preface

The first and foremost concrete fact which every one will affirm to belong to his inner experience is the fact that consciousness of some sort goes on.[1]
—William James, 1893

We are witnessing today a mounting interest among behavioral and biological scientists in problems long recognized as central to our understanding of human nature, yet until recently considered out of the bounds of scientific psychology and physiology. Sometimes thrown into the heading of "altered states of consciousness," this growing research bears directly upon such time-honored questions as the nature of conscious experience, the mind–body relationship, and volition. If one broadly views this research as encompassing the two interrelated areas of consciousness and self-regulation, one can find many relevant contemporary examples of creative and experimentally sophisticated approaches, including research on the regulation of perception and sensory experience, attention, imagery and thinking, emotion and pain; hypnosis and meditation; biofeedback and voluntary control; hemispheric asymmetry and specialization of brain function; drug-induced subjective states; and biological rhythms. Because the material is spread over many different kinds of publications and disciplines, it is difficult for any one person to keep fully abreast of the significant advances. The overall aim of the new Plenum Series in *Consciousness and Self-Regulation: Advances in Research* is to provide a scholarly forum for discussing integration of these diverse areas by presenting some of the best current research and theory.

It is our hope that these volumes will enable investigators to

[1] William James, *Psychology: Briefer Course* (New York: Henry Holt and Company, 1893), p. 152.

become more well-rounded in related areas of research, as well as provide advanced students with a ready means of obtaining up-to-date, state-of-the-art information about relevant problems, theories, methods, and findings. By selecting significant developments in theory and research, we also hope that over the years the series can help legitimate the field as a scientific venture as well as delineate critical issues for further investigation.

Psychology and biology are going through a reawakening, and research on the issues to which this series is devoted is helping to bring these fields closer together. History tells us that Wundt founded psychology as the science of consciousness, and James expanded it to encompass "such things as sensations, desires, emotions, cognitions, reasonings, decisions, volitions and the like."[2] But these ideals could not be achieved, or so it seemed, and psychology turned away from questions of experience and volition, as well as from biology, and was replaced with behaviorism. The transformation was arduous, and it required a certain allowance for inconsistency. For example, Edmund Jacobson, one of the pioneers in the psychophysiology of higher mental processes, recalled, "Lashley told me with a chuckle that when he and Watson would spend an evening together, working out principles of behaviorism, much of the time would be devoted to introspection."[3]

In *William James: Unfinished Business* (1969), Mandler summarized the good points, and the bad points, of this era of psychology in his "Acceptance of Things Past and Present: A Look at the Mind and the Brain." He aptly noted:

> I think the Watsonian behaviorist development was inevitable—I think it was even healthy—if we learn not to do it again. Watson and the behaviorists did, once and for all, clean up the problem of the proper data language for psychology. In that sense, we are all behaviorists. The behaviorists inveighed against an establishment which imported theoretical notions and hypotheses into purely descriptive realms of psychology. They successfully excluded vague notions about the causes of behavior— the introspective statements—from the facts of psychology. But in the process the Watsonians felt called upon to do the reverse and to remove complex and imaginative models from psychology. . . . Behaviorism has been one of the most antitheoretical movements in science. . . .

[2] Ibid., p. 1.
[3] Jacobson, "Electrophysiology of Mental Activities and Introduction to the Psychological Process of Thinking." In F. J. McGuigan and R. A. Schoonover (Eds.), *The Psychophysiology of Thinking* (New York: Academic Press, 1973), p. 14.

> . . . I submit that it was this antitheoretical stance that prevented any close attention to physiology. . . . If the mechanisms we postulate are "like" physiological mechanisms, then we will have heeded James in modern terms. But if we are, as we were, afraid to postulate complex mental mechanisms, we will never find the corresponding complex physiological mechanisms.[4]

This series is dedicated to William James, emphasizing the integration and patterning of multiple processes, coupled with the most significant advances in methodology and knowledge. Some of the chapters will be broad-based and theoretical; others will focus on specific research problems or applications. Inclusion of material in all cases is determined by the investigator's focus on or concern with consciousness and related processes, whether in normal or in abnormal populations. While the editors have a decided bias toward biologically oriented approaches to consciousness and self-regulation, papers that deal primarily with cognition or self-report are included when of particular significance to these topics. Since important findings in this area are often derived from the study of clinical populations and are of direct relevance to the assessment and treatment of psychological and psychophysiological disorders, chapters dealing with basic research are interwoven with chapters of more clinical concern. In this way it is hoped that the series can provide a fertile interchange between the basic and applied sides of this area. To help the reader understand the perspective and rationale for the diverse selections comprising a given volume, a brief overview of each volume is presented by the editors.

The impetus for and organization of the series grows out of student response to our interdisciplinary seminars at Harvard on the psychophysiology of consciousness, emotion, and self-regulation, coupled with the enthusiasm and support of Seymour Weingarten, Executive Editor of Plenum. Their input, and prodding, is gratefully acknowledged.

GARY E. SCHWARTZ
DAVID SHAPIRO

---

[4] G. Mandler, "Acceptance of Things Past and Present: A Look at the Mind and the Brain." In R. B. MacLeod (Ed.), *William James: Unfinished Business* (Washington, D.C. American Psychological Association, 1969), pp. 13, 14.

Overview of Volume 2

In "The Human Brain and Conscious Activity," A. R. Luria defines consciousness as the "ability to assess sensory information, to respond to it with critical thoughts and actions, and to retain memory traces in order that past traces or actions may be used in the future." Drawing heavily from the Soviet work of Vygotskii, Luria argues that consciousness is a complex neuropsychological structural system with semantic function. Insights from observations with patients having brain damage in selective regions lead Luria to the conclusion that "all attempts to seek some special formation or some special cell group in the brain as the 'organ of consciousness' are meaningless from the very beginning." Luria illustrates how "localization of a symptom" does not by any means imply "localization of a function." Rather, Luria illustrates in great detail how the three major functional systems of the brain—involving subcortical structures, sensorimotor cortex, and frontal cortex—interact in unique ways to create the emergent experience of consciousness.

The relationship between sensory, cognitive, and motor processes in consciousness is illustrated in the chapter by F. J. McGuigan on "Imagery and Thinking: Covert Functioning of the Motor System." McGuigan presents the thesis that much of ongoing thought involves the cortical regulation of motor processes, which can be seen at the periphery by the recording of small changes in patterned muscle activity. The role of bodily processes in thought have been noted by such eminent researchers as Titchener, Watson, Jacobson, and Hebb, but according to McGuigan, some of the strongest statements of this position are to be found in the Russian literature, for example, by Sechenov, who held that "all the endless diversity of the external manifestations of the activity of the brain can be finally regarded as one phenomenon—that of muscular movement . . . therefore, all the external manifestations of brain activity can be attributed to muscular movement." Furthermore, he held that "the time must come when people will be able to analyze the external manifestations of the activity of the brain just as easily as the physicist now analyzes a musical chord or the phenomena presented by a falling body." McGuigan discusses four methodological criteria for evaluating somatic concomitants during the "silent performance of various types of cognitive tasks" and critically reviews the available research in six categories: (1) problem solving, (2) imagination, (3) silent reading, (4) speech perception, (5) learning, and (6) sleep–dreams. McGuigan concludes with a detailed analysis of the possible role of "oral" and "nonoral" motor activity as feedback to the brain of its cognitive processes.

Kenneth S. Pope and Jerome L. Singer, in their chapter on "Regulation of the Stream of Consciousness: Toward a Theory of Ongoing Thought," illustrate how the material of consciousness has long been present in the arts and sciences, yet until very recently has received "rough treatment at the hands of twentieth-century American psychology." In an attempt to identify and discuss some of the fundamental factors that regulate our moment-to-moment awareness, Pope and Singer discuss 10 interrelated areas of research, including work on the bias favoring sensory input; the effects of predictable, dull, or barren environments; the matching function; and the set toward internal processing. Pope and Singer view the brain as a "continually active working organ," seeking and selecting external stimuli and generating its own. Pope and Singer are careful to emphasize the important role that emotion plays in modulating conscious experience. Based on the theory of Silvan Tomkins, they view emotion as a neuropsychological motivational system. A number of methods for studying the nature of ongoing thought are illustrated, including the use of lateral eye movements to examine possible hemispheric differences in the processing and regulation of verbal and spatial imagery.

The capacity of the brain to process and respond to information that it is not consciously aware of is addressed in the chapter by Harold A. Sackeim and Ruben C. Gur on "Self-Deception, Self-Confrontation, and Consciousness." Sackeim and Gur develop the thesis that the brain's tendency to consciously register information from the outside environment, or consciously perceive its own cognitions and beliefs, is in part determined by motivational factors. Drawing on the clinical literature of defense mechanisms and depression, Sackeim and Gur relate these ideas to the experimental social psychology literature on self-deception and self-confrontation. Building upon the fact that self-confrontation is often aversive and leads to increased physiological responding, Sackeim and Gur describe the results of a creative experiment demonstrating that the subject's autonomic reactions more closely mirror the presence or absence of a relevant stimulus (in their case, the auditory presentation of the subject's name) than the subject's conscious perception of the stimuli. Sackeim and Gur illustrate that this research meets four necessary criteria for arguing that self-deception is "an experimentally real phenomenon." They conclude that parallels between the research on self-deception and repression and current work on lateralization of brain function provide a possible direction for future work on the mechanisms underlying these effects.

György Ádám, in his chapter "Visceroception, Awareness, and Behavior," deals with a related problem in the area of consciousness, the perception of visceral activity. Ádám argues that although much of the feedback emanating from the viscera does not result in conscious sensations, this feedback nonetheless can modulate ongoing behavior and electrical activity of the brain. Furthermore, these effects appear to depend on specific parameters of the feedback. For example, Ádám presents data from his laboratory in Hungary suggesting that "under physiological conditions a weak train of impulses (below the viscero-somatic threshold) elicits synchronization and sleep, a more intense train evokes arousal." After reviewing a series of studies on learned discrimination of visceral feedback, Ádám hypothesizes that conditioning procedures can be used to render unconscious visceral stimuli conscious. In one experiment, using female subjects, stimulation of the cervix uteri using a verbal feedback procedure not only led to increased awareness of these sensations but also appeared to be effective in the treatment of some cases of infertility. Recognizing both the theoretical and the practical implications of this work, Ádám concludes that "we must be extremely careful and cautious . . . the application in therapy of any visceral learning procedure must be preceded not only by intensive research in this field but also by careful investigation of human typology (personality)."

The interaction of visceral feedback, perception, and self-regulation is discussed in the chapter by Judith Rodin on "Stimulus-Bound Behavior and Biological Self-Regulation: Feeding, Obesity, and External Control." According to Rodin, "One challenge of contributing to this series is that it provides the incentive to try to reconceptualize work on the eating behavior of humans in terms of consciousness and self-regulation. In animals, eating is one behavioral component of long-term weight regulation and energy balance and, as such, is part of an exquisitely precise biological feedback system. However, in humans, eating often occurs for reasons other than the regulation and maintenance of body weight, and thus the biologically determined system can be overcome or at least disturbed." Rodin describes a series of ingenious experiments that investigate how external stimulation of relevant food cues differentially influences the regulation of eating behavior in obese and normal subjects and, furthermore, how obese and normal subjects differ in their response to other stimuli in the environment (e.g., distractors). Interestingly, these relationships do not seem change when obese subjects lose weight *per se*. Rather, Rodin argues, for example, that "While obese dieters continued to find sweet-tasting substances more palatable than normals after weight loss, obese patients who lost weight as the result of surgical reduction of their intestine began to show responsiveness to sweet taste that essentially resembled normal weight curves." Rodin provides an extensive review of current studies on the role of various neurophysiological feedback mechanisms in the regulation of eating behavior in animals and man and their relationship to conscious processes.

The complexities involved in the study and understanding of self-regulation of autonomic processes, especially in animals, is addressed in the chapter by Larry E. Roberts on "Operant Conditioning of Autonomic Responses: One Perspective on the Curare Experiments." Writing from the perspective of learning theory, Roberts has prepared an extensive chapter whose major goal is to "review recent efforts to obtain operant conditioning of autonomic responses in the curarized rat and to consider the interpretation of the original studies that seems to be necessitated by repeated failures to obtain learning." A further goal is to "discuss the implications of these developments for the study of operant autonomic conditioning and self-regulation." Roberts illustrates how the initial theoretical impetus for using the curarized rat preparation as a means of studying visceral learning was oversimplified and incorrect. Furthermore, he illustrates how "the more important reason for the impact of the curare literature on research biofeedback concerns the rather remarkable properties that were evidenced by visceral operants in the curarized rat." Roberts argues that the initial enthusiasm for the seemingly powerful and selective learning seen in the curarized rat blinded researchers to the tremendous complexities involved in conducting, interpreting, and replicating these findings. Based on an extensive presentation of a series of studies conducted in his laboratory as well as in others, Roberts concludes that "The phenomena reported in these experiments are unlikely to have been a product of learning and provide little if any information pertaining to the plasticity and organization of the autonomic nervous system." Roberts speculates on how inadvertent experimenter bias may have influenced the early studies and cites a similar example from a colleague whose enthusiasm for an initial discovery led him to fail to question the adequacy of the methods used until subsequent failures of replication emerged.

The question of visceral self-regulation is addressed further by Wesley C. Lynch and Uwe Schuri in their chapter on "Acquired Control of Peripheral Vascular Responses." Lynch and Schuri review the basic anatomy and physiology of the peripheral vasomotor system with special interest in uncovering "particular variables that may inadvertently affect vascular response, making the results of psychological studies difficult to assess." These authors review the literature on acquired self-regulation from the perspective of learning theory, evaluating the classical and instrumental approaches to visceral learning. The interaction of awareness and learning is shown to exist within the classical conditioning paradigm, but the authors question whether the results reflect the role of consciousness *per se*, or whether awareness interacts with motivation and thereby influences vasomotor learning. Data on vasomotor self-regulation using biofeedback procedures are also reviewed and critically evaluated. Whereas studies by Lynch and Schuri themselves failed to obtain vasomotor self-control in adults, the authors do present positive results in children. However, Lynch and Schuri suggest that these observed changes in vasomotor activity were secondary to learned control of hand isometric-muscle tension. They conclude that much is to be learned about the mechanisms by which persons can learn to self-regulate vasomotor activity and about the limitations of this control.

Martin T. Orne and Stuart K. Wilson, in their chapter "On the Nature of Alpha Feedback Training," raise similar theoretical and practical issues with regard to the learned self-regulation of EEG alpha rhythms. Orne and Wilson critically evaluate the early observations of Brown and Kamiya suggesting that alpha biofeedback training was associated with pleasant, relaxed feelings. They seriously question whether alpha biofeedback is a "method by which modern man might achieve direct control over his anxiety and dysphoria," and they evaluate "the disparate scientific observations that made this dream plausible." Based on a detailed presentation of their own series of studies on the regulation of EEG alpha, as well as a review of the findings of other investigators, Orne and Wilson conclude that many of the initial assumptions about the relationship of alpha abundance to subjective state and their mechanisms of self-regulation are incorrect. Regarding potential clinical applications, Orne and Wilson suggest that "once novelty and visuomotor effects are eliminated, alpha augmentation may be the product of relaxation in one individual and hyperarousal in another, while a third may show little relationship between subjective state and alpha density." Emphasizing the need for a closer scrutiny of individual differences, Orne and Wilson suggest potential directions for future EEG biofeedback research, including the need to examine specialized areas of the brain and the patterning of physiological changes. They conclude that "A new integration of basic neurophysiological and neuropsychological perspectives may yet permit a more scientifically mature and fruitful second approach to the use of this elusive method of interacting with man's neurophysiological self."

Charles F. Stroebel and Bernard C. Glueck compare and contrast EEG and other types of biofeedback with meditation training in the regulation of stress in their chapter "Passive Meditation: Subjective, Clinical, and Electrographic Comparison with Biofeedback." Their chapter is based on a summary of studies that they have conducted since 1970 of a "variety of self-responsibility techniques that alter consciousness to create states that are incompatible with the fight-or-flight response to stress." For example, based on an analysis of reaction times of different physiological parameters, Stroebel and Glueck conclude that "parallel proprioception (biofeedback) probably should not be instantaneous; instead, a time lag should be introduced into the extrinsic feedback circuit that is suitable for the function in question." After reviewing research on various biofeedback and meditation techniques, they discuss their findings on the use of transcendental meditation with psychiatric inpatients and the problems of differential dropout rates in various self-regulation therapies. They emphasize that whereas "compliance is very high for EMG-thermal biofeedback applied to *specific* psychosomatic problems where symptom relief is self-reinforcing, as in reduction of headache pain, compliance is much lower for conditions with relatively "silent" symptoms, such as hypertension."

Stroebel and Glueck present preliminary data suggesting that there are EEG similarities and differences between various types of relaxation procedures. They speculate that "during passive meditation, the usual affective outflow from limbic structures is diminished with enhanced transmission of signals between the hemispheres via the corpus callosum or other commissures." Stroebel and Glueck conclude by arguing that "we need to recognize more widely that there is a large domain of our physiological functioning that is responsive to behavioral stimuli, is potentially adaptive, and is vulnerable to disregulation (Schwartz, 1977) as well as voluntary self-regulation. This behaviorally modifiable physiological domain is becoming known as behavioral medicine in formal recognition of the interaction of physiology and behavior."

Contents

4   Self-Deception, Self-Confrontation, and
Consciousness   139

HAROLD A. SACKEIM AND RUBEN C. GUR

8   Acquired Control of Peripheral Vascular Responses   321

Wesley C. Lynch and Uwe Schuri

9   On the Nature of Alpha Feedback Training   359

Martin T. Orne and Stuart K. Wilson

10   Passive Meditation: Subjective, Clinical, and Electrographic Comparison with Biofeedback   401

Charles F. Stroebel and Bernard C. Glueck

1 *The Human Brain and Conscious Activity*

A. R. Luria

I

The relationship between consciousness and the brain, never absent from the pages of the philosophical and psychological literature, has become the topic of particularly active discussion in recent decades. It has been the subject not only of individual investigations but also of complete major international symposia, attended by the leading representatives of psychology, neurology, and physiology[1]; eminent neurophysiologists, morphologists, and clinicians return to it time and time again.

This revival of the problem of the brain mechanisms of consciousness can be attributed to a whole group of factors. First, its discussion has been reinvigorated by advances in neurosurgery and psychopharmacology, which have made possible observations on fluctuations of sleep and wakefulness during actual brain operations and active interference with human conscious behavior. Second, the revival of interest in this problem is intimately connected with the impetus given to investigation of levels of wakefulness by the discovery of the brain-stem reticular formation, by action upon which it is possible to raise or lower the state of wakefulness of an animal, and the development of microelectrode techniques, by means of which action potentials can be recorded from discrete groups of neurons, whereby it is possible to study how these groups of neurons (or even single

[1] The relations between the brain and consciousness have been examined in books such as those by Sherrington (1934, 1940) and Eccles (1953) and also in the proceedings of international symposia, including: "Brain Mechanisms and Consciousness" (directed by E. Adrian, F. Bremer, and H. Jasper), Oxford (1954), "The Nature of Sleep" (directed by G. Wolstenholme and M. O'Connor), London (1960); "Mechanisms of the Brain" and "Progress in Brain Research" (directed by G. Moruzzi, A. Fessard, and H. Jasper), Amsterdam (1963), and finally, "Brain and Conscious Experience" (directed by J. Eccles), Berlin (1966).

A. R. Luria · Late of the Department of Sociology, University of Moscow, Moscow, USSR.

1

neurons) respond to information reaching the animal and what artificially evoked sensations or emotions arise during their stimulation.

However, a factor of special importance in this revival of discussion of relations between the brain and consciousness was that despite great interest in this problem, it remained just as unclear as ever and its solution still eluded the investigator's grasp.

The reason for the difficulties hindering the solution of this problem lay largely in the mainly theoretical approach to consciousness that determined the course of all the principal attempts to find its "brain mechanisms." Following the traditions of classical idealistic philosophy, formulated by Ernst Mach at the beginning of this century, physiologists and neurologists when discussing the problem of relations between brain and consciousness persisted in understanding consciousness as a primary subjective quality, incapable of further subdivision, that a person experiences directly and in relation to which the outside world is secondary, a reality derived from consciousness. "Because conscious experience is the immediate and absolute reality, it is necessary that I base my account of it on my own experience, adopting a purely personal or egocentric method of presentation, which may be called methodological solipsism," wrote the eminent physiologist Eccles. ". . . it is only because of and through my experience that I come to know of a world of things and events . . . this external world has the status of a second-order or derivative reality" (Eccles, 1966, pp. 315–316). The positions adopted by some authors have led them to make the remarkable statement that: "Even today we still have to retain Plato's ideas on conscious events as different from everything that takes place in the outside world" (Kneale, 1962).

Such a definition of consciousness as a directly perceived primary reality naturally compels the investigator to turn to the fundamental question that determines the direction of his efforts: What corresponds in the nervous system to this primary subjective experience? Where, in what part of the brain, does the subjective quality that constitutes the basis of consciousness first appear? What nerve cells or structures can be regarded as its carriers? It is thus quite clear why all the efforts of those investigators who, as one of them had stated, "grew up in the traditions of Mach's philosophy" (R. Granit, 1966) are directed not toward analysis of the historical quality of consciousness, examination of the basic forms of conscious reflection of the world, and description of its complex, changing structure but toward finding mechanisms of consciousness inside the brain, distinguishing the brain formations or neuronal structures by stimulation of which the simplest manifestations of conscious experiences could be obtained or by the destruction of which the quality of "subjective experience" could be removed from human behavior.

These searches for the brain mechanisms of consciousness "without quality" have assumed a different character in the hands of different workers. Some have directed their attention to the reticular formation in the brain stem. Its isolation from the cortex causes the subject to lose consciousness and to fall into deep sleep. On the basis of this fact, it is postulated that it is not the cerebral cortex (destruction of which can disturb certain forms of behavior but never leads to the loss of consciousness and never produces "direct" subjective experience) but the "centrencephalic system" located in the depth of the brain that is the true brain organ of conscious experience (Penfield, 1958, 1966). Other workers, not content with a description of the function of whole brain systems, have directed their efforts toward the analysis of single neurons, and profiting by recent advances in microelectrode techniques, they have begun to look for tiny synaptic formations, action upon which either leads to the appearance of very simple subjective states or converts indefinite and random forms of motion of molecules into organized, orderly systems characterizing the appearance of the events of consciousness (Eccles, 1953, 1966; Gomes, see Eccles, 1966). Finally, a third group of workers, considering that consciousness is always a single entity and cannot be separated or divided, has begun to look for neuronal systems that determine the unity of brain activity and whose destruction leads unavoidably to the disintegration of conscious experience (see Sperry, 1966), or they abandon concrete investigations of the brain and build cybernetic models that lend themselves to the postulating of "metaorganized" systems that control the course of all other processes and determine the unity, the self-estimation, and the self-regulation that characterize the state of consciousness (MacKay, 1966).

There are no grounds for supposing that the efforts of neurologists and physiologists, so diverse in their character, will not yield as by-products discoveries of the utmost importance: the theory of the reticular formation, facts showing the high specialization of functions of single neurons, new data on the structure of synapses, descriptions of the subject's responses to stimulation of various parts of the brain, experiments involving separation of the two hemispheres by complete division of the fibers of the corpus callosum—all these are among the extremely important achievements of modern neurology and neurophysiology. However, we must recognize that all these investigations leave the question of the cerebral basis of conscious activity completely unsolved and that—as has frequently been pointed out—we know just as little about the relations between consciousness of the brain today as we did in the past.

II

Why is it that these tremendous efforts by leading specialists in neurology and physiology, which have yielded such a mass of new information, have proved so unproductive as regards the solution of this fundamental problem?

Failure can confidently be attributed to a mistaken approach to the underlying theoretical problem and, hence, misdirection of the basic search.

Is consciousness really a primary state, without quality, given to each one of us directly? Is it a simple and indivisible state, devoid of all history, in the course of which it could be formed gradually? Must consciousness in fact be understood as a primary "inner state" and must its roots be sought inside the organism, in the depths of the "mind" or in the neuronal structures of the brain?

All that we know from the development of modern materialistic science and from the basic propositions of modern materialistic philosophy compels us to express grave misgivings on this matter and to adopt a different, opposite standpoint.

Consciousness never was a primary "inner state" of living matter; psychological processes arose not "inside" the living cell but in its relations with the surrounding medium, on the boundary between the organism and the outside world, and it assumed the forms of active reflection of the outside world that characterize every vital activity of the organism. As the form of life became more complex, with a change in the mode of existence and with the development of a more complex structure of organisms, these forms of interaction with the environment or of active reflection changed; however, the basic features of this reflection, as well as its basic forms as established in the process of social history, must be sought not within the nervous system but in the relations toward reality that are established in successive stages of historical development.

Despite the rapid development of modern ethology—the science of the basic forms of animal behavior—we still know very little about the laws on which their psychological activity is based; however, the fact that the character of behavior of animals depends on their mode of life rather than on the structure of their nervous system, so well known to ethologists, and the fact that different ecological conditions can lead to the development of different forms of behavior in animals of closely similar species, or that behavior of similar structure can be seen in animals with different types of nervous system (a description of the types of behavior of animals with a "hunting" or a passive, "gathering" mode of life was given many years ago by Buitendijk and more recently by ethologists) confirms the view that differences in psychological activity are determined by different forms of existence, giving rise to new functional systems that lie at the basis of behavior, rather than by the inner properties of neurons.

Modern scientific psychology, resting on a philosophical basis of scientific materialism and the theory of reflection, has introduced radical changes into our views of consciousness.

The classical idealistic theory of consciousness understood it as a direct primary gift, as an experience of the "ego" inherent in the subject from the beginning, which—after the time of Plato and Descartes—was contrasted with the objectively existing outside world.

Modern scientific psychology sets out from the opposite position. Having received a powerful stimulus from the work of Vygotskii (1934, 1958, 1960), it has from the very beginning rejected the meaningless notion of consciousness as an invariant subjective quality, as the scene against which the meaningful events are played, or as an epiphenomenon accompanying human behavior.

Vygotskii set out from the position, perfectly logical for the philosophy of Marxism, that consciousness, which is "life made aware," is always meaningful and subjective in character.

The basic assumption of Mach's philosophy, according to which sensations of elements of consciousness are merely awareness of the function of the sense organs themselves, is false for the simple reason that physiological processes taking place in the organism as a rule are not perceived, and the function of the brain itself (which, as an organ, is without sensation[2]) and physiological processes taking place in the receptors remain unperceived. It is not inner processes in the receptor structures that are reflected in consciousness, but always the external objective world. That is why consciousness, as a reflection of objective reality, has an essential biological function, enabling the organism to find its bearings, to analyze incoming information, and to store traces of it, and as V. M. Bekhterev pointed out originally, it leads to the "correct assessment of external impressions and to the goal-directed choice of movements in conformity with that assessment."

For that reason, consciousness is ability to assess sensory infor-

---

[2] Because of this special feature of the brain, operations can be performed on it even without anesthesia, for they evoke no sensation in the patient.

mation, to respond to it with critical thoughts and actions, and to retain memory traces in order that past traces or actions may be used in the future.

Vygotskii's hypothesis that consciousness is a structural system with semantic function and the idea of its gradual and continuous development closely connected with him are important contributions of Soviet psychological science to the theory of consciousness.

Even if human consciousness is primarily a reflection of the outside world (and, in the last resort, awareness of self and of one's own actions, although this appeared only relatively late), it must not be forgotten that at different stages of development it differs in its semantic structure and that different systems of psychological processes are involved in its operation. After the work of Piaget, Vygotskii (1958, 1960), and Wallon (1925, 1942), there was no doubt of the radical differences that exist between the consciousness of the young infant and that of the adult or between the psychological mechanisms responsible for this difference.

The infant at the "sensorimotor" stage of mental development cannot yet distinguish himself from the surrounding world, and the reflection of direct stimuli received by him does not go beyond elementary impressions or diffuse motor responses. In the child just before school age, these primitive forms of consciousness are replaced by more complex forms of analysis of information, formed with the development of manipulative actions and the perception of objects that arises on their basis, with the features of selectivity and the constancy characteristics of such perception. It is in this important period of the child's development that we find the initial forms of distinction of self from the surrounding world and the appearance of self-awareness (connected with the phenomena of the "crises" at the ages of 3 and 7 years so familiar to specialists in child psychology) and the primary forms of conscious voluntary control of movement, the stages of development of which have been described in detail in modern psychology (Zaporozhets, 1959).

It is quite certain that this whole process cannot be entirely the result of simple maturation of neurons or steady and spontaneous development (as it appeared at one time to the theoreticians of mental development, such as Bühler). From the very earliest stages, the child's mental development takes place not only under the influence of objective reality (itself the result of social history) but also under the constant influence of communication between the child and adults. This communication, requiring the close participation of language, leads to the formation of speech in the child, and this causes a radical reorganization of the whole structure of his psychological processes.

Having learned the speech of adults and then having learned to form his own speech, with its aid the child starts to recode incoming information; when naming objects and classifying them on the basis of the verbal system, which Pavlov (1949, Vol. 3) deliberately distinguished as the "second signal system of reality," he begins afresh to analyze and classify impressions obtained from the outside world and to analyze incoming information. Perception mediated through speech appears (see Vygotskii, 1960; Rozengardt-Pupko, 1948); a new structure of memory, becoming logical and voluntary in character is formed (Leont'ev, 1959); and new forms of voluntary attention (Vygotskii, 1956) and new forms of emotional experience of reality arise (Wallon, 1942; Vygotskii, 1960).

Finally, as research in the last two decades has shown, it is on the basis of speech that complex processes of regulation of man's own actions are formed (Luria, 1956, 1958); although initially a method of communication between the child and adults, speech thus gradually becomes converted into a form of organization of human psychological activity.

There is every reason to suppose that analysis of this type will provide the pathway for a new scientific approach to such difficult problems as self-awareness, which in classical idealistic philosophy was regarded as a direct "quality," incapable of further subdivision, but which from these new standpoints must be regarded as a complex product of evolution, a special "contracted" form of what was previously expanded mental activity, taking place with the close participation of internal speech and fully amenable to scientific analytical investigation (see Gal'perin, 1959).

From these basic principles, Vygotskii concluded that human consciousness, in the various stages of development, not only differs in its semantic structure but operates by means of different systems of psychological processes; whereas in the first stages of its formation the leading role in the structure of consciousness is played by direct emotional impressions, in the later stages the decisive role is taken over first by complex perception of and manipulation with objects and in the final stages by a system of abstract codes, based on the abstracting and generalizing function of language.

Human consciousness, formed on the basis of manipulative activity, naturally acquires a new character, radically different from the psychological processes of animals; Vygotskii was thus perfectly right to insist that words, as elements of speech, are correlates of consciousness, the basic units of human consciousness, rather than correlates of thinking (Vygotskii, 1958).

It will be clear how the concept of consciousness as formulated in

modern psychology differs radically from previous views of a primary,
subjective state, devoid of concrete content and of historical development.

III

If consciousness has a complex semantic and system-based structure, if conscious activity in its different stages is carried out by a
variety of functional systems, changing in the course of successive
moments of our conscious life, changing depending on the level of
wakefulness and on man's immediate aims and purposes, it will be
perfectly clear why all attempts to seek some special formation or some
special cell group in the brain as the "organ of consciousness" are
meaningless from the very beginning. Attempts to find an organ
generating consciousness in the depth of the brain would be just as
senseless as were the attempts within our own lifetime to seek the
"seat of the soul" in the pineal gland, in support of the naive
hypotheses of Descartes. The search for the "brain apparatus of
consciousness," proceeding along these lines, could at best lead to the
recognition of the systems in the brain responsible for wakefulness (as
did those workers whose research led to the discovery of the brain-
stem reticular formation, maintaining the alert state of the cortex and
thereby creating optimal conditions for the cortical cells); however,
this search did not contribute in any way to the solution of the
problem of the brain structures responsible for conscious reflection of
reality or the complex and variable forms of conscious activity.

This view that consciousness is semantic and system-based in
structure, that psychological processes are complex and variable in
structure, as a result of which the specifically human forms of active
reception of reality and conscious control over human behavior
become possible, demands a radical redirection of our attempts and of
the attention of the research worker toward the identification of the
system of brain mechanisms, each component of which contributes to
human conscious activity.

There is no need to say that such an approach has nothing in
common with the correct but empty assertion that "the brain works as
a whole" and that the "whole brain" is the organ of consciousness.
Without pursuing this theme that consciousness is a function of mass
action of the brain, the parts of which exhibit "equipotentiality" (such
views are nowadays rejected by all progressive neurologists; see
Eccles, 1966, pp. 553–554), we must direct our attention to the analysis
of the concrete contribution made by each brain system to human

conscious activity so that we can analyze the integral pattern of those systems whose combined function makes these highly complex forms of vital activity possible. Our support must be restricted to those writers who, after pointing out that neurons at all levels of the nervous system from the spinal cord to the cortex have the same structure (see Eccles, 1966, p. 49ff), consider that attempts to find the brain substrate responsible for conscious processes must be carried out not at the neuronal or molecular level but at the level of analysis of the architecture of the major brain systems that constitute the units of the working apparatus controlling behavior as a whole (views similar to these have been expressed by Anokhin, 1955, and Bernshtein, 1947, 1957).

Those workers who have set out to study the cerebral basis of conscious activity (even if they still continue with their efforts to analyze the work of individual groups of neurons and their connections) are in fact adopting this standpoint if, rejecting the view of consciousness as an internal subjective state, they give it a more complex definition and understand it as the organization of integrated behavior. Such a course was followed, for example, by the physiologist Bremer, who defined consciousness as "a specific property of brain activity characterized by increased selective reactivity and the harmonious organization of all behavioral acts responsible for correct adaptation to the current situation," and the same view is held by a leading authority such as Jasper (see Eccles, 1966, p. 257); the Italian physiologist Moruzzi, whom I have mentioned earlier and who defines consciousness as a process by means of which sensory information is evaluated and responded to critically with thoughts and actions, with the accumulation of appropriate memory traces, adopts the same standpoint (see Eccles, 1966, p. 345); so also, finally, do those workers who refuse to regard consciousness as the "subjective side" of physiological processes and who try to discuss the mechanisms that lie at the basis of "conscious experience" or "conscious activity."

These definitions of consciousness, no longer regarding it as an epiphenomenon but adopting the new approach to it as a complex form of organization of activity, naturally pave the way to the analysis of its concrete cerebral mechanisms and to the search for the components of the functional systems responsible for its course.

A concrete investigation aimed at discovering the role of particular brain regions in the construction of conscious activity can be carried out by methods that have proved themselves in the history of science. They include: comparative anatomy, comparing the structure of the brain and behavior of animals; stimulation of individual areas of the brain (a procedure that has developed rapidly in recent years with the introduction of methods of microphysiological investigation), analyzing changes in conscious activity that arise in response to stimulation of these areas; and finally, destruction of brain areas, a method which was successfully combined by Pavlov some years ago with conditioned-reflex investigations and which is the basis of neuropsychological analysis of patients with local brain lesions.

The first of these methods, that of comparative anatomical investigation, has already yielded a wealth of information in the study of animal behavior, but it is hardly suitable for the analysis of the brain mechanisms of human consciousness. As has often been pointed out, the human brain does not function through the creation of new morphological organs reflecting progress in psychological activity but through the formation of new functional systems (or, to use Leont'ev's expression, "functional organs"), and the enormous progress made in the forms of human mental activity observable throughout the course of history is hardly likely to be reflected in morphological changes in the brain (see Teilhard de Chardin, 1959).

The second method, that of electrophysiological investigation, one that nowadays has a very large following, also has only limited importance. Although experiments involving stimulation of the human cerebral cortex, made possible through recent advances in neurosurgery, have enabled surgeons such as Penfield (1966; Penfield and Jasper, 1954; Penfield and Roberts, 1959) to amass a wealth of data of the utmost interest, electrical stimulation of the cortex must increasingly be regarded as an unnatural form of brain stimulation that evokes artificial analogues of experiences or elements of movement of minor importance in the study of the real contribution made by a particular brain zone to concrete forms of behavior rather than units of purposive psychological activity (see the remarks by Phillips in Eccles, 1966, p. 391). Electrophysiological investigations at the single-neuron level are equally limited in the contribution they can make to the study of human conscious activity. Although they yield extremely valuable information on the functional properties of single neurons and thus help to clarify and enrich our ideas of the structure and functional role of the various brain systems (ideas of decisive importance where the analysis of the cerebral substrate of psychological processes is concerned) and although they serve to study the intimate mechanisms of excitation, by their very nature they are confined to the neuronal level and they can yield only indirect conclusions on the importance of individual brain structures in the general regulation of human conscious activity.

More direct results for our purpose can be expected from the third method, the analysis of changes in behavior arising as a result of local brain lesions. This method, the basis of neuropsychology, consists essentially of the psychological analysis of changes observable in conscious activity in patients with local brain lesions, and it has already yielded much information of value to the analysis of the role of individual cortical zones and individual brain systems in the structural behavior. There are solid grounds for saying that by far the greater part of what we now know of the cerebral basis of psychological activity has been obtained by the neuropsychological investigation of patients with local brain lesions. By studying the changes in complex human psychological activity following the destruction of particular brain zones, we can obtain invaluable information that shows the role of the corresponding brain zone in the structure of any, including conscious, human activity (see Luria, 1966, 1973).

However, at the outset it is essential to specify the limitations of this method also.

The disturbance of a psychological activity by a local brain lesion does not necessarily mean that the corresponding "function" is localized in the destroyed area. To speak in this way would imply *localizing* the movement of a clock in the broken pendulum or in damage to some other part of the clockwork mechanism. Classical neurologists for that reason stated many years ago that "localization of a symptom" does not by any means imply "localization of a function." Disturbance of a complex form of human activity by a certain local brain lesion indicates that that particular brain zone is important for the normal activity of the whole functional system, and if that part of the brain is destroyed, the functional system begins to seek ways around the difficulty and works differently. Investigators using the neuropsychological method must therefore always endeavor not to concentrate on the description of psychological "functions" that are "lost" in the presence of a certain local brain lesion but to analyze what changes take place in the higher forms of conscious activity when the functional systems of the brain have to function as best they can without support from the corresponding brain area affected by the pathological focus. However, an investigation of this type is an invaluable component of the psychological analysis of functional systems; once he knows the "intrinsic function" of particular brain areas (as revealed by other—comparative anatomical or electrophysiological—data), the investigator can judge the contribution made by each brain system to the general structure of functional systems; in other words, he can assess the part it plays in the functional architecture of brain activity, and this is information of decisive importance to the problem we are discussing.

The use of local brain lesions for neuropsychological analysis has another limitation that should not be forgotten. The pathological process not only excludes a certain component from its participation in the functional systems of brain activity, but it has its own intrinsic pathophysiological features that lead to essential changes in the course of brain processes. A pathological focus, however circumscribed it may be, significantly alters the hemodynamics of the brain and the flow of cerebrospinal fluid; it causes marked perifocal changes; and it may sometimes alter the normal function even of distant parts of the brain. This last fact, described originally by Monakow (1914) under the name *diaschisis,* has more recently been confirmed by the observations of Moruzzi and the experiments of Jasper, who showed that an epileptic focus causes substantial changes in the symmetrically opposite zones of the other hemisphere and that these changes in the "mirror focus" can persist for many months after removal of the primary focus (see Jasper, 1966). Pathophysiological changes (a pathological increase in external inhibition, a decrease in mobility of the nervous processes, etc.) characterizing the function of an affected brain tissue are also known to lead to the appearance of behavioral changes that have no analogy in the normal course of psychological processes. All these facts naturally add greatly to the difficulty of using clinical data for the deduction of conclusions relating to normal psychophysiology.

However, despite all these limitations, the facts obtainable by analysis of changes in human conscious activity in local brain lesions—the basis of the new science of neuropsychology—still remain the chief source of information that can be used, with good prospects of success, for the concrete analysis of this problem of the cerebral basis of human conscious activity.

IV

No lesion of the cerebral hemispheres, however large and however massive the disturbance of individual functions that it causes, can lead to loss of the waking state or to a disturbance of the unity of the personality; "loss of consciousness" arises only after operations on the brain stem so that impulses running to the cortex from the brain-stem reticular formation are blocked, with a sudden consequent fall of cortical tone. This fact led the workers who first described it to regard the brain-stem reticular formation as the apparatus of wakefulness (Magoun, 1958), and some of them have actually gone so far as to postulate that the "centrencephalic system" of the brain stem is the true supreme brain level, with the role of controller of human conscious life (Penfield, 1957, 1966).

The fact that the brain-stem reticular formation, with its ability to modulate cortical tone, regulates the state of wakefulness is no longer in any doubt. However, the view that lesions of certain portions of the cerebral hemispheres, although not reflected in the waking state of the cortex, leave consciousness completely unaffected seems to the writer to be deeply mistaken.

If we accept the definition of consciousness given above and regard it as a specially complex form of brain activity—permitting the analysis of incoming information, the evaluation and selection of its significant (useful) elements, the use of memory traces, control over the course of goal-directed activity, and, finally, evaluation of the results of its own activity and the correction of any mistakes made—it will be easy to see that the elements of this complex system must inevitably suffer in local brain lesions; moreover, what is particularly important, they do not always suffer in the same way, but they are disturbed very selectively in brain lesions in different situations.

These arguments lead to a conclusion that is to some extent opposite to the one generally held, for we must suppose that the integrity of consciousness in patients with massive local brain lesions, to which many writers have referred, is a purely apparent phenomenon, and in reality massive lesions of the cerebral hemispheres, although not causing loss of wakefulness, do nevertheless evoke substantial disturbances (but differing in different cases) of conscious activity, which call for special analysis and precise qualification in each case.

This proposition, which invariably arises if we accept the concept of the semantic structure of consciousness, necessitates rejection of the simplified, purely quantitative approach to consciousness that amounts to nothing more than the mere statement of the presence or absence of consciousness (or at best, references to clear, incomplete, or confused consciousness) and replaces it with the more concrete task of describing exactly what changes in the structure of conscious activity can be found in brain lesions in different situations. It is only by this approach—one that does not rest on subjective methods of assessment but requires the objective, structural analysis of the patient's activity—that we can obtain truly scientific information on the role of the various zones or systems of the brain in human conscious activity.

Modern views on the structure of activity—as developed previously by individual workers (Bernshtein, 1935, 1947; Anokhin, 1935; Leont'ev, 1959; Miller, Galanter, and Pribram, 1960) and that at the present time, with the development of the study of self-regulating systems, are shared by virtually everybody—regard human conscious activity as consisting of a number of major components. These include the reception and processing (recoding) of information, with the selection of its most important elements and retention of the experience thus gained in the memory; enunciation of the task or formulation of an intention, with the preservation of the corresponding motives of activity, the creation of a pattern (or model) of the required action, and production of the appropriate program (plan) to control the selection of necessary actions; and finally, comparison of the results of the action with the original intention (the *"Ist-Wert," "Soll-Wert"* of Bernshtein or, in Anokhin's expression, mobilization of the "action acceptor" apparatus), with correction of the mistakes made. All these components of conscious activity, modeled in dozens of schemes suggested by different workers, are carried out in man with the closest participation of external and internal speech: not merely for the encoding of information reaching the subject, but also for storing the experience obtained, abstracting from direct influences and the creation of behavior programs, and thus participating both in the regulation of conscious activity and in the assessment of its results and correction of mistakes.

This model of complex human conscious activity gives much greater precision to our search by confining it to the problem of which component of conscious activity is disturbed as a result of the destruction of particular cortical zones (or particular brain systems) and how the changes in the structure of this activity arise under these circumstances.

Enunciation of the problem in this way must replace the naive (and usually subjective) assessment of "state of consciousness" that serves as the starting point for most philosophers, psychologists, and physiologists concerned with the study of the relation of consciousness to the brain.

V

Let us now review the facts relating to the various forms of disturbance of conscious activity at our disposal.

Lesions of the primary (projection) cortical areas—or as they are now generally called, *intrinsic areas*—disturb neither the complex forms of information processing nor the programming and monitoring of personal actions nor the selectively organized course of psychological processes; in other words, they do not in any way disturb conscious behavior.

According to views that have developed in neurology, these areas are merely the "ways in or ways out" of the cerebral hemispheres or, as some writers prefer to express it, the "posterior and anterior horns of the brain" (Bernshtein, 1947). A lesion of these zones causes partial or complete interruption of the arrival of information (visual in the case of an occipital lesion, tactile in the case of a postcentral lesion, and auditory in lesions of the medial zones of the temporal region) or a similar partial or complete cessation of the flow of impulses from the brain to the muscles (lesions of the precentral gyrus). In all these cases, a patient partially deprived of incoming information at the "input" or with impairment of the flow of efferent impulses from the "output" can easily compensate for his defects with the aid of intact cortical zones, by reorganizing the work of the affected system or replacing the nonfunctioning system by another that is intact.

That is why at this stage we can say no more about disturbances of conscious activity than we can about disturbances of peripheral receptors or muscles. The picture is different with lesions of the secondary (projection-association) cortical zones, which include the secondary areas of the visual (occipital), auditory (temporal), or tactile (parietal) cortex and, stretching the point a little, the more complex "overlapping zones" of the posterior portions of the hemispheres (the parieto-temporo-occipital region), usually classified for good reason as "tertiary" zones, but belonging in principle to that same group of complex afferent systems of the cortex that I have just mentioned.

These zones (composed mainly as regards their structure by interneurons or association neurons of the second and third layers of the cortex) have functions that differ significantly from those of the "primary" zones. After dozens of investigations in recent years, as before we still have no reason to doubt that these zones form the cortical apparatus for further processing of information, as a result of which incoming stimuli are integrated and encoded. The fact that these cortical zones receive impulses not only from the "primary" cortical areas but also from nuclei at a lower level in the thalamus and from cortical areas belonging to other systems (an example of this is the connections of the superior temporal region with the lower zones of the premotor and postcentral cortex described by Blinkov) introduces a fresh factor into their activity in the modifying and recoding of incoming information.

Lesions of these cortical areas naturally lead to a disturbance of the encoding of information and to difficulty with the selection of the "useful cues" and to changes in the selective, organized structure of perception that distinguish the various forms of visual, auditory, and tactile agnosia.

From two features that distinguish these lesions, it can, however, be considered that disturbances of conscious activity in these cases also remain very limited, if not absent altogether.

First, in all these cases the disturbance of processing or encoding of information is restricted to one modality (visual with lesions of the occipital cortex, auditory with lesions of the temporal, and tactile-kinesthetic, with lesions of the parietal cortex). A subject with a local lesion of one of the "secondary" areas of the posterior parts of the cortex can thus still substitute other intact systems for a disturbed source of information; he can still compensate for his defective visual perception of objects by tactile perception or for his defective auditory perception (for example, the auditory evaluation of the sounds of speech) by visual or kinesthetic (for example, lip reading) perception. It must simply be noted that the more important the place of the corresponding brain system in the general structure of behavior, the more severe the disturbances produced in conscious activity by a lesion of one of the "secondary" (perceptual) areas. That is why a lesion of the olfactory system in man may be almost unnoticed, whereas a lesion of the auditory-speech system, preventing the normal perception of speech, which plays a decisive role in human conscious activity, renders the patient helpless. It must also be noted that, as Vygotskii pointed out, a lesion of the "secondary" (perceptual) zones in the child can give rise to immeasurably more severe disturbances of conscious activity than a similar lesion in the adult: in this case, the disturbance of encoding of acoustic information results in a disturbance of the whole development of complex forms of psychological activity based on the normal processing of incoming information, and the partial defect of information processing that can be easily compensated in the adult by systems formed previously gives rise to gross impairment of psychological development in the child (Vygotskii, 1934, 1960).

The second reason that partial disturbances of information processing arising in lesions of the "secondary" (perceptual) cortical zones do not give rise to massive disturbances of conscious activity is that the anterior brain zones (the functions of which I shall deal with below), if left intact, leave unimpaired the patient's ability to form intentions and programs of behavior, to assess the defects of his actions, and to take steps to compensate for them. That is why patients with such lesions clearly recognize their shortcomings and strive diligently to compensate for them by resorting to special methods and using brain systems that are still intact. The presence of at times surprising tenaciousness (an absolutely essential condition) rules out any possibility that these lesions, which restrict the inflow of encoded information, cause a disturbance of conscious behavior.

A similar place is occupied by the cases mentioned above of lesions of the "overlapping zones" or "tertiary zones" of the posterior parts of the hemispheres (the parieto-temporo-occipital zones of the cortex). The distinguishing feature of these cases is that the disturbance of information synthesis is more massive and more complex in character. I have described elsewhere (Luria, 1966, 1973) the disturbance of spatial syntheses that arises in these patients and their inability to convert successively incoming information into simultaneously surveyable schemes, a basic feature of these disorders. These disturbances, manifested equally in the analysis of visual, tactile, and auditory information, are to some extent "supramodal" in character; this characteristic is reflected in the difficulties encountered by these patients in their intellectual "symbolic" activity, for they are no longer able to understand or operate with the ordered structure of number or with complex logical-grammatical relations, and they find it completely impossible to grasp immediately complex systems of relations between individual elements. In such cases, there are good grounds, therefore, for suggesting a disturbance of conscious activity, but it must be recalled that the difficulties are "operative" in character or— as psychopathologists frequently say—are difficulties confined to the instrumental or effector component of conscious activity. It must not be forgotten that in these cases the integrity of the anterior brain zones—responsible for the stability of intentions, the precision of programming of actions, and a clear understanding of defects that arise—leaves the goal-directed activity of these patients unimpaired and so ensures the logical and critical character of their behavior.

Lesions of the "secondary" zones of the anterior regions of the hemispheres occupy a special place. I have described in detail elsewhere the disturbances of higher cortical functions arising in such cases (Luria, 1966, 1973), and for that reason I shall mention them here only very briefly.

Lesions of the premotor zones of the cortex (Brodmann's area $6a\beta$) give rise to no appreciable disturbances of the encoding of information, but they render the patient unable to create the motor schemes enabling "kinetic melodies" to be performed smoothly or, in other words, enabling the motor plan to be converted into a smooth chain of consecutive movements. Whereas lesions of the "tertiary" zones of posterior cortical regions impair the conversion of successive items of incoming information into simultaneous schemes, in the cases we are now considering the disturbance is opposite in character, for the patient's "simultaneous scheme" cannot develop into a cycle of serially organized, successive movements. Even here, however, the disturbance affects only the effector (operative) component of motor behavior, and we can speak of a disturbance of conscious activity in these cases only in a very limited and conventional context.

Patients with lesions of the posterior frontal zones of the dominant (left) hemisphere (or those with the closely similar picture of
lesions of the anterior zones of the speech area), of which I have made
a special analysis elsewhere (Luria, 1966, 1969), are much more
interesting.

Disturbances of the conversion of the original plan into a successive kinetic melody, such as are found in these patients, affect a
special section of motor processes, namely, speech; their dominant
manifestation is that although the patient completely understands
speech and can name objects easily, he has great difficulty in converting an original thought into a fluent utterance. He will state that he
knows what he wants to say but that the thought will not evoke
coherent speech; images and words flashing separately in his consciousness are not converted into fluent, coherent expression. Many of
these patients are quite unable to form a continuous expression, and
they complain of a feeling of "empty-headedness" or the random
flashing of disconnected thoughts. "For all of you Friday comes after
Thursday," said one such patient trying to put his defect into words,
"but for me there is nothing."

Phenomena of this type, based in all probability on a disturbance
of specifically verbal motor schemes embodied in the form of internal
speech (Vygotskii, 1934, 1956), naturally involve something much
closer to disturbances of conscious activity, although even in such
cases conscious activity is disturbed not so much in the creation of
intentions or formulation of programs as in their performance (in
other words, in their effector or operative component). Inability to
contract such an extended action or to convert a thought into an
extended utterance—a characteristic feature of these forms of "dynamic aphasia," which I have analyzed elsewhere (Luria and Tsvetkova, 1967)—is not limited in such cases to the narrow phenomena of
speech, but it also leads to considerable disturbance of "spontaneity,"
which most investigators unhesitatingly regard as a defect of conscious activity. Because of this fact, the disturbances I have just
described begin to assume a completely different place in the pattern
of disturbances of human conscious activity in local brain lesions that
we are now discussing.

VI

I have examined the characteristics of those cortical zones whose
lesions either leave the course of conscious activity unaffected or

disturb only its effector (operative) component, leaving the structure of conscious activity itself intact.

We must now go a step further and consider the function of brain areas whose lesions cause substantial impairment of the structure of conscious processes.

An examination of the definitions of conscious activity shows that many authorities regard as its most important feature the ability "to use the past to regulate the future," "to select information received," and "to subordinate behavior to conscious aims." These factors, which play an essential role in the organization of conscious behavior, are largely dependent on integrity of the frontal lobes and are severely impaired in patients with lesions of that region.

The frontal lobes, which increase considerably in size in the course of evolution and in man occupy one-third of the total mass of the hemispheres, are not directly concerned with the reception of information or with the dispatch of efferent impulses to the periphery. Belonging structurally to the typical "tertiary" cortical zones (or the intrinsic areas), they play an important role in the formation of programs of conscious activity, in ensuring the dominant role of these programs (formed in man with the close participation of speech) in the course of movement and actions, in inhibiting all interfering impulses, and in enabling continuous comparison to be made between the action as performed and the original intention, or in other words, ensuring control over the course of activity.

The function of the frontal lobes in the regulation of conscious activity has been the subject of many of the writer's earlier investigations (Luria, 1966, 1969, 1973; Luria and Khomskaya, 1966), and I shall therefore dwell only very briefly here on the conclusions drawn from work that has taken place elsewhere over a number of years.

Extirpation of a large area of the frontal lobes in animals, as many workers have shown, causes no significant disturbance of elementary forms of conditioned-reflex activity; however, it does prevent the formation of complex conditioned-reflex (or "pretrigger") syntheses, controlling the behavior of the normal animal, and it prevents the normal comparison of the results of action with the original intention and, consequently, prevents the correction of inadequate or incorrect actions (Anokhin, 1949); that is why a dog without its frontal lobes substitutes for an adequate system of motor responses inertly repeated motor stereotype, unable to inhibit movements that have long ago lost their adaptive role (Shumilina, 1966). Numerous investigations also have shown that extirpation of the frontal lobes in animals (monkeys) seriously affects the integrity of complex "plans" of behavior, so that

delayed responses become impossible; programs of behavior elaborated in these animals are replaced by uninhibitable orienting reflexes
or by involuntary responses to irrelevant stimuli (Malmo, 1942; see
also Warren and Akert, 1964). These observations have led many
investigators to suggest that in higher animals the frontal lobes play
an important role in the complex process of differentiating the dominant systems of connections (Pribram, 1966) and inhibiting irrelevant
responses (Konorski and Lawicka, 1964), disturbance of which has the
invariable result that "the animals do not assess their actions as they
should, they do not establish definite relations between the imprints
of new impressions and the result of previous experience, and they do
not direct their movements and actions to their individual advantage"
(Bekhterev, 1907).

Whereas the essential role of the frontal lobes in the creation and
maintenance of complex behavioral programs was already apparent in
higher animals, in man their importance in the organization of
complex (in this case, conscious) activity is many times greater and
has acquired new qualitative features.

We now know the decisive role played in the formation of human
conscious activity by external—and later by internal—speech, by
means of which a person can analyze the situation, distinguish its
important components, and formulate programs of necessary actions.
Modern psychology has described with sufficient clarity the organizing role of speech for the formation of consciousness (Vygotskii, 1934,
1958) and has traced the stages of development of its regulating
function (Luria, 1956, 1958). There is every reason to suppose that it is
"thanks to speech, which was an inter-psychological function shared
by two people, but later became an intra-psychological form of
organization of human activity" (Vygotskii, 1958) that man was able to
rise above the level of impulsive responses to direct environmental
situations and that his behavior began to be determined by the
"internal semantic field" that reflects in general form the environmental situation, formulates the motives that lie at the basis of behavior,
and gives human activity its conscious character. Numerous observations confirm that this complex regulation of motivated behavior by
speech can take place successfully only with the participation of the
frontal lobes and that it is substantially disturbed in patients with
lesions of them.

I can illustrate this important conclusion by a number of observations and experiments of a model character that I have specially
analyzed elsewhere (Luria, 1966, 1969, 1973; Luria and Khomskaya,
1966); they show clearly the difficulty experienced by a patient with a
massive bilateral lesion of the frontal lobes in creating a stable

intention and the ease with which the performance of a complex behavioral program is disturbed by other interfering factors.

1. In a patient with a massive bilateral lesion of the frontal lobes, one can easily evoke a simple direct response to a stimulus—for example, by instructing him to lift his hand or shake the doctor's hand.

If, however, the patient's hand is under the blanket and the instruction "raise your hand" has to be subdivided into a series of subsidiary programs (take your hand from under the blanket, then raise your hand), the patient cannot follow the instruction and just goes on looking helplessly at the physician, unable to proceed.

Similar difficulties arise if such a patient is given the complex instruction "Shake my hand three times," requiring subdivision into the following subprograms: (shake my hand, count "one," shake my hand, count "two," shake my hand, count "three," and then stop the action). In this case also, the patient cannot obey the instruction but (still retaining the spoken instruction) continues to perform the undivided program and does not stop the action at the required moment.

2. In a patient with a massive bilateral lesion of the frontal lobe, an echopraxic response can easily be evoked by an instruction to repeat a movement demonstrated by the examiner. If, however, a verbal instruction is given that conflicts with the direct perception of the signal (for example, if he is asked to raise his finger in response to being shown a clenched fist, and to clench his fist in response to being shown a finger, or if he has to respond to one tap by two taps and to two taps by one tap), performance of the action in such cases becomes impossible. Although he can easily retain and repeat the spoken instruction, the patient begins to subordinate his real action to the visually perceived signal, and his performance becomes the echopraxic repetition of the movement of the examiner.

3. In a patient with a massive bilateral lesion of the frontal lobes, it is relatively easy to evoke the performance of a simple action (such as drawing a figure or a group of figures, to repeat a given rhythm, and so on); however, if the patient is then called upon to perform another similar action (for example, to draw another figure or group of figures, to repeat another given rhythm, and so on), switching the action into the performance of the new program may be difficult (or sometimes even impossible), and instead of the new action the patient continues inertly to repeat the earlier stereotype, although he can retain and can readily repeat the new verbal instruction. This time, the conscious performance of the necessary action is interrupted by pathological perseveration of the previous program, which was ade-

quate at the time when the action began but ceased to be adequate with the switch to the new instruction.

The instability of the goal-directed, conscious behavior of patients with frontal lobe lesions and the ease with which the conscious performance of actions (governed by the internal program) is replaced either by the more elementary "field" action (subordinated to direct external situations) or by perseverating inert stereotypes can be seen also in the behavior of such patients in a natural setting. I cannot forget a patient with a massive (traumatic) lesion of the frontal lobes who, when trying to find his way out of the clinic, yielded to the impression made by the first staircase he found in his way and went up it instead of down it, or who went through the open door of a cupboard instead of leaving the room (B. V. Zeigarnik's case), or a patient who, when asked to fetch some cigarettes from a ward situated at the end of the corridor, met some patients coming in the opposite direction and turned back after them (although he remembered the instruction quite clearly). I remember a similar patient who, after a severe wound of the frontal lobes, was discharged from hospital and, having been given a railroad ticket to her home town, broke her journey where she had to change trains and settled down there without ever reaching her destination. Finally, I recall a patient with a massive wound of the frontal lobes who, when instructed to plane a piece of wood, continued the action inertly until most of the wood had been planed away.

In all these cases, the patients' conscious behavior was disturbed on the same principle: the verbal expression of the intention (or instruction) could be retained for a long time but it lost its regulatory influence; once the patient had ceased to behave in accordance with the internally formulated plan, his behavior fell under the influence of direct impressions or of inert stereotypes.

The disturbance of conscious activity arising in patients with passive lesions of the frontal lobes may assume a different character and be manifested at different levels of psychological activity. In lesions of the basal zones of the frontal lobes (for example, in tumors of the olfactory fossa), they assume the character of uncontrollable, impulsive actions, arising whenever the task is made more difficult, whereas in lesions of the lateral zones of the frontal region, they assume the form of gross simplification of motor programs and pathological inertia of earlier stereotypes. In patients with massive bilateral frontal lobe lesions, they may assume the form of disintegration of the patient's behavior, whereas in milder forms of the "frontal syndrome," disturbances arise only during complex forms of intellectual activity (Luria and Tsvetkova, 1966).

However, despite the diversity of manifestations of the behavioral disturbances in lesions of the frontal lobes, as a rule two essential features are preserved. First, the patient's behavior ceases to be controlled by a motivated verbal program, falls under the influence of interfering factors, and becomes more primitive in character. Second, even when the patient retains the correct verbal formulation of the instruction (it becomes distorted or disappears only in patients with the severest type of frontal lobe lesions), as a rule he can never compare his actual performance with the original intention, is unaware of mistakes he makes, and makes no attempt to correct them himself.

In lesions of the frontal lobes, the disturbance of conscious activity thus has a precise structure: complex programs of actions disintegrate, on the one hand, and monitoring of the action during performance (the "action-acceptor" apparatus) is disturbed, on the other hand.

These two distinguishing features were familiar to psychiatrists, who described the "aspontaneity" and "disturbed critical attitude" of a patient with a frontal lobe lesion (Kleist, 1934). More recent neuropsychological studies have simply filled in some of the details of the mechanisms at the basis of these defects.

In the cases described above, can we speak of a disturbance of conscious activity?

If we restrict our understanding of the term *consciousness* to evidence of the presence of a waking state or unity of the personality, then of course we cannot. If, however, we adopt the view, which the writer accepts, that consciousness is semantic and system-based in structure, the cases I have described not only fully justify the conclusion that conscious activity is disturbed, but they also point to a definite structure of that disturbance.

Clearly, the state of wakefulness, like the unity of the personality, remains intact in these cases; the effector (operative) aspects of conscious activity, which are disturbed in patients with lesions of the secondary zones of the posterior areas of the cortex, likewise remain intact. However, the fact that an intention once adopted or a program once assigned through a spoken instruction is so easily abandoned and so easily disintegrated by interfering factors clearly points to a disturbance of conscious control over the patient's activity, a definite, although admittedly only partial, manifestation of a disturbance of conscious activity. If we add the fact that patients of this group are still able to assess mistakes made by another person but are unable to evaluate their own mistakes critically (see Luria, Pribram, and Khomskaya, 1966; Lebedinskii, 1967), it becomes increasingly evident that a partial disturbance of conscious activity exists in patients with frontal lobe lesions.

As we have seen, disturbances of consciousness are complex in character and are least in accordance with the "all-or-nothing" principle; they cannot be expressed on a quantitative scale, starting with complete preservation and ending with complete loss of consciousness. A careful description of the disturbance of the various components of conscious activity and the various types of disturbance of its structure must therefore demand our closest attention.

VII

So far we have dealt with brain zones whose lesions either do not disturb conscious activity or disturb it partially, by interfering with the performance of programs of conscious action and preventing a critical attitude toward its defects.

We must now turn to the analysis of cases in which a brain lesion causes disturbances that all observers describe as changes in consciousness but whose brain mechanisms have remained obscure or difficult to describe for a long time.

In all the cases I shall now discuss, disorders of brain activity were connected with disturbances of memory, and the connection is often so close that it is sometimes difficult to draw a line between the disturbance of consciousness and the disturbances of memory.

Local lesions of the posterior zones of the hemispheres, restricting the processing of incoming information, often may also be accompanied by definite disturbances of memory. However, these disturbances of memory are strictly modality-specific in character and never lead to changes in consciousness.

We know, for example, that lesions of the middle zones of the left temporal lobe, which do not cause marked defects of phonemic (verbal) hearing may lead to definite disturbances of audioverbal memory; the patient is unable to retain audioverbal series and cannot repeat the names of objects as easily as he should. A characteristic feature of these disturbances (I have analyzed them in detail elsewhere: Luria, 1947, 1966; Luria and Rapoport, 1962) is, however, that the memory defects in these cases are limited to the audioverbal sphere only, and visual or kinesthetic memory is never disturbed. There is reason to suppose that the opposite relations apply in lesions of the occipitoparietal zones of the cortex, when changes in visuospatial memory (intimately connected with disturbances of visuospatial analysis) leave audioverbal memory intact and may actually be partly compensated with its aid.

Disturbances of a similar type arise in lesions of the medial zones of the temporal cortex, adjacent to or even involving structures of the hippocampus. These lesions, which have been studied closely in the literature and specially described in the writer's laboratory (Luria, 1974–1975), are characterized by the same features, for they lead primarily to disturbances of auditory memory, and it is only in cases of bilateral lesions of the "hippocampal circle" that they produce more diffuse disturbances, bordering in the most severe cases on Korsakov's syndrome.

A characteristic feature of all these cases, however, is that in all forms of these "primary" disturbances of memory, the selective, goal-directed character of the activity remains unaffected, as also does the patient's critical attitude toward his defects and his attempt to compensate for them.

Patients with lesions of this type retain their ideas of events in the distant past but exhibit loss of short-term memory. Traces of incoming information are not consolidated, or they are subjected to pathologically increased retroactive inhibition: the preceding link in the chain of excitation is inhibited by the succeeding link, so that if a series of words, numbers, movements, or pictures is presented to the patient, he often retains only the last member of the series and is quite unable to recall the previous members (Luria, 1974–1975). These disturbances are seen particularly clearly in special tests during which, having just repeated two short series consisting of a few elements (words, numbers, movements), the patient is instructed to recall a previous (the first) series (Luria, 1974). It soon becomes clear in tests such as these that although the patient previously repeated this first series without difficulty, now, after being given a second similar series, he cannot recall the first until a long interval has elapsed, when he does so by reminiscence.

However, the memory disturbances in such cases remain disturbances of one of the effector (operative) components, and they do not lead to general disturbance of consciousness or of conscious activity.

The pattern is completely different in massive lesions of the brain stem or hippocampal circle, blocking the normal flow of impulses from the reticular formation to the cortex, and in particular, in cases when the pathological focus involves the limbic region and the medial zones of the frontal lobes.

In such cases, normal cortical tone falls sharply. The cortex is in an inhibitory, "phasic" state and unable to distinguish between strong, dominant foci of excitation and foci induced by weak, interfering stimuli. Because of this state of affairs, a physiological interpretation that was given originally by Pavlov, traces of strong and weak excitation become equalized, and the distinction between important, essential (biologically strong) and secondary, irrelevant (biologically weak) foci disappears. Besides a disturbance of the imprinting (consolidation) of traces in such cases, a disturbance of the selectivity of connections arises and becomes the most important feature of these states, leading to a disturbance of consciousness.

Normal consciousness, as we know, is characterized by strict selectivity of connections, which fall into clearly demarcated systems, sometimes with an hierarchic structure. The sphere of things connected with the family do not mix with the sphere of things connected with work or with scientific knowledge; the sphere of what constitutes the subject of an activity in which a person is engaged at a particular moment is separated strictly from the sphere of interfering influences or "noise." However, this selectivity of psychological processes, typical of normal consciousness, is what is disturbed in pathological states of the cortex used by the lesions I have just mentioned.

In the most severe cases (they can be observed in extended form during the early period after closed head injury, leading to clear changes in cortical-brain stem relations, or in the initial state of diencephalic or frontodiencephalic brain tumors), the patient's behavior begins to show marked evidence of confusion (see Luria, Konovalov, and Podgornaya, 1970; Luria, 1974-1975). The patient loses the precise orientation in space and, in particular, in time; he considers that he is in some indefinite place: "in hospital," "at work," or "at the station." Sometimes this primary disturbance of orientation is compensated by naive, uncontrollable guesses: seeing the white gowns and white hats of the physicians, the patient declares that he is "at the baker's," "at the barber's." His orientation in time is totally disturbed, and he cannot tell the month, the year, or the time of day. Because of the added severe disturbances of memory, such a patient cannot answer when he is asked where he was the same morning or the night before, and the irrepressible traces of past experience lead him to fill this gap with confabulations: he says he was "at work," or "walking in the garden," and so on. Recognition of other people is seriously impaired: an approaching physician is identified as a "work mate" or a "friend of the family." The patient's attitude toward himself is also profoundly upset: sometimes he considers that he is fit and well, at other times that he has just been visiting "this place" (the nature of which he also is not quite sure about). The contradictions between his assessment and the real situation cause such a patient little confusion because the rapidly disappearing traces of his impressions do not provide an opportunity for reliable, critical comparison.

A characteristic feature of these cases is that for all his confusion, the patient frequently can still perform certain formal operations: he can read a text offered to him, write a sentence from dictation, and carry out simple arithmetical operations (not requiring retention of intermediate components in the memory); sometimes he can interpret the meaning of a thematic picture. I shall never forget one case, that of a highly educated person who, as a result of an automobile accident, suffered a very severe closed head injury with petechial hemorrhages into the brain stem and diencephalon and who remained confused for a long time but could easily converse with the physician in four languages, had no difficulty in switching from one to the other, and never mixed these systems, which were firmly consolidated in his past experience.

Consequently, there are no grounds for considering that the picture in such cases is to any extent the opposite of that I described above, namely, that in local lesions of the lateral zones of the cortex, direct orientation and the unity of the personality remain intact, whereas the effector (operative) aspect of activity is severely disturbed.

The picture I have just described of a state of confusion arising in the acute period of a closed head injury or in massive brain-stem tumors is a familiar one in clinical practice. Some degree of novelty is introduced by the fact that similar signs of a disturbance of the selectivity of psychological processes and, consequently, changes in conscious activity can be seen in patients with lesions of the medial zones of the frontal lobes (tumors) or aneurysms of the anterior communicating artery.

Changes in psychological processes in such cases (Luria, Khomskaya, Blinkov, and Critchley, 1967; Luria, Konovalov, and Podgornaya, 1970; Luria, 1974–1975) are essentially as follows. The patients of this group may show no sign of depression or exhaustion, so very characteristic of the patients in the acute period after trauma or of patients with deep brain tumors and increased intracranial pressure. A general oneiroid state of consciousness with hallucinations and general confusion may be completely absent. Often they are completely wide awake, so that it may be wrongly concluded that the disturbances of their consciousness are less severe than is actually the case.

The central phenomenon characteristic of these patients is, however, a profound disturbance of conscious activity manifested in the sphere of orientation in their immediate surroundings, of experiences, of memory, and of complex intellectual processes rather than in the sphere of movement and actions, and it is manifested as a marked disturbance of selective systems of connections. A characteristic feature of such cases is that although individual operations can still be performed normally, a confused state of consciousness may suddenly arise when the patient loses his correct orientation in his surroundings, begins to confabulate, and assesses the situation quite incorrectly. In one such case (with a tumor of the medial zones of the frontal lobes), that of a research worker, the illness showed itself when, while engaged on a mission, he suddenly began to behave oddly, inquired if his father (who was long since dead) had come to see him, and wrote a letter to his home full of imaginary, confabulatory events (Luria et al., 1967). Another such patient (with an aneurysm of the anterior communicating artery and hemorrhage into the medial zones of the frontal lobes) suddenly started to utter confabulatory statements, saying that he had gone on a long journey but that at the same time, he was in Moscow, where he had had "an operation on his head." Subsequently, these phenomena may either change to more severe confused states or regress, but the mingling of actual perceptions and imaginary experiences in the record of recent events remains a noticeable feature for quite a long time.

Objective neuropsychological tests reveal a unique picture in these patients: motor processes sometimes remain completely intact; usually there are no disturbances of visual, auditory, or spatial gnosis; and all complex forms of speech and logical operations are intact, in sharp contrast to the disturbance of assessment of the surroundings and of the patient's own state.

The disturbances of memory are a central feature of these patients and are coupled with reduced activity and an insufficiently critical attitude toward defects, which assumes the form of a disturbance of the selectivity of particular systems of connections. This last symptom, as observations have shown, is the earliest to appear and the one that persists the longest, and frequently it can be found early on in the illness, before there is any severe disturbance of orientation in the surroundings.

Distinct manifestations of this disturbance of selective systems of connections (presumably attributable to the "equalization" of excitation of different strengths already referred to) appear when the patient, who has been given certain information—series of words or sentences, an action or story (Group A)—is later given similar information (Group B) and is then instructed to recall the first information (Group A). As a rule, in such cases the traces of Group A are retroactively inhibited to some extent, and during attempts to recall them, they become mixed with the traces of Group B, thus giving rise to contamination, or the selectivity of recall is lost and a mass of interfering associations—which the patient cannot inhibit and which deprive the recalling of traces of necessary selectivity—begins to be interwoven into it (Luria, 1974-1975).

Characteristically, in all these disturbances, the patient does not display the necessary critical attitude toward these phenomena of contamination or intermingling of interfering associations; he makes no attempt—in the course of his defects of memory he cannot—to compare the material reproduced with the traces of that given previously; and he is quite unaware that his answers are incorrect.

The value of these tests is that they reveal, as it were, a model of the processes that, as the disease develops further, may assume the form of marked confusion and gross disturbances of consciousness.

There is no doubt that all these phenomena belong to a sphere that, without any qualification or restriction, can be classed as disturbances of consciousness arising in local brain lesions. The interest of the facts I have given above (and the study of which is still in its earliest stages) is, however, that they enable us to distinguish another, qualitatively distinctive structure of disturbances of conscious activity by linking it with specific disturbances of memory and by indicating the importance of lesions of specific brain structures in its pathogenesis.

VIII

I have completed this survey of my views on the brain systems that lie at the basis of human conscious activity, and I can now draw certain conclusions.

Most attempts to study relations between consciousness and the brain have set out from the notion that consciousness is not qualitative, that it is a subjective experience bestowed *ab initio* on man, incapable of further analysis into components, totally devoid of both history and structure, and fundamentally different in principle from all the rest of the (especially external) material world. These dualistic views led inevitably to a search for the location in the brain where, as Sherrington put it, "consciousness enters the brain," or the most elementary brain formations in which consciousness is "generated." Despite the fact that research into this problem, with the most sophisticated methods of studying the precise functional structure of neurons and synapses, has yielded rich and important information as a by-product, the view that consciousness does not possess quality must be regarded as theoretically sterile and practically unrewarding.

Modern psychology makes a different approach to consciousness and to conscious activity.

By understanding consciousness as a complex form of active reception of reality, modern psychology adopts the position, formulated some time ago by Vygotskii, that consciousness is semantic and system-based in structure, and is thus amenable to true scientific investigation.

According to this view, human consciousness, which is the result of complex activity and whose function is concerned with the highest form of orientation in the surrounding world and the regulation of behavior, has been formed during man's social history, in the course of which manipulative activity and speech developed, and its mechanism requires their close participation. By reflecting the outside world indirectly through speech, which plays an intimate role not only in the encoding of incoming information but also in the regulation of his own behavior, man is able to carry out both the simplest forms of reflection of reality and the highest forms of regulation of his own behavior. Impressions reaching him from the outside world are subjected to complex analysis and are recoded in accordance with categories that he has learned and acquired as a result of the entire historical experience of mankind, and his reflection of the outside world becomes abstract and generalized in character, changing at each successive stage of psychological development. At the same time, man is able to formulate complex intentions, to prepare complex action programs, and to subordinate his behavior to these programs, distinguishing the essential impressions and associations incorporated into this program and inhibiting impressions and associations that do not correspond to these programs or are interfering or distracting. He is able to compare the actions he has performed with his original intentions and to correct mistakes he has made.

Naturally, all these processes are carried out by complex psychological symptoms that change at each successive stage of development, and the "architecture" of the functional systems lying at the basis of conscious activity does not remain constant. Vygotskii rightly pointed out that whereas in the early (sensorimotor) stages of development of behavior direct impressions (often emotionally tinged) play the leading role in these functional systems, in the later stages the task of reflecting reality and regulating behavior begins to be taken over by systems of "interfunctional relations," in which the leading role is subsequently assumed by perception of objects, concrete memory, and, finally, speech activity, on which basis all other psychological processes are reconstructed.

There is every reason to suppose that the great majority of

psychological processes that have hitherto been regarded as "primary" and "bestowed *ab initio*" (including "experiences of the ego") are in fact the condensed and "interiorized" result of the development of this complex, system-based activity.

This view regarding the semantic and system-based structure of consciousness determines the direction of the search for the brain mechanisms that lie at its basis.

Attempts to seek the material substrate of consciousness at the single-unit or synaptic level (a level that, of course, plays a most important role in the basic physiological mechanisms essential to all psychological activity) thus begin to be seen as completely hopeless. The cerebral basis of man's complex, semantic, system-based conscious activity must be sought in the combined activity of discrete brain systems, each of which makes its own special contribution to the work of the functional system as a whole. It is only through these complex and highly differentiated functional systems that man can carry out the highly complex processes of the recoding of information, the formation of action programs with selection of the essential connections and inhibition of interfering factors, and, finally, a comparison of the effect of his action with the original intention, which are the characteristic features of conscious activity. The intimate participation of speech processes in human conscious activity makes this system more complex still.

As a result of research, much of which is devoted to the analysis of changes arising in human conscious activity as a result of local brain lesions, we can take the first step toward clarification of the role played by individual units of the brain system in the mechanism of conscious activity.

The facts show that changes in conscious activity in patients with lesions of the brain and its individual systems are by no means homogeneous but are characterized by a highly differentiated structure; different components of the functional systems may be affected, and the resulting disturbances of conscious activity may thus differ in structure.

Disturbance of the normal connection between the brain-stem reticular formation, lowering cortical tone and the level of wakefulness (a constant field for research in recent decades), is an important but special case of the whole field of possible changes in conscious activity. Consequently, the brain-stem reticular formation is only one (important, but special) component of the functional systems of the brain concerned in the mechanism of conscious activity.

An important role in the formation of conscious activity is played by the secondary zones of the posterior (afferent) cortical areas that play an active part in the recoding of incoming information. However, a lesion of these brain zones gives rise to disturbances of recoding and storage of information that are limited and modality-specific in character; they do not affect systems responsible for the formation of intentions and action programs, and they are therefore reflected only in the effector (operative) section of conscious activity and can easily be compensated.

A more important role in the formation of conscious activity is played by the frontal lobes. With their intimate participation in the formation of intentions and of action programs, subordinating activity to the dominant focus and inhibiting interfering factors, and enabling the results of actions to be compared with the original intentions, the frontal lobes play an essential role in the conscious regulation of behavior and in ensuring the stable selectivity of human goal-directed activity. The fact that massive frontal lobe lesions make the inhibition of interfering factors impossible and thus lead to the collapse of goal-directed behavior, replacing it by elementary "field" or perseveratory acts, simply confirms this conclusion.

A particularly important role in the mechanism of conscious activity is played by the medial zones of the frontal lobes. By intimately connecting the most complex brain structures with the older limbic cortex and diencephalic formations, according to all the evidence, they participate intimately in the regulation of cortical tone and thus in the preservation of selective memory traces. Facts obtained in recent years showing an essential disturbance of the selectivity of memory traces and, consequently, gross disturbances of the subject's direct orientation in his surroundings, observed in patients with lesions of the medial zones of the frontal lobes and with frontodiencephalic lesions, have shed light on a new and very important aspect of the brain mechanisms of conscious activity.

The neuropsychological study of the brain systems lying at the basis of human conscious activity is still only in its infancy.

However, there is no doubt that modern views on the complex semantic and system-based structure of consciousness are pointing out the right road for the search for its brain mechanisms and that future generations of researchers will make an essential contribution to the solution of this type of problem.

References

Anokhin, P. K. *The problem of center and periphery in the physiology of nervous activity.* Gorki: Gosizdat, 1935.

ANOKHIN, P. K. *Problems in higher nervous activity.* Moscow: Izd. Akad. Med. Nauk, SSSR, 1949.

ANOKHIN, P. K. New data on special features of the afferent apparatus of the conditioned reflex. *Voprosy Psikhologii,* 1955, No. 6.

ANOKHIN, P. K. *Biology and physiology of conditioned reflexes.* Moscow: Meditsina, 1968.

ANOKHIN, P. K. *Essays in systemic analysis of physiological processes.* Moscow: Meditsina, 1975.

BEKHTEREV, V. N. *Fundamentals of the study of brain functions,* No. 7. St. Petersburg, 1907.

BERNSHTEIN, N. A. The problem of relations between coordination and localization. *Arkhiv Biologicheskikh Nauk,* 1935, *38,* No. 7.

BERNSHTEIN, N. A. *The structure of movement.* Moscow: Medgiz, 1947.

BERNSHTEIN, N. A. Some growing problems in the regulation of movement. *Voprosy Psikhologii,* 1957, No. 6.

BERNSHTEIN, N. A. *The coordination and regulation of movements.* Oxford: Pergamon Press, 1967.

BLINKOV, S. M. *Structural characteristics of the human brain.* Moscow: Medgiz, 1955.

BREMER, F. Neurophysiological correlates of mental unity. In J. Eccles (Ed.), *Brain and conscious experience.* Berlin–New York: Springer, 1966, pp. 283–287.

ECCLES, J. *The neurophysiological bases of mind.* Oxford: Clarendon Press, 1953.

ECCLES, J. (Ed.). *Brain and conscious experience.* Berlin–New York: Springer, 1966.

ECCLES, J. *Facing reality.* Berlin–New York: Springer, 1970.

GAL'PERIN, P. YA. The development of research into the formation of intellectual actions. *Psychological Science in the USSR.* Moscow: Izd. Akad. Pedagog. Nauk RSFSR, 1959.

GRANIT, R. Consciousness: discussion. In J. Eccles (Ed.), *Brain and conscious experience.* Berlin-New York: Springer, 1966, p. 255.

JASPER, H. H. Brain mechanisms and states of consciousness. In J. Eccles (Ed.), *Brain and conscious experience.* Berlin–New York: Springer, 1966, p. 562.

KLEIST, K. *Gehirnpathologie.* Leipzig: Barth, 1934.

KLIMKOVSKII, M., LURIA, A. R., AND SOKOLOV, E. N. *Mechanisms of audioverbal memory,* 1976, in press.

KNEALE, W. *On having a mind.* Cambridge: Cambridge University Press, 1962.

KONORSKI, J., AND LAWICKA, W. Analysis of errors by prefrontal animals on the delayed-response test. In J. M. Warren and K. Akert (Eds.), *The frontal granular cortex and behavior.* New York: McGraw-Hill, 1964.

LEBEDINSKII, V. V. Performance of symmetrical and asymmetrical programs by patients with frontal lobe lesions. In A. R. Luria and E. D. Khomskaya (Eds.), *The frontal lobes and regulation of psychological processes.* Moscow: Izd MGU, 1966, pp. 554–578.

LEONT'EV, A. N. *Problems in the development of the mind.* Moscow: Izd. Akad. Pedagog. Nauk RSFSR, 1959.

LEONT'EV, A. N. The struggle for consciousness in the formation of Soviet psychology. *Voprosy Psikhologii,* 1967, No. 2.

LURIA, A. R. *Traumatic aphasia.* Moscow: Izd. Akad. Med. Nauk, 1947.

LURIA, A. R. (Ed.). *Problems of the higher nervous activity of the normal and abnormal child,* Vols. 1 and 2. Moscow: Izd. Akad. Pedagog. Nauk, 1956, 1958.

LURIA, A. R. *The human brain and psychological processes,* Vols. 1 and 2. Moscow: Izd. Akad. Pedagog. Nauk 1963, 1970. (English edition of Vol. 1, New York: Harper & Row, 1966.)

LURIA, A. R. (Ed.). The frontal lobes and regulation of behavior. *Symposium of the 18th International Psychological Congress,* Moscow, 1966a.

LURIA, A. R. *Higher cortical functions in man.* New York: Consultants Bureau, 1966b.

LURIA, A. R. *Higher cortical functions in man,* second edition. Moscow: Izd. MGU, 1969.

LURIA, A. R. *Traumatic aphasia.* The Hague: Mouton and Cie, 1970.

LURIA, A. R. *The working brain.* New York: Basic Books, 1972.

LURIA, A. R. *Fundamentals of neuropsychology.* Moscow: Izd. MGU, 1973.

LURIA, A. R. *Neuropsychology of memory,* Vols. 1 and 2. Moscow: Pedagogika, 1974–1975. (English edition, Washington: Scripta Technica.)

LURIA, A. R., AND KHOMSKAYA, E. D. (Eds.). *The frontal lobes and regulation of psychological processes.* Moscow: Izd. MGU, 1966.

LURIA, A. R., KHOMSKAYA, E. D., BLINKOV, S. M., AND CRITCHLEY, M. Impaired selectivity of mental processes in association with a lesion of the frontal lobe. *Neuropsychologia,* 1967, 5, 105–117.

LURIA, A. R., KONOVALOV, A. N., AND PODGORNAYA, A. YA. *Disorders of memory in patients with aneurysms of the anterior communicating artery.* Moscow: Izd. MGU, 1970.

LURIA, A. R., PRIBRAM, K. N., AND KHOMSKAYA, E. D. An experimental analysis of the behavioral disturbances produced by a left-sided arachnoidal endothelioma. *Neuropsychologia,* 1964, 2, 257.

LURIA, A. R., PRIBRAM, K. N., AND KHOMSKAYA, E. D. Impairment of the control of motion and activity in association with massive lesions of the left frontal lobe. In A. R. Luria and E. D. Khomskaya (Eds.), *The frontal lobes and regulation of psychological processes.* Moscow: Izd. MGU, 1966.

LURIA, A. R., AND RAPOPORT, M. Y. Regional symptoms of disturbance of higher cortical functions in intracerebral tumors in the left temporal lobe. *Voprosy Neirokhirurgii,* 1962, No. 4.

LURIA, A. R., SOKOLOV, E. N., AND KLIMKOVSKII, M. Toward a neurodynamic analysis of memory disturbances with lesions of the left temporal lobes. *Neuropsychologia,* 1967, 5.

LURIA, A. R., AND TSVETKOVA, L. S. *The neuropsychological analysis of problem solving.* Moscow: Prosveshchenie, 1966.

LURIA, A. R., AND TSVETKOVA, L. S. *Solution des problèmes au course des lesions du lobe frontaux.* Paris: Gautier-Villars, 1967.

LYUBLINSKAYA, A. A. *Essays on the psychological development of the child.* Moscow: Izd. Akad. Pedagog. Nauk RSFSR, 1959.

MACKAY, D. M. On the logical intermediation of the free choice. *Mind,* 1960, 69.

MACKAY, D. M. Cerebral organization of the conscious control of action. In J. Eccles (Ed.), *Brain and conscious experience.* Berlin–New York: Springer, 1966, p. 422.

MAGOUN, H. W. *The waking brain.* Springfield: C. C Thomas, 1958.

MALMO, R. B. Interference factors in delayed response in monkeys after removal of the frontal lobes. *J. Neurophysiol.,* 1942, 5, 295–308.

MILLER, G. A., GALANTER, E., AND PRIBRAM, K. *Plans and the structure of behavior.* New York: Holt, 1960.

MONAKOW, V. *Die Lokalisation im Grosshirn.* Wiesbaden: Bergmann, 1914.

PAVLOV, I. P. *Complete collected works.* Moscow–Leningrad: Izd. Akad. Nauk SSSR, 1949.

PENFIELD, W. Consciousness and centrencephalic organization. *Le Congrès Intern. Scientif. de Neurol. Bruxelles,* 1957.

PENFIELD, W. *The excitable cortex in conscious man* (The Sherrington lecture). Liverpool: Liverpool University Press, 1958.

PENFIELD, W. Speech, perception and the uncommitted cortex. In J. Eccles (Ed.), *Brain and conscious experience.* Berlin–New York: Springer, 1966.

PENFIELD, W., AND JASPER, H. H. *Epilepsy and the functional organization of the brain.* Boston: Little, Brown, 1954.

PENFIELD, W., AND ROBERTS, L. *Speech and brain mechanisms.* Princeton: Princeton University Press, 1959.

PHILLIPS, C. G. Precentral motor area. In J. Eccles (Ed.), *Brain and conscious experience.* Berlin–New York: Springer, 1966.

POPOVA, L. T. *Memory and its disturbances in local brain lesions.* Moscow: Meditsina, 1967.

PRIBRAM, K. N. Recent studies of the function of the frontal lobe in monkeys and man. In A. R. Luria and E. D. Khomskaya (Eds.), *The frontal lobes and regulation of psychological processes.* Moscow: Izd. MGU, 1966.

ROZENGARDT-PUPKO, G. L. *Speech and the development of perception in early childhood.* Moscow: Izd. Akad. Med. Nauk SSSR, 1948.

SHERRINGTON, C. S. *The brain and its mechanisms.* Cambridge: Cambridge University Press, 1934.

SHERRINGTON, C. S. *Man on his nature.* Cambridge: Cambridge University Press, 1940.

SHUMILINA, A. I. The functional role of the frontal region of the cortex of the brain in the conditioned reflex activity of dogs. In A. R. Luria and E. D. Khomskaya (Eds.), *The frontal lobes and regulation of psychological processes.* Moscow: Izd. MGU, 1966.

SPERRY, R. W. Brain bisection and consciousness. In J. Eccles (Ed.), *Brain and conscious experience.* Berlin–New York: Springer, 1966, p. 298.

TEILHARD DE CHARDIN, P. *The phenomenon of man.* New York: Harper, 1959.

VYGOTSKII, L. S. Psychology and the localization of function. *Proceedings of the 3rd Ukrainian Conference of Psychoneurologists,* Kiev, 1934a.

VYGOTSKII, L. S. *Thought and speech.* Moscow: Sotsekgiz, 1934b.

VYGOTSKII, L. S. *Selected psychological investigations.* Moscow: Izd. Akad. Pedagog. Nauk RSFSR, 1958.

VYGOTSKII, L. S. *Development of higher mental processes.* Moscow: Izd. Akad. Pedagog. Nauk RSFSR, 1960.

WALLON, H. *L'enfant turbulent.* Paris: Alcan, 1925.

WALLON, H. *De l'act à la pensée.* Paris: Flammarion, 1942.

WARREN, J. M., AND AKERT, K. (Eds.). *The frontal granular cortex and behavior.* New York: McGraw-Hill, 1964.

ZANGWILL, O. L. *Cerebral dominance and its relation to psychological function.* London: Oliver & Boyd, 1960.

ZANKOV, L. V. *The memory of the school child.* Moscow: Uchpedgiz, 1944.

ZAPOROZHETS, A. V. *The development of voluntary movement.* Moscow: Izd. Akad. Pedagog. Nauk RSFSR, 1959.

2   *Imagery and Thinking: Covert Functioning of the Motor System*

F. J. McGuigan

I. Bodily Systems Implicated in Thought

In numerous studies, it has been found that a variety of bodily systems are covertly activated during cognition. Excellent accounts of brain functioning during thought may be found in Delafresnaye (1954), Eccles (1966), and more recently Young (1970). An instance of a strong centralist position is that of Lashley (1958), in which it is held that thought occurs *exclusively* within the cerebrum (the "Donovan's brain theory," cf. McGuigan, 1973b). The eye also has ranked high in importance among bodily systems that have been empirically implicated in the silent performance of cognitive tasks. Hebb (1968), for instance, in analyzing perception and imagery, held that peripheral activity, especially eye movement, is essential during the formation of images. A general treatment of visual system functioning during cognition may be found in Chase (1973). Visceral activity has been empirically and theoretically implicated in cognitive processes in a variety of ways; we should especially mention work on the esophagus (e.g., Jacobson, 1929), on intestinal activity (e.g., Davis, Garafolow and Gault, 1957), on electrodermal responding (e.g., Grings, 1973), and on the autonomic system in general (e.g., Lacey and Lacey, 1974). Finally, we may note that the skeletal musculature has, since the time of the ancient Greeks, been held to perform critical functions during thought (cf. Langfeld, 1933, and Smith, 1969). The importance of cognitive motor responding was particularly emphasized in Russia and in the United States during the latter part of the 19th and 20th centuries. It was Sechenov (1863/1965) who was most responsible for a

F. J. McGuigan · Performance Research Laboratory, University of Louisville, Louisville, Kentucky.

long line of cognitive psychophysiological theorizing and empirical research in Russia. Sechenov held that "all the endless diversity of the external manifestations of the activity of the brain can be finally regarded as one phenomenon—that of muscular movement . . . therefore, all the external manifestations of brain activity can be attributed to muscular movement." Furthermore, he held that "the time must come when people will be able to analyze the external manifestations of the activity of the brain just as easily as the physicist now analyzes a musical chord or the phenomena presented by a falling body" (1965, pp. 309-310). Sechenov's line of reasoning has been carried on into contemporary Soviet psychology, especially through the works of Pavlov (1941), Bechterev (1923), Leont'ev (1959), Vigotsky (1962), and Gal'perin (1959).

In the United States Titchener (1909) placed great emphasis for the development of meaning on the skeletal musculature by means of his context theory of meaning, though the early behaviorists (e.g., Dunlap, 1922; Hunter, 1924) probably constituted the primary force in perpetuating theoretical conceptions of thought in which muscle responding was critical. Watson, the leading spokesman for the early behaviorists, defined thinking as implicit language behavior (e.g., Watson, 1930). Implicit language behavior, though, was not confined to the speech musculature—while it is often said that Watson held that thought was laryngeal or subvocal responding, he actually stated that manual (nonoral skeletal muscle) responses were also necessary components of an implicit language habit. An example might be that an external conditional linguistic stimulus (e.g., "Eiffel Tower") evokes localized conditional muscle response patterns in the eyes, in the speech musculature, and in the viscera too. Indeed, Watson and the other early behaviorists vigorously promoted the position that one thinks with his entire body. Nonoral behavior was so critical for Watson's theory of thinking that he held that nonoral (as well as oral) responses were necessary for thought. As he put it:

> This line of argument shows how one's total organization is brought into the process of thinking. It shows clearly that manual and visceral organizations are operative in thinking even when no verbal processes are present—*it shows that we could still think in some sort of way even if we had no words!* We thus think and plan with the whole body. But since . . . word organization is, when present, probably usually dominant over visceral and manual organization, we can say that *"thinking"* is largely *subvocal talking*—provided we hasten to explain that it can occur without words. (1930, p. 267-268)

The confusion about Watson's theory of thinking on this point probably came about because people abstracted only the abbreviated statement that thinking goes on largely subvocally.

More contemporary representation of the behaviorist position that thinking occurs throughout the body comes from the work of Skinner (e.g., 1957). Following Watson rather closely, Skinner has also included nonverbal components of thought:

> The simplest and most satisfactory view is that thought is simply *behavior*—verbal or nonverbal, covert or overt. It is not some mysterious process responsible for behavior but the very behavior itself in all the complexity of its controlling relations, with respect to both man the behaver and the environment in which he lives. The concepts and methods which have emerged from the analysis of behavior, verbal or otherwise, are most appropriate to the study of what has traditionally been called the human mind.
>
> The field of human behavior can be conveniently subdivided with respect to the problems it presents and the corresponding terms and methods to be used. A useful distinction may be made between reflexes, conditioned or otherwise, and the operant behavior generated and maintained by the contingencies of reinforcement in a given environment. Tradition and expedience seem to agree in confining the analysis of human thought to operant behavior. So conceived, thought is not a mystical cause or precursor of action, or an inaccessible ritual, but action itself, subject to analysis with the concepts and techniques of the natural sciences, and ultimately to be accounted for in terms of controlling variables.
>
> The emphasis upon controlling variables is important. A practical consequence is that such a scientific account implies a technology. There is no reason why methods of thinking and of the teaching of thinking cannot be analyzed and made more effective. (1966, pp. 17–18)

With this introduction to the view that cognitive processing involves a number of bodily systems, let us now turn to a consideration about how those systems might interact.

II. NEUROMUSCULAR CIRCUIT MODELS OF THOUGHT

Early conceptions of brain functioning held to a "center" model in which there was extreme cerebral localization, such as advocated by Gall and Spurzheim (1809). Neurophysiology has since advanced from "center" models to those of systems (circuits, loops). Historically interesting circuit conceptions in which thought occurs when loops are activated were summarized by Dashiell (1949) as of two kinds: (1) thought consists strictly of the activation of intracerebral circuits: or (2) thought is the activation of circuits between the brain and various peripheral systems (Figure 1). Dashiell pointed out that the motor representation A is an oversimplification in part because it represents thought as a simple serial-order process. I know of no serious thinker who ever conceived of thought as a single-channel linear process, certainly not Watson. For instance, note his complex multichannel interaction representation on page 266 of his 1930 edition.

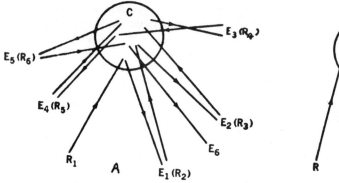
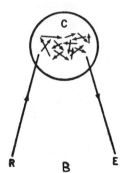

Figure 1. Two extreme views of the role of the brain in thinking. In an extreme motor theory (A) "the original stimulations from a problem situation playing upon receptor R_1 evoke an abbreviated response at effector E_1. This in turn serves to excite receptor R_2 (kinesthetic or other) which evokes a response at effector E_2. And so the nascent abbreviated symbolic responses continue until the thinking eventuates in an overt act, as performed by effector E_6. . . . The neural counterpart of each idea was an excitation in a local spot (cell-cluster) in the brain [B]; and the transitions from idea to idea were referable physiologically to the passage of a neural impulse or train of impulses from cell-cluster to cell-cluster. Now this shooting around of neural currents within the cerebrum is as grossly oversimplified an account as is the story of receptor–effector arcs told above and suggested in part A of the figure" (Dashiell, 1949, pp. 588–589).

Jacobson's pioneering work (e.g., 1932) empirically confirmed the importance of neuromuscular circuits between the brain and the skeletal musculature during higher mental processes. Lilly's interpretation of Jacobson's early studies was that Jacobson proved "that the brain had no closed circuits when it came to mental activity" (Jacobson, 1973, p. 8).

There probably are strictly intracerebral circuits such as those hypothesized by Hebb (1949) in his conceptions of cell assemblies, as well as central-peripheral ones—with the amazing complexity of the interconnections of some 10 billion cerebral neurons, one would be surprised if there were not some strictly transcortical and cortical-subcortical circuits. Nevertheless, such cerebral circuits would no doubt themselves interact with peripheral mechanisms both afferently and efferently, as considered in the above discussion of Sechenev. While Hebb too has emphasized the great importance of central processes for cognitive activity, he has also held that activated cell assemblies result in efferent neural volleys to the musculature and that feedback from muscle activity is of great importance in directing the onflowing circuits of cell assemblies. Whether or not there are closed circuits within the brain that do not interact in any sense with the external musculature is an empirical question (regardless of Sechenov's position) that will probably not be decided within the foreseeable future. The important point for us here is that the early theorizing of central–peripheral circuits (as in Figure 1, though with many simultaneous channels) was empirically confirmed by Jacobson in his classic measurement of mental activities in terms of neuromuscular activity. Jacobson's work and that of later researchers has thus provided us with a sound empirical basis for concluding that the several classes of covert processes discussed in the introduction occur during the silent performance of cognitive tasks (also cf. McGuigan, 1966, 1970, 1973b). These psychophysiologically measured covert events are widespread throughout the body, extremely complex, and often of very low amplitude, and many occur with great rapidity (muscle responses of special interest to us frequently are of but several msec in duration and of less than 1 μV in amplitude).

Much contemporary research is directed toward the specification of functions for these covert processes; of special prominence are processes designated as the contingent negative variation (CNV or "expectancy wave"), evoked brain potentials, galvanic skin responses, heart responding, and covert skeletal muscle activity. Our model has been one in which these brain, muscle, and glandular events are all critical components of neuromuscular circuits that function in highly complex internal information-processing systems within humans. More particularly, we have hypothesized that these covert processes form: (1) intracerebral circuits within various brain regions and (2) circuits between the brain and peripheral mechanisms (the eyes, the skeletal muscles in the neck, arms, tongue, etc.). When activated, these neuromuscular circuits may serve cognitive functions by generating and transmitting verbal codes (cf. McGuigan, 1970, 1973a,b). In Figure 2, we represent a model by which various bodily systems interact during internal information processing. We also indicate complex circuits between the cerebrum and autonomic systems that are assumed to add emotional tone to the linguistic input. These autonomic circuits are extremely slow, perhaps involving seconds, in contrast to the neuromuscular circuits above, which involve but a few msec.

This model is more extensively discussed, together with some of the data on which it is based, in McGuigan (1976). With regard to skeletal muscle data, we have critically summarized data that implicate the speech muscle components of these circuits (McGuigan, 1970) but have not done so for the somatic musculature. In view of our discussion above that covert nonoral responses generated by the

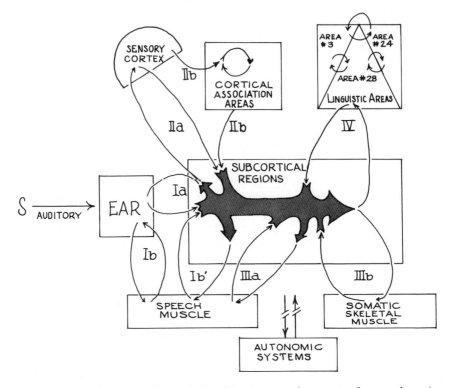

FIGURE 2. Once the external linguistic signal impinges on the receptor (here on the ear), circuits of the class Ia and Ib are simultaneously activated. Circuit class Ib directly functions with the speech musculature, while in circuit Ia information enters the subcortical regions of the brain, whereupon the receptor is modulated by feedback. Next the information is processed between the speech musculature and the subcortical regions (circuit class Ib'). The incoming information is directed to the sensory cortex for integration from the two separate receptors by circuit class IIa. Cortical-subcortical circuits are also activated through the cortical association areas (wherein there are transcortical reverberating circuits) through circuit class IIb. Following this initial processing, cerebral to skeletal muscle circuits are activated (IIIa) for the speech musculature and (IIIb) for the nonoral skeletal muscle; the function of circuit class III is in the generation and transmission of verbal coding for lexical-semantical processing in conjunction with the three major linguistic regions of the brain through circuit class IV.

somatic skeletal muscle systems are also important components of cognitive neuromuscular circuits, we shall now assess the data on which such a conclusion could be based. To do this, we shall critically summarize findings (principally electromyographic ones) during the silent performance of language tasks that have been referred to with such cognitive terms as *imagination* and *thinking*. This step, laborious though it may be, is necessary in order to assure us that there *is* sufficient empirical justification for the position that the motor system serves important functions during imagery and thought. Assuming a positive answer, next is the extremely difficult question of specifying possible cognitive functions of the nonoral skeletal musculature.[1]

III. Methodological Criteria

To assess the research on nonoral, somatic responses during the silent performance of various kinds of cognitive tasks, we will evaluate each study by four general criteria. The first two criteria will allow us to determine whether or not the response actually occurred, and if so whether it was a function of the condition of interest (an experimental treatment, or whatever). The second two criteria are designed to help us ascertain the function of somatic responses by providing an index of the degree of general bodily arousal during the condition or the experimental treatment. If the response is a localized, relatively unique occurrence, it is more likely to serve an information-processing function within neuromuscular circuits. However, if it is accompanied by many other responses, it probably is but one aspect of a state of generalized bodily arousal, perhaps serving only an energy expenditure function. Jacobson (1932) emphasized the importance of the empirical finding that instructions to imagine certain acts resulted in localized versus generalized responses. When Jacobson, for instance, asked subjects to imagine lifting a weight with the right forearm, he found increased electromyographic activity concentrated in the right forearm musculature, leading to the important conclusion that image-produced responses are similar to stimulus-produced responses. Jacobson (1967) commented on the importance of finding localized neuromuscular patterns as follows. He recalled that, starting in the early 1920s, Hans Berger and he were unknowingly engaged in a race with each other to be the first to measure brain voltages. At that time, both assumed that there was an identifiable specific brain pattern characteristic of each mental act. Jacobson eventually doubted this assumption. As he later said:

> Instead, as the result of experiments of others and of myself . . . I am inclined to the opposite belief, surprising as this may at first seem. According to the ultrasensitive measurements during mental activities which have been continued almost daily in my laboratory these past thirty-five years, a specific neuromuscular pattern marks the character of each

[1] Eye activity is so important for cognition that we need to treat it separately (McGuigan, 1978). Consequently, nonoral eye skeletal muscle responses are excluded from this review.

and every moment of their occurrence. The assumption that there is an equally specific and as readily recordable central pattern has not borne fruit, excepting in a minority of recordings. No one has produced such recordings in convincing measure. . . . In every mental activity what is specific is the neuromuscular pattern. (Jacobson, 1967, p. 118)

Davis (1939) also emphasized the importance of the empirical finding of localized covert EMG responding to external stimuli during thought when he summarized and interpreted a variety of findings in terms of his principles of focus of muscular responses. This principle, applicable for the inhibition as well as for the excitation of muscular activity, states that for any psychological process, there is a certain bodily region in which there is a relatively high degree of muscular activity. Furthermore, the amplitude of the response activity decreases as the bodily distance from the focal point increases. Finally, Greenwald (1970) found the following empirical support for his image approach to instrumental conditioning. In various researches when subjects imagined stimuli that would involve localized movement if the act were performed overtly, there was covert movement of the same muscles.

Criterion 1. To determine that a response actually occurred, it is necessary to ascertain whether the measure employed by the researcher systematically changed. One method for determining whether or not the measure systematically changed is for the researcher to have first established a stable, resting baseline condition, following which he administered the experimental treatment (or whatever). The question is whether some kind of measure of the nonoral musculature changed from the resting baseline condition to the period of administration of the experimental treatment. If the researcher followed this procedure and did determine that his covert response measure systematically changed from baseline, then we marked "yes" in Column 1 of Table 1. If the experimenter followed this procedure but reported that there was no systematic change in his measure, then we marked "no" in Column 1 of Table 1. Finally, if the researcher did not compare his covert response measure during the period of the experimental treatment with a previous resting baseline condition, we marked "?" in Column 1 of Table 1, indicating that the experimenter did not successfully employ this criterion as to whether or not the response occurred.

An asterisk in Table 1 indicates that the researcher employed a statistical test and found a significant effect—in the case of Criterion 1, an asterisk indicates that the covert response reliably changed from the baseline resting condition.

Incidentally, some researchers satisfied Criterion 1 in principle,

TABLE 1
Summary of Nonoral Skeletal Muscle Activity during Cognitive Tasks

Task and experimenter	Did the specified muscle response:			
	(1) change from baseline?	(2) vary as a function of conditions?	(3) occur independently of other covert processes?	(4) specifically relate to a cognitive aspect?
Problem solving:				
Golla (1921)	Yes (arm)	Yes	?	Yes
Tuttle (1924)	Yes (patellar reflex)	Yes	?	Yes
Bills (1927)	Yes (general)	Yes*	?	No
Golla and Antonovitch (1929)	Yes (arm, leg, patellar reflex)	No		No
Freeman (1930)	Yes (leg)	Yes	Yes (respiration)	Yes
Freeman (1931)	Yes (arms and legs)	?	?	No
Max (1933)	Yes (arm and hand)	Yes	?	No
Clites (1936)	Yes (rt. arm)	?	?	Yes
Davis (1937)	Yes* (rt. arm)	?	?	Yes
Max (1937)	Yes (arms)	Yes	Yes (leg)	Yes
Davis (1938)	Yes* (rt. arm)	Yes*	No (neck)	Yes
Davis (1939)	Yes (leg, arms)	Yes	Yes (arms, leg)	Yes
Ellson et al. (1952) Exp. 8	Yes* (rt. arm)	Yes*	?	Yes
Reuder (1956)	Yes* (rt. arm)	Yes*	?	Yes
Stennett (1957)	Yes* (arms)	Yes*	No (palmar conductance)	Yes
Leshner (1961)	Yes* (arms)	Yes*	?	Yes
Novikova (1961)	Yes (hand and tongue)	?	?	No
Pishkin (1964)	? (preferred arm)	?	?	Yes
MacNeilage (1966)	Yes* (forehead and rt. arm)	Yes*	Yes and no (see text)	Yes
Pishkin and Shurley (1968)	Yes* (forehead)	Yes*	No (GSR)	Yes

(continued)

TABLE 1. (Continued)

Task and experimenter	Did the specified muscle response:			
	(1) change from baseline?	(2) vary as a function of conditions?	(3) occur independently of other covert processes?	(4) specifically relate to a cognitive aspect?
Problem solving: *(continued)*				
Vaughn and McDaniel (1969)	Yes* (frontalis)	Yes*	?	Yes
McGuigan (1971)	Yes* (left arm)	Yes*	No* (lip EMG, EEG) Yes (leg EMG, respiration rate)	Yes
Imagination:				
Jacobson (1927)	Yes (biceps)	?	?	Yes
Jacobson (1930a)	Yes* (rt. biceps)	Yes	?	Yes
Jacobson (1930b)	Yes (rt. arm)	Yes	?	Yes
Jacobson (1930c)	Yes (rt. arm)	Yes	?	Yes
Jacobson (1931a)	Yes* (rt. biceps)	Yes		Yes
Jacobson (1931b)	Yes (left arm)	Yes	Yes (eye)	Yes
Shaw (1938)	Yes* (various)	No	No (rt. arm)	No
Shaw (1940)	Yes (rt. arm)	Yes	?	Yes
Wolpert (1960)	No (various)	?	?	No
Silent reading:				
Jacobson and Kraft (1942)	Yes (leg)	?	?	Yes
Strother (1949)	Yes* (arms and legs)	Yes*	Yes (right arm)	Yes
McGuigan and Rodier (1968)	No (left arm)	No		No
Hardyck and Petrinovich (1970)	Yes (right arm)	Yes*	No (chin–lip and laryngeal EMG)	

Speech perception:				
Smith et al. (1954)	Yes (arms, neck, and fore head)	Yes*	No (arms and chin) Yes (neck, forehead)	Yes
Wallerstein (1954)	Yes* (forehead and arms)	Yes*	Yes (chin, forehead, and arms are independent)	Yes
Bartoshuk (1956)	Yes* (forehead and arms)	Yes*	Yes (chin, arms, and fore head EMGs are independent) No (frontalis and EEG)	
Learning:				
Travis and Kennedy (1947)	Yes (brow)	Yes	?	Yes
Berry and Davis (1958)	Yes* (forehead and left arm)	Yes*	No (masseter) Yes (forehead and masseter)	?
Berger, Irwin, and Frommer (1970)	Yes (rt. wrist and arm)	Yes*	?	Yes
Petrinovich and Hardyck (1970)	Yes (laryngeal, chin–lip and rt. arm)	Yes*	?	?
Beh & Hawkins (1973)	Yes (arm)	?	?	
Sleep–dreams:				
Max (1935)	Yes (arms)	Yes	?	Yes
Stoyva (1965)	Yes (arm)	Yes	No (EOG)	Yes
Wolpert & Trosman (1958)	Yes (general)	?	?	Yes*
Wolpert (1960)	Yes (wrist)	Yes (?)	No (EEG, EOG)	Yes*
Jacobson et al. (1964)	Yes (29 muscle groups)	?	(various)	Yes
Baldridge et al. (1965)	Yes (hand, foot)	?	No (eye)	Yes
Sassin & Johnson (1968)	Yes (arm & leg)	?	No (EEG)	?
Larson and Foulkes (1969)	Yes (forehead)	?	No (EOG, EEG)	Yes
Pessah and Roffwarg (1972)	Yes (middle ear muscle)	Yes*	No (EOG)	Yes
Gardner et al. (1973)	Yes (various)	—	No (EOG)	Yes

though they did not employ a resting baseline condition. We will mention such variations in the application of this criterion as appropriate when we discuss the experiments below.

Criterion 2. If it is established by Criterion 1 that the response did occur, a researcher could have ascertained whether or not the response occurred because of an experimental treatment *per se*; that is, while one might establish that a response changes from baseline, such a change could have occurred as a function of essentially any stimulation or activity and not because of what was specifically done to or by the subject. Criterion 2 may be satisfied if it is shown that the covert response systematically changes as a function of two (or more) experimental conditions; for example, one might show that electromyograms from the preferred arm are greater when the subject imagines lighting a cigarette than when he imagines looking at the Eiffel Tower (Jacobson, 1932). A particularly valuable control in this regard is one in which the response is measured during some nonlinguistic condition and compared with that during a linguistic condition. For example, subjects might have nonlinguistic trials of listening to white noise (McGuigan and Rodier, 1968) or meaningless changing tones (McGuigan and Pavek, 1972) for a comparison of response values under those conditions with measures during the condition of special interest. Obviously, if a subject makes a certain response during a linguistic condition that he does not make during a nonlinguistic condition, that response is less likely to be a component of a general arousal pattern, and the probability is thereby increased that the response is serving some internal information-processing function.

The same notation as for Column 1 is used for Criterion 2 in Column 2 of Table 1, viz., if the experimenter studied the covert response measure as a function of two or more conditions and found that his measure systematically varied, "yes" is written in Column 2; if he found that the measure did not systematically vary as a function of conditions, "no" is written in Column 2. A question mark indicates that the experimenter did not study the covert response as a function of two or more conditions.

We may note that Criterion 2 is more powerful than Criterion 1 for demonstrating that a response actually occurred. That is, Criterion 2 could substitute for Criterion 1 because a second experimental treatment (or control condition) may serve the same function as that of a baseline measure (and more). To elaborate on this point, a subject told to rest in order to establish a baseline is not "in a vacuum." Rather, he is in some cognitive state unknown to the experimenter. Hence, rather than allowing the subject to be under his own internal stimulus control ("choosing" his own "cognitive activity") for a baseline condition, the experimenter can bring the subject under external stimulus control by administering an experimental treatment of his own selection. An experimental treatment that is common among subjects should thus produce more uniform behavioral effects than would instructions to rest (in which state the "mind wanders"). Nevertheless, the more powerful experimental design is one in which it is possible to determine whether or not a response changes: (1) from a baseline condition and (2) as a function of two or more experimental treatments.

Criterion 3. To determine whether a given response is a unique, localized bodily event, it should be shown that the response occurs independently of other covert processes. For this, concomitant measures should be made from a sample of bodily regions or systems. If the researcher successfully employed this criterion and did find that the response was independent of some other bodily reaction(s), a "yes" is marked in Column 3 of Table 1. If he employed the criterion but found that the response was not independent of the other measure(s) taken, "no" is entered in Column 3. In either case, the concomitant measure taken is specified. If the researcher did not simultaneously record other reactions, a question mark is entered for Criterion 3.

Criterion 4. A final probabilistic indication that a response is a localized event would be the specification of a relationship between a response parameter and a specific aspect of cognition (the latter determined by verbal reports about the subject's "experience," by systematic variation of the subject's conditions or characteristics, etc.). Such specific relationships indicate the intimate involvement of the response with the cognitive activity; for example, Jacobson (1932) showed that the eyes move upward when one is told to imagine the Eiffel Tower in Paris. We should add, though, that this is a rather "loose" criterion, and we will take some considerable liberty in specifying the kinds of variables involved in specific relationships—the nature of the studies to be considered are so diverse that it is probably best for us to be flexible in applying this criterion during this exploratory phase of research evaluation. Perhaps after this initial step, we will learn how to improve our application of Criterion 4, the results of which are summarized in the appendix. With these four criteria, we shall now summarize and evaluate relevant empirical research. The studies that we shall consider fall into six categories, as follows: (1) problem solving; (2) imagination; (3) silent reading; (4) speech perception; (5) learning; and (6) sleep-dreams. Readers who are specializing in this research area will probably wish to study the empirical section in detail. Others may merely wish to use it as a reference section, in which case they might choose to skim the following studies merely in order to form an empirical basis for the interpretation to be considered at the end.

IV. Empirical Studies

A. *Problem Solving*

Although he was primarily concerned with the physiology of neurosis, Golla (1921) also reported data relating changes in muscle activity to cognition. In the first study (McGuigan, 1970), a subject was instructed initially to sing up and down an octave and then to imagine the same activity. Phasic changes of the front neck musculature (hence laryngeal movements associated with thyroid cartilage movement) were measured by a system of tambours and an optical lever. Sample records showed that muscle activity during imagination was of lesser amplitude but in the same pattern as that observed during actual performance of singing. In the second, more directly relevant study, tonic muscle activity of an unspecified forearm was measured by a similar apparatus during a mental arithmetic task. Records obtained from one "unsophisticated" subject indicated that muscle tonicity increased during the task and was positively related to the difficulty of the problem. Golla concluded that such muscle activity may not only be a manifestation of cerebral activity but a necessary concomitant of it. In Table 1, because the arm measure changed from baseline, we enter "yes" in Column 1 (the lack of an asterisk indicating that no statistical test was applied.) The "yes" in Column 2 is indicative of Golla's finding that muscle tonicity increased as a function of a difficulty of the problem, this specific relationship also accounting for the "yes" in Column 4. The question mark in Column 3 indicates that no other bodily measures were concomitantly made with arm activity.

Tuttle (1924) tapped subjects' patellar tendons with a constant force at constant intervals and obtained measures of muscle tonus during conditions of rest, problem solving, and conversation. Muscle tonus was measured as the distance of leg deflection during the knee jerk. The records from all subjects showed that mental activity increased muscle tonus, with reflex activity being highest during problem solving, next highest for conversation, and lowest for the relaxation condition. Agreeing with A. P. Weiss, Tuttle concluded that "attention" is increased tonicity of the muscles which adjusts the body for the favorable reception of stimuli. Furthermore, the amount of muscle tonus seemed to be positively associated with the degree of attention. Because the assessments in Table 1 for each article should be fairly apparent from this point on, the reader should be able to relate each study to the four criteria without further comment here except as necessary.

Bill's (1927) approach was unique. He asked, "Will an increase in the total amount of muscular tension in the body increase mental efficiency?" and thus reversed the usual order of dependent and independent variables in the experiment. Muscle tension was increased by having the subjects squeeze a spring dynanometer, and the increased tension was confirmed by kymographic records. Mental work included the learning of nonsense syllables, the learning of meaningful paired associates, the adding of columns of numbers, and a rapid perception task. Learning efficiency (average learning time) was measured under normal and increased muscular tension. During all types of mental work, learning efficiency was significantly greater under increased muscular tension, with no sizable differences among the various mental tasks.

The effect of fatigue upon adding numbers and upon the perception task indicated that learning speed was less susceptible to decrement under increased muscular tension than under normal tension, however, the decrement in accuracy of performance did not differ during fatigue between the two muscle conditions. After a thoughtful analysis of various ways in which heightened muscular tension might facilitate mental work, Bills implied a confirmation of Washburn's (1916) hypothesis that motor innervations are not mere accompaniments of directed thought but are essential parts of the cause of directed thought. Bills also presented a most interesting historical summary of previous research on the influence of muscular tension on the efficiency of mental work, citing the positive findings of Lombard in 1887, Dresslar in 1891, and so forth. The "yes" in Column 1 for this study may be somewhat misleading because Bills employed degree of muscle tension as the independent variable, thus intentionally increasing tension from a resting condition. In Column 2, the "yes" indicates the successful use of a control (normal muscle tension) condition, and the "no" in Column 4 reflects the finding that there were no sizable differences in learning efficiency as a function of the various mental tasks. (This same comment applies to several other studies too, particularly to Smith, Brown, Toman, and Goodman, 1947, and to Beh and Hawkins, 1973).

Golla and Antonovitch (1929) measured tonus or arm and leg extensor muscles and the patellar reflex by means of an optical myograph while subjects performed various cognitive tasks (mental arithmetic, pursuit tasks, etc.). In general, there was an immediate rise of tonus or reactivity at the inception of mental work, an increase that remained for a brief period before returning to the original level. No relation between efficiency or task difficulty and amount of muscle activity was found. Golla and Antonovitch concluded that these *involuntary* responses serve a preparatory function in the performance of cognitive tasks. The inconsistency between these results and those summarized by Bills (1927) that show that increased muscular tension improves mental efficiency may be due to the fact that the previous work dealt with voluntary innervation and thus may have no direct bearing on the involuntary responses studied by Golla and Antonovitch.

Two experiments in which muscle tension changed with the performance of "mental work" were reported by Freeman (1930). In the first experiment, tension of the quadriceps muscle group of the right leg was measured during conditions of rest and during various counting operations that varied in difficulty. Tension was measured with an optical lever attached to the patellar tendon; a beam of light was reflected from the lever upon a millimeter scale so that the higher the reading, the greater the quadriceps tension. The result was that tension increased upon presentation of the problem and decreased as the task was completed. Tension during the first part of the problem varied directly as a function of task difficulty. Diminution of the tension in this muscle group appeared to be a positive function of the correctness of the response.

In a second and similar experiment, subjects were interrupted during the performance of their tasks. The findings were in accord with those of the first experiment, though there were additional tension increments following task interruption. Freeman concluded that increased muscle tonus occurs during mental work because it has been previously reinforced by the successful completion of the task.

In further work, Freeman (1931) obtained records of muscle thickening of the arms and legs while his subjects engaged in a mental arithmetic task. The subjects sat in a device resembling a pillory or "stock," and displacements of levers resting on the arm and leg muscles were photographically recorded. The data indicate that muscle thickening increased from baseline during performance of the task, although the loci of these movements varied from subject to subject. Freeman concluded that the peripheral neuromuscular "flux" during this cognitive activity provides evidence of the general fertility of a motor theory of consciousness.

Using deaf-mute subjects, Max (1933)[2] recorded covert (electromy-

---

[2] These data are further described in Max (1935).

ographic—EMG) contractions of the arm and hand muscles during "simpler types of consciousness" (sleep, dreams, and sensation) and during thought problems (verbal, visual, kinesthetic, and arithmetic). The results indicated (1) that arm and hand action-currents increase during dreams; (2) that sensory stimulation is associated with action-current responses of the peripheral musculature; (3) that the subjective experience of a kinesthetic image is a correlate of actual muscular contraction; and (4) that in deaf subjects, responses in the hand muscles are associated with thinking and appear to be present during vocalization by deaf subjects able to speak. Max stated that hand EMG varies with the type of problem; hence the "yes" in Column 2.

Clites (1936) examined the relation between involuntary muscle contractions, grip tension, and action potentials during successful and unsuccessful problem solving. Grip tension, as measured by an arrangement of tambours and a kymograph, and right forearm muscle action potentials (EMG) were recorded during periods of relaxation and during attempts to solve the second water-dipping problem of the Binet test. Comparisons of performance between successful and unsuccessful subjects indicated that successful subjects showed significantly greater right-forearm EMG and significantly less overt movement of the arm; they also manifested greater relaxation of the grip, but this change was not significant. Unsuccessful subjects exhibited relatively consistent forearm EMG, grip pressure, and overt movement from rest periods to solution periods. Disregarding task performance, no significant correlations were found between EMG, grip tension, and overt involuntary movement of the arm. Clites concluded that the superior performance of the successful subjects may be attributed to increased muscle activity. The general conclusion from his entire series of studies was either that muscle activity is increased during problem solving or that problem solving is identical with increased muscle activity. Either explanation is offered as a substitute for the hypothesis that there is a mere "overflow" of efferent impulses from the brain.

Davis (1937) investigated the relationship between "mental work" and muscular phenomena (EMG recorded from the right forearm with an electron oscillograph). Three types of "mental work" were studied: memorization of poetry, rotational addition, and multiplication. Baseline action potentials were obtained during relaxed rest preceding each task. Significant EMG increases from baseline were found during poetry reading and multiplication. During addition, there was also an EMG increase, but the effect was not statistically significant. No EMG comparisons were made as a function of type of mental work. For all three types of "mental work," there tended to be a negative correlation between the amount of right arm action potentials and the amount of work accomplished.

Investigating the motor theory of consciousness (in which cognitive activity is related to motor activity of the linquistic apparatus), Max (1937) hypothesized that the activity of the linguistic mechanisms of deaf sugjects should increase relative to that of hearing subjects during the solution of "thought problems." His measure was EMG activity of the musculature of both forearms that controlled finger movements (the locus of the subject's "speech"). A response was implicitly defined as any measurable voltage during problem solving; response amplitude ranged between 0.1 and 9 μV (microvolts). Max found that abstract thought problems elicited action-current responses more frequently and to a greater extent in the arms of the deaf individuals than in the legs. Some particular findings were as follows: (1) the subjective experience of a kinesthetic image was accompanied by peripheral EMGs in 73% of the instances for hearing subjects and in 88% for deaf subjects; (2) for deaf subjects, abstract thought problems produced heightened EMGs in 84% of the cases as compared with 31% for hearing subjects; (3) simultaneous recording of EMGs from the arms and legs of the deaf produced 73% positive responses in the arms and 19% in the legs; (4) for deaf subjects, simple silent reading and repetition of verbal material produced smaller and less frequent EMGs than reading with the intent to remember or engaging in relatively complex thought problems; (5) in general, the more intelligent and better educated the deaf subjects, the less the EMG response to problem situations; (6) vocalized speech was accompanied by manual currents more frequently in deaf than in hearing subjects. Max's conclusion was that these manual responses in the deaf are more than adventitious effects of irradiated tensions and that they have some specific connection with the thinking process. His results thus lent support to the behavioristic form of the motor theory of consciousness.

Davis (1938) recorded muscle action potentials from the right forearm and side of the neck near the thyroid gland while his subjects mentally solved five series of graded number problems. Baseline recordings were obtained. Preceding and following each series, the subjects relaxed. Forearm EMG was significantly lower than neck EMG during the baseline period. Both significantly increased during problem solving from the baseline levels. Forearm EMG exhibited a significantly greater percentage of increase than neck EMG, although Davis suggested that this difference may be attributed to a greater sensitivity of the arm apparatus. Although no differential EMG responses were associated with success or failure, there was a corresponding increase in action potentials of the arm and neck as task difficulty increased. Davis concluded that these results confirm the hypothesis that muscular tensions form a part of the ordinary psychological processes and that further attempts should be made to relate such processes and muscle action.

In further work, Davis (1939) had two independent groups of subjects engage in mental arithmetic and in memorizing nonsense syllables, respectively. EMGs were recorded from the left and right forearms and from the calf of the left leg. The subjects worked under normal conditions and also with instructions to relax the right arm. There were increases (as measured by percentage of increase during work relative to resting) that were not statistically evaluated in all three bodily locations during normal work conditions. During multiplication, the focus of activity was in the right arm (with the least activity in the leg), while in the learning of nonsense syllables, neither arm dominated the other. The subjects spontaneously reported that there was a strong tendency to write during multiplication but not while memorizing nonsense syllables. There was little difference during the learning of nonsense syllables among these three locations, leading Davis to speculate that activity during the nonsense-syllable condition was concentrated in some other part of the body, such as in the speech musculature. Instructions to relax the right arm during work reduced EMG activity in all three bodily regions for both conditons. Furthermore, there was "definite evidence" that work output decreased when the subjects tried to keep the arm relaxed.

Interpreting his own current and previous findings, and also the work of Shaw (1938) and others, Davis put forth a "principle of focus of muscular responses," applicable to both the inhibition and the excitation of muscular activity. The principle is that for any psychological process, there is some region in which there is a relatively high degree of muscular activity. A corollary of this principle is that the amplitude of activity decreases as the bodily distance from the focal point increases.

In their eighth experiment, Ellson, Davis, Saltzman, and Burke (1952) recorded EMGs from opposed muscle groups in the arm during "lying" and "nonlying." The subjects were provided the opportunity to take 50 cents in various coin denominations. During a subsequent interrogation period, crucial questions were presented visually concerning the denominations of the particular coins taken. Subjects then responded to these questions by making "yes" or "no" movements of a key. They were instructed that they could keep the money if they successfully escaped detection. The results indicated that EMG response *amplitude* did not significantly discriminate lies from truths. However, EMG response *latencies* were significantly shorter for critical lying responses than for critical nonlying responses. Ellson *et al.* concluded that the temporal order of responses to questions may provide a useful means of detecting deception.

In the following three studies, the investigators attempted to manipulate the subject's subjective approach to the problem-solving task in order to assess the relationship of this variable to the degree of covert muscle activity occurring during the task. The focus of these studies is upon general bodily arousal, rather than on localizing specific bodily areas of responding.

Reuder (1956) studied the differential effects of ego- and task-orienting instructions on muscle tension during problem solving. She factorially combined two types of instruction (ego-orienting versus task-orienting) with two levels of difficulty of mathematical progressions. Right forearm EMGs were obtained during rest, presentation of instructions, and problem solving. The results indicated that no significant increases in EMGs from initial rest occurred during instruction or interproblem rest periods but that right forearm EMG did significantly increase during the problem solving. The effect of increased problem difficulty significantly increased EMG activity. A significant instruction-by-difficulty interaction indicated that task-oriented subjects exhibited higher EMG levels on the more difficult problems than they did on the easy problems, whereas the ego-oriented subjects showed higher EMG levels for the easy problems than for the difficult ones. Reuder concluded that ego- and task-orienting instructions interact with task difficulty and therefore that this experimental variable must be considered in the design of experiments relating muscle tension and performance.

The hypothesis that an inverted-U relationship exists between level of arousal and performance on an auditory tracking task was tested by Stennett (1957). As a measure of arousal, right and left arm EMGs and palmar conductance were recorded during a baseline condition of rest and during the performance of the tracking task under various incentive conditions. Incentive was varied widely from one condition in which the subject thought performance was not recorded, to another, in which performance determined the avoidance of a 100–150 V shock. The results indicated that the hypothesized relation between performance and arousal was generally appropriate, regardless of the measure considered. Stennett concluded that incentive is the most important experimental variable determining the steepness of the EMG gradient during task performance. The "yes" in Column 4 refers to the relationship between levels of incentive and arousal. It could be argued, that this is not a specific cognitive relationship and should therefore read a "no" for this study.

Leshner (1961) studied the effects of levels of aspiration on muscle action potentials during a problem-solving task. Subjects were assigned to four groups designated as "Expect–Success," "Hope–Success," "Expect–Failure," and "Hope –Failure." All groups were given figure-pattern problems during two task sessions, which were preceded and separated by rest periods. "Expect" groups stated aspirations in terms of scores they expected to obtain; "Hope" groups stated the scores they wanted to achieve. Following the task, half of each group were given fictitious scores and norms indicating that they had failed, while the other half received fictitious information indicating success. EMGs from both forearms were recorded throughout the entire experimental session. The results indicated a general (though nonsignificant) trend for all groups of an increase in EMGs above resting levels during aspiration periods, followed by a further increase during the task. Muscle activity decreased from the task level when subjects were informed of their success or failure. A significant aspiration by achievement interaction indicated that for subjects who failed, the rate of tension increase was greater for subjects who stated expectations than for those with unrealistic aspirations; but for subjects who succeeded, EMGs of the unrealistic were significantly higher than those of the realistic. Regardless of aspiration, EMGs during work significantly decreased among successful subjects and significantly increased among those who failed.

Seeking to localize covert responding in deaf-mutes during problem solving, Novikova (1961) recorded (unspecified) arm and tongue EMGs as the subjects solved mental arithmetic problems. Sample records showed increased EMGs from both regions above rest while the subjects were engaged in the tasks. The same phenomenon was reported for normal subjects who were proficient in manual speech. Novikova concluded that a single functional system develops that apparently includes control of both fingers and the tongue.

Using chronic schizophrenics, Pishkin (1964) investigated the intercorrelations between concept-identification performance, number of trials to criterion, time per response, learning rate, and EMG, with the focus on the relationship between EMG and concept-identification performance. Subjects categorized geometric patterns as "A" or "B," following which a light came on above either A or B to indicate correct response. There was a significant positive correlation between preferred-arm EMG amplitude and learning rate, and a negative correlation between preferred-arm EMG amplitude and time per trial. These relationships suggested that some motivational influence was involved and that the general tension level was lower in those subjects who produced more errors.

Although specifically interested in studying changes in EEG amplitude, MacNeilage (1966) also obtained records of various other indices of activation, including right-arm and forehead EMG, EKG, and palmar conductance during a spaced auditory serial addition task. Baseline recordings were taken during rest; following that, there were two experimental conditions in which the subjects simply wrote numbers or silently performed serial addition of numbers that were auditorially presented. These two conditions were then repeated and followed by a final rest period. The results showed that all indices of activation significantly increased from rest during both of the experimental conditions, but no reliable differences were found between the two experimental conditions. Difficulty of the serial addition task (varied by speed of presentation), significantly increased only forehead and right-arm EMG in the first part of the experiment; however, in the second part of the experiment, the difficulty of the task significantly increased heart rate, respiration, and right-arm EMG, while significantly reducing EEG alpha. Forehead EMG was not significantly affected by task difficulty in the second part. A description of the within-trials effects for the addition task indicated that as percentage of correct responses, EKG, and palmar conductance decreased, the EEG alpha amplitude increased. However, arm and forehead EMG showed no similar gradients. MacNeilage concluded that all measures excepting EMG show a high concordance and that this exception presents difficulty for an activation theory of mental performance.

Pishkin and Shurley (1968) studied the effects of cognitive stress upon subsequent performance of a concept-identification task and on level of arousal. Three levels of task complexity were factorially combined with two sets given to the subjects (solvable and unsolvable). The concept-identification tasks required the subjects to classify geometric patterns in accordance with the relevant dimension (size, color, or shape) by pressing one of two response keys. In the first stage of the procedure, the subjects were given a set task that established either a solvable or an unsolvable set. For the solvable set, subjects received accurate feedback. In the unsolvable set, subjects were given incorrect feedback on 50% of the trials. In the second stage of the experiment, the subjects were presented a similar series of concept-identification problems while spontaneous GSR and forehead EMG were recorded. The results were that task complexity and the effects of cognitive stress induced by the unsolvable set significantly increased the number of errors on the concept-identification task and forehead EMG, while spontaneous GSR significantly decreased. Significant task-set interactions indicated that increases of muscle tension and number of errors and decreases in spontaneous GSR are of lesser degree for the unsolvable than for the solvable conditions. Correlational analyses showed a significant positive relationship between EMGs and number of errors and significant negative relationships between these measures and the GSR. Pishkin and Shurley interpreted these data as indicating that increased muscle activity is associated with the inability to process information, while spontaneous GSR indicates successful information intake.

Vaughn and McDaniel (1969) recorded frontalis muscle activity ("forehead" EMG) during a match-to-sample visual discrimination task. Control recordings during relaxation, viewing a sample stimulus, and performance of the manual response were followed by six experimental trials. The results showed a significantly higher EMG amplitude associated with correct responses than with incorrect responses, with attentuation of muscle tension following errors for all but the first and last trial. Phasic EMG responses were typically superimposed on a progressively rising and then falling gradient of frontalis muscle activity. Vaughn and McDaniel concluded that these data support Sokolov's (1963) conception of the orienting reflex, in that phasic increments and decrements are dependent upon tonic adjustments. Thus, habituation of the phasic orienting reactions explains the downward trend of this response during the final trials.

Max's classical conclusion that covert finger movements occur in deaf subjects during thinking was tested by McGuigan (1971) using six subjects who were proficient in manual speech and who were learning oral speech. It was found that amplitude of left-arm and lip EMG significantly increased during problem solving. Left-arm EMG increased significantly more during problem solving than during a nonverbal control task; integrated EEG from the left motor area decreased significantly more during the problem solving. No significant differences occurred for leg EMG, but respiration rate increased significantly during all tasks. In conformity with the findings of Max (1937) and Novikova (1961), McGuigan (1971) concluded that the manual and oral regions were covertly functioning as a single linguistic system during thinking.

B. Imagination

The classical work in this section has been conducted primarily by Jacobson. Further on we discuss Jacobson's development of this research area—perhaps a review of that section would facilitate the reader's perspective of the following articles. Principally, Jacobson was interested in the psychophysiological measurement of mental activities, as a basic science endeavor and for clinical application (the measurement of progressive relaxation and the elimination of phobias).

Jacobson (1927) reported the effects of progressive relaxation training on various conscious processes including imagery, attention, reflection, and emotion. His observations indicated that extreme relaxation was incompatible with the simultaneous presence of these activities. To test this conclusion using another approach, Jacobson employed a string galvanometer to measure electrical activity of brachial–biceps muscles of the arm while the subject imagined activities using the same arm. Nonamplified readings from this instrument indicated that muscle action potentials increased from rest during the period of imagination. Jacobson suggested that a clear-cut interpretation of these preliminary data would require recordings from several muscle groups during a variety of tasks. Jacobson (1930a) conducted an experiment to determine if imagination of a specific motor act is associated with an increase of muscle action potentials (EMG) of the muscles that would be involved in the overt performance of that act. EMGs were recorded from the right biceps–brachial muscles of the arm by use of a string galvanometer and vacuum tube amplifiers. The subjects first relaxed and then, at a tone signal, imagined that they voluntarily flexed their right arm. For control conditions, subjects either were presented the tone signal and instructed not to imagine or were asked to imagine movements of the body other than the right arm. The results indicated that during imagination of right arm flexion, 96% of the (141) tests were associated with EMG increments from the right arm; whereas 93% of the (149) control tests of imagination of other than right arm movement showed no increase of right arm EMG. Additionally, EMG levels during imagination of right arm flexion were consistently above relaxation levels and of the same form and duration but lower in amplitude than during actual overt right-arm flexion. Jacobson concluded that imagination of voluntary movement is associated with neuromuscular activity in the locale of the imagine act.

The next report in this series by Jacobson (1930b) replicated and extended his previous finding that localized EMG increments accompany imagination of voluntary motor acts. The subjects were instructed to imagine various acts commonly performed with the right arm: "Imagine lifting a cigarette to your mouth"; "Imagine throwing a ball"; "Imagine pulling on your socks." EMGs were recorded from the right arm during the experimental conditions as well as during control periods of relaxation, when subjects were under instructions either not to imagine at all or to imagine performing motor acts with the *left* arm following the auditory signal. The results indicated that EMG increments of 186–550% above resting baseline occurred in 159 of 163 tests. All control tests were negative. In a second part of the experiment, subjects were asked to recollect any previous muscular acts commonly performed with the right arm. Recording and control procedures were similar to those of the first experiment. EMG increments were found in 60 of 90 experimental tests. Postsession interviews indicated that some subjects recalled these past experiences *visually*, hence, Jacobson reasoned that the negative instances in the right arm may have been accompanied by increases in other body locations (e.g., the eyes), thus accounting for this relatively low percentage of positive findings. In any event, Jacobson did extend the base for his general conclusion that imagination and recollection of voluntary acts are accompanied by localized electrical changes in appropriate neuromuscular regions.

In a replication of previous procedures (1930a, 1930b), Jacobson (1930c) used platinum iridium wire electrodes for more precise measurement of muscle action potentials. Electrode insertion was in the biceps muscle of the right arm. EMG records were made during baseline relaxation, while the subjects imagined lifting a 10-pound weight in the right hand and while they imagined lifting the weight in the left hand (control tests). To corroborate the EMG data, a mechanical device composed of a system of levers was attached to the supported right forearm, allowing the measurement of microscopic flexions. All records obtained during experimental conditions of imagined movement of the right arm did show a correspondence between microscopic flexion and increased muscle action potentials. The 19 control tests (imagining lifting the weight with the left hand) were all negative for both measures of muscle activity. To further specify the relation between muscular activity and imagination, subjects were instructed to cease imagining or to relax upon hearing an auditory signal. Comparisons of records for each condition showed that both instructions returned muscle activity to resting levels, suggesting to Jacobson that muscle activity is required for imagination. In another procedure, subjects were instructed to relax the right arm and simultaneously imagine lifting a weight with the same arm. In one condition, the instruction was added that if this was impossible then the subject should engage in imagination; in the other condition, the subject was instructed to relax if he could not perform the simultaneous tasks. EMG records showed that all subjects in the first condition had increased muscle activity, whereas subjects in the second condition showed resting levels of right arm activity. Jacobson concluded that imagination of movement of a part of the body cannot occur if the muscles of that area are relaxed. Generally, these data confirm previous findings of Jacobson (1930a, 1930b) that contraction of specific muscles occurs following instructions to imagine an act that involves those muscles during overt performance.

Jacobson (1931a) further examined the differential activity of arm and ocular muscles during imagination by instructing relaxation-trained subjects either to "imagine" or to "imagine visually" lifting a weight with the right arm. EMGs were recorded by use of inserted electrodes during the experimental conditions and also during a control condition in which subjects were instructed not to imagine following the signal. After the instructions simply to imagine the action, all subjects showed EMG increases from rest of the right biceps muscle, whereas instructions to imagine the action *visually* produced increased biceps activity in only 1 of 17 tests. When EMG was simultaneously recorded from the ocular region following instructions to imagine visually, voltage changes from rest were observed in 29 of 31 tests. No changes from rest of arm or ocular muscle activity were recorded during the control condition. Further tests indicated that subjects instructed to "imagine" the arm action consistently showed increased biceps activity and occasionally showed ocular muscle activity. Jacobson concluded that imagination involves specific neuro-muscular activities and that the locus of this activity is dependent upon the type of imagery (i.e., visual versus nonvisual).

Jacobson (1931b) conducted a series of tests to determine if a subject could imagine flexion of a left arm amputated 32 years previous to the experiment. EMG during instructed imagination of left-hand flexion was recorded from the partly amputated biceps muscle and from the muscles that flex the right hand. When the subject was instructed to imagine left-hand flexion, the biceps stump EMG showed increased activity in 13 of 14 trials, while recordings of right arm EMG showed increases in 6 of 6 cases. Control tests in which the subject was instructed to imagine nothing showed no increased activity from either electrode placement. In other control tests, the subject was instructed to overtly bend the left and right foot or the right arm. Unlike in normal subjects, left-arm EMG was usually found to increase during imagination of these activities.

These latter data suggested to Jacobson that activities of the arms were not clearly dissociated in this subject. However, of particular interest was the voluntary report of the subject at the conclusion of the experiment that he could not imagine left-hand activity independent of the right hand. That is, no independent imagination apparently existed for this subject's left hand. Jacobson concluded that imagination or recalled use of the lost muscles that flex the left hand are associated with a "substitute reaction" of the corresponding muscles of the right arm or in the remnant muscles of the upper left arm. It would be of interest to conduct further work with more recent (or double) amputees, since building up substitute circuits presumably takes time.

In work that is related closely to Jacobson's, Shaw (1938) investigated the distribution of muscle activity during various tasks of imagination to determine if there was a localization in the muscle groups involved in the actual performance of the imagined activity. EMG was recorded from those muscle groups expected to increase in activity during imagination of various tasks, including typing, singing, playing a wind instrument, and squeezing a hand dynamometer. The results indicated that there were significant increments in EMG for all subjects, although localization was not always consistent. Furthermore, there was an absence of increased EMG in subjects unable to imagine the instructed actions. Shaw concluded that muscle activity is a necessary concomitant of the imagination of various activities.

In subsequent work, Shaw (1940) studied the relation between muscle action potentials and imagination by instructing subjects first to lift a series of weights with the right arm and then to imagine lifting the same weights with the same arm. At no time was the subject allowed to see the weights. Action potentials were recorded from the right forearm during actual and imagined lifting. The results indicated that increments in right arm EMG occurred during actual and imagined lifting of the weights and that the magnitude of the muscle response in *both* conditions increased linearly with the magnitude of the weight. Of particular importance is that these muscle responses did not decrease with repeated imaginations—since the responses did not habituate, they are more likely to be critical for the imagination process. Shaw concluded that muscular activity during imagination appears to increase with the amount of difficulty associated with the imagined task.

Wolpert (1960) recorded EMG from a variety of electrode placements while subjects imagined actions that had, upon previous overt performance, yielded measurable potentials. No increased EMG responses were noted during imagination. Wolpert attributed his failure to confirm Jacobson's (1932) findings to his use of surface electrodes (rather than needle electrodes) and to the use of subjects untrained in progressive relaxation. These nontrained subjects were probably tenser than trained, relaxed subjects, so that the small potentials that accompanied thought may have been swamped by generalized tension potentials generated by nervous subjects anticipating instructions.

C. Silent Reading

Jacobson and Kraft (1942) electromyographically measured muscle activity of the leg (right quadriceps femoris) with wire electrodes while (100) subjects engaged in a task of silent reading. The results indicated that the mean leg EMG curve ran between the values of 1.5 and 2.0 μV for the duration of the 30-min reading period. The highest levels occurred during the first 2 min of reading and during the last 4 min of reading; the lowest EMG level occurred during the interval of 16–18 min of reading. Post-experimental-session recordings indicated that the average EMG level of the quadriceps muscle dropped to less that 0.5 μV during relaxation. Jacobson and Kraft concluded that the level of quadriceps EMG during reading is consistently above the level of rest.

Strother (1949) monitored arm and leg EMGs while subjects read interpretive material expressive of happiness, hate–anger, tranquility–reverence, and fear. Half of the subjects had electrodes placed on the left arm and the left leg, while the other half had electrodes placed on the right arm and the right leg. The results showed that regardless of location, muscle activity differed significantly as a function of the four different kinds of emotional material read. The order of EMG magnitude for the different emotions were (in descending order): fear, hate–anger, happiness, and tranquility-reference. Strother studied the difference between subjects trained and untrained in dramatic reading, a contrast that does not concern us here. For his untrained subjects, however, he concluded that the *right* arm gave consistently the highest level of activity, with a degree of consistency that led him to argue for its acceptability as a conclusion, though the number of subjects was too small to lend itself to statistical treatment.

In two experiments, McGuigan and Rodier (1968) systematically manipulated the amplitude of covert oral behavior during silent reading. There were four reading conditions: (1) silence, (2) auditory presentation of prose, (3) backward prose, and (4) white noise. Oral activity (chin and tongue EMG) generally increased under the reading conditions, as did breathing rate. However, nonoral responding was inconsistent: left arm EMG increased slightly in 13 statistical tests (only 1 of which was significant), decreased in 4 tests (none of which was significant), and did not change in 1.

Hardyck and Petrinovich (1970) studied the relationship of subvocal speech to difficulty of reading material and to comprehension. Three groups of subjects read two passages, varied as to level of difficulty, while laryngeal, chin–lip, and right forearm flexor EMGs were recorded. Subjects in the *normal* group simply read the passages, whereas in a laryngeal *feedback* group, subjects heard a tone following any increase in the amplitude of the integrated laryngeal EMG. To control for the added complexity of this task, a *control* group received the same tone if the right forearm flexor EMG exceeded a predetermined relaxation level. All measures of EMG activity were found to increase from baseline during the reading tasks, although no statistical analyses were conducted.

All three EMG measures did significantly increase as the difficulty of the prose read increased. There were also two significant interactions: experimental condition interacted with muscle group, and difficulty level interacted with muscle group. Specifically, laryngeal EMG increased for "easy" versus "hard" reading material for the normal and control groups but remained near zero for the feedback group, whereas chin–lip and forearm flexor activity showed no systematic change in relation to the experimental condition. The interaction between difficulty level and muscle group indicated that laryngeal and chin–lip activity were correlated with difficulty, while the forearm flexor group showed little change. Comprehension was significantly and inversely related to difficulty, with the feedback condition exhibiting a significantly greater decrement in comprehension relative to the experimental and control conditions. Hardyck and Petrinovich concluded that subvocal speech serves as a vital stimulus input capable of mediating a cognitive response—an extension of a proposal by Osgood (1957).

D. Speech Perception

The internal processing that occurs during listening is no doubt unique in some important respects. By systematically recording various covert processes, we should be able to specify the critical neuromuscular circuits that function during speech perception. Unfortunately, as we shall see, much additional research is necessary on this important problem. Neck, forehead, chin, and both forearm EMGs were recorded from subjects during listening and talking by Smith, Malmo, and Shagass (1954). Two groups of subjects—psychiatric patients and college students—heard a tape-recorded article on sleep. Subsequently, they were asked to recall verbally what the article was about. EMG activity was recorded during a period of quiescence both preceding and following the tape recording. No sizable differences in amount of muscle tension were measured between the periods before and after listening. However, significant increases in muscle activity were found in both forearms and the chin during listening. During talking, significant increases in EMG activity occurred at all sites monitored. When amount of muscle tension between the patients and the students was compared, the patients showed a significantly higher amount of tension in the chin only during both reading and talking. These muscle tension changes were thought to be related to attention. However, the tape recording the subjects listened to sounded in places "like a bad radio," so that the subjects evidently had generally to strain to be able to comprehend the words; consequently, the EMG changes in this study are not unequivocally related to the process of speech perception and should be evaluated with that caution in mind.

Wallerstein (1954) recorded EMG from the chin, the forehead, and both forearm extensors during tasks of attentive listening that were varied in ease of comprehension. His subjects listened to a detective story ("easy") and then to a philosophical essay ("difficult") of about 10 minutes' length. Each was preceded and followed by rest (baseline) intervals, and each was repeated three times. The results indicated that frontalis EMG significantly increased from the baseline during all listening periods, whereas a significant increase in chin EMG was found for only the second and third hearings of the story, but not similarly for the essay. During the listening period, frontalis EMG exhibited a nonsignificant rising gradient of tension, while chin EMG showed no clear pattern. Wallerstein concluded that rising gradients of muscle tension reflect the amount of information processed, rather than task difficulty or level of arousal. Theoretically (after Hebb, 1949), these gradients may be viewed as the interaction of central and motor events constituting the thought process.

Wallerstein also found that prerest tension of the frontalis significantly decreased from the first to third hearings of the story and the essay, while a similar pattern for chin EMG was not significant. Right and left arm EMGs were not observed to vary systematically during the rest and listening periods.

Examining the relationship between motivation (as indicated by the slope of EMG gradients) and arousal (measured by EEG amplitude), Bartoshuk (1956) obtained frontalis, chin, and both forearm entensor EMG as well as EEG recordings preceding, during, and following three successive auditory presentations of a story. Significant frontalis EMG gradients above baseline occurred during all three presentations; the EMG slope and EEG amplitude were inversely related for the first presentation only. Recordings from the chin revealed positive EMG gradients above baseline in approximately half the subjects, whereas the forearm extensors showed a significant decrease from baseline during the initial hearing. Both chin and forearm EMGs were independent of EEG voltage. Considering the data of his experiment together with those of the similar one by Wallerstein (1954), Bartoshuk provided three empirical conclusions: (1) positive frontalis EMG gradients are significantly associated with listening to either a story or an essay; (2) the slope of the frontalis EMG gradient is positively associated with interest in the material listened to, suggesting that this gradient is indicative of motivation to listen; and (3) frontalis EMG is more closely associated with listening than are either forearm or chin EMG. In both studies, forearm entensor EMG failed to show positive gradients during listening; although positive chin EMG gradients did appear during the three listening sessions, they were found to be unrelated to interest, frontalis EMG, and EEG amplitude.

E. Learning

Travis and Kennedy (1947) studied the effect of external feedback from supraorbital ("brow") muscle tension during a simulated "look-out" task in which the subjects signaled the perception of visual or auditory stimuli. Visual or auditory stimuli were presented contingent upon the reduction of supraorbital muscle tension (EMG), with the criterion being successively reduced as a function of trials. The results showed that rate and amplitude of supraorbital EMG and reaction time are inversely related. The authors noted that alertness often decreased to the point of somnolence. Travis and Kennedy concluded that this technique may be practically applied to maintain alertness. We indicate in Column 2 of Table 1 that there was a change of brow EMG from baseline during the task; this conclusion seems reasonable because the procedure used produced EMG decrease, though this is not a typical baseline procedure.

Berry and Davis (1958) recorded EMGs from the right forearm extensor, the masseter (jaw), and the frontalis muscles of subjects engaged in a serial learning task. Nonsense syllables were presented so that there was a 3-sec information interval and a 3-sec intersyllable interval. A learning score was computed as the total number of correct responses for 20 trials. The results indicated that the sum of jaw and forehead EMGs for response and information intervals was significantly and nonlinearly related to learning scores. The best and poorest learners had higher potentials than mediocre learners. For an assessment of the differential behavior after right and wrong resposnes, a measure representing the difference between the drop in EMG following a right response and the drop following a wrong response was computed for each subject. It was found that these changes were also nonlinearly related to learning scores, the differences being larger for the best and the poorest subjects. For all analyses, arm EMG and learning scores were not significantly related. Berry and Davis noted that the nonmonotonic relations between muscle tension and learning are more complex than usually thought and therefore require further study before firm conclusions may be arrived at. Their preference, however, was for the following interpretation. The muscle activity recorded during superior learning represents responses such as pronunciation of the syllable vocally and subvocally. This type of action would favor learning, especially as there was more of it following an incorrect response that needed to be replaced than following a correct response that did not need to be replaced. For poor learners, the heightened EMG represented tendencies to escape, to make subvocal ejaculations of surprise or dismay, or other indiscernable activity; thus, when the subject is shown to be wrong, such responses probably interfere with learning.

Berger, Irwin, and Frommer (1970) measured EMGs during two different observational learning tasks: (1) learning eight hand signals from the manual alphabet for the deaf by observing pictorial models; and (2) memorizing eight word-number pairs presented on a card. EMGs were recorded from the right wrist and the right forearm flexor positions during the two learning periods. Baseline recordings were taken during rest periods preceding each observational learning task. The results indicated that muscle activity at both electrode placements was significantly greater during the hand-signal task than during the word-number task. No tests of differences between baselines and experimental periods were reported. Berger *et al.* concluded that their data supported previous results relating localized muscular activity and cognitive activity.

Petrinovich and Hardyck (1970) studied the relative amount of generalization of an instrumental response from words to pictures and from pictures to words. The picture and word training stimuli were presented to subjects who were instructed to press a key when each stimulus appeared. During the test series, each subject pressed the key only when a slide that had been included in the training series was detected. During testing, EMGs were recorded from the muscle group active in the performance of the overt response (*viz.*, forearm flexor). Consequently, overt and covert EMG response records were obtained.

Considering only overt responses, the results indicate that retention for the picture stimuli was significantly higher than that for the words, that the retention for both pictures and words was significantly higher than for the generalization from either words to pictures or from pictures to words, and that there was no significant difference between the number of generalized responses from either words to pictures or from pictures to words. A similar analysis of overt *and* covert responses yielded the same results, except that the mean number of generalized responses from pictures to words was significantly higher than from words to pictures. Petrinovich and Hardyck suggested that the relatively higher generalization from pictures to words was possible because subjects verbally coded the name of the object shown in the picture when the training slide was presented. Thus, the greater generalization during testing may be understandable because the relevant covert response was made earlier, during training.

In a procedure reminiscent of Bill's (1927), Beh and Hawkins (1973) examined the effect of induced muscle tension on the acquisition and retention of a serial list of 12 words. They used four groups of subjects in a 2 × 2 factorial design of tension–relaxation during acquisition and tension–relaxation during recall. Tension was induced by the use of a hand dynamometer with an EMG feedback system that signaled the subject when the prescribed level of tension had not been achieved. The results indicated that the subjects who learned under tension required significantly fewer trails to learn the list; furthermore, groups who learned under tension demonstrated significantly better recall one week after training. Beh and Hawkins concluded that their data were in essential agreement with those reported by Bills (1927). An increase in arm EMG is indicated in Column 2 of Table 1, although, because it was induced by the dynamometer, this is not a typical response increase over baseline.

F. Nocturnal Dreams

Mental activity occurs throughout sleep, being most vivid during dreams. While the eyes have been the major focus of study during dreaming, nonoral muscle responding has received attention too. Max (1935) conducted an experimental study of the motor theory of consciousness by recording EMGs from the arms and legs of "deaf-mute" subjects during sleep, dreaming, and external stimulation during sleep. Since "speech" was produced by activity of the hands and arms of his deaf subjects, Max hypothesized that increased EMGs in these regions would be associated with dreaming and with consciousness in general. The records showed that the transition from the waking to the sleeping state was associated with a progressive diminutive of arm EMGs for both deaf-mute and normal subjects. When the subjects were awakened from periods of increased arm EMG activity, it was found in 30 of 33 instances that the subjects reported dream activity. There was no leg EMG response during dreaming. As a control, deaf subjects were also wakened during periods of electrical "silence," and for only 10 of 62 such awakenings were dreams reported. Similar procedures for hearing subjects indicated that although dreams were reported, arm EMG activity remained constant throughout sleep. When other stimuli were presented during sleep, it was found that they elicited increased arm EMG activity more frequently for deaf subjects than for normal subjects. Max concluded that the dreams of deaf-mute subjects appear to be associated with increased EMG activity of the arm and are therefore consistent with the motor theory of consciousness. The increase from baseline in Table 1 is interpreted here as an observation that was monitored by Max and related to dream reports; it is thus atypical in that it was not produced by an experimental treatment. The same reasoning applies to most of the other articles in this section on sleep research.

Stoyva (1965) repeated Max's (1935) study on the association between finger activity and mental activity during the sleep of deaf subjects. EEG, eye movements (EOG), and finger EMG were recorded from deaf and normal hearing subjects during sleep. The subjects were awakened for dream-narrative collections following bursts of finger activity or prolonged quiescence in the EMG record. The results showed that the mean rate of finger EMG bursts for deaf and hearing subjects during REM (rapid eye movement) and non-REM (NREM) sleep was essentially the same. A replication of these procedures employing more sensitive apparatus and scoring techniques yielded similar results. Stoyva concluded that these data fail to confirm Max's (1935) earlier findings and therefore refute the motor theory of thinking in which cognitive activity is related to motor activity of the linguistic apparatus.

In the evaluation of Stoyva's (1965) study, it should be pointed out that he employed an ink-writing polygraph for recording EMG, a technique that is probably not as sensitive as that used by Max. Furthermore, let us examine Stoyva's conclusion that there was "no difference between deaf and normal subjects with respect to amount of finger EMG activity in any stage of sleep. Accordingly, finger movements during sleep on the part of deaf persons cannot be taken to substantiate the motor theory of thinking", (p. 348). This conclusion is based on the assumption that the fingers of normal hearing dreamers are inactive during the mental activity of dreaming. But we have noted in this chapter considerable evidence that the arms (including finger activity) are quite active during thought. Hence, we take Stoyva's findings to confirm a motor theory in that he found, on the average, heightened finger EMG during dreaming in all subjects (both those who could hear and those who were deaf). Finally, it should be noted that Stoyva used a measure called "mean rate of finger EMG bursts," based only on whether an amplitude of 20 μV was exceeded, thus ignoring responses of smaller amplitude. Many of the covert responses that we measure have amplitudes of less than 1 μV, so that perhaps Stoyva missed the critical responses by this technique.

Wolpert and Trosman (1958) recorded eye movements (EOG), frontal and parietal EEG, and gross body movements (as EEG artifacts) of 10 subjects over 51 nights of experimental sleep. The results indicated that detailed dream recall occurred significantly beyond chance when the subjects were awakened during gross body movements of Stage 1 sleep. Wolpert and Trosman concluded that sleep researchers should awaken subjects for narrative collection during periods of gross body movement rather than REM in order to obtain maximum recall of completed dream episodes. These researchers did not, however, present a comparison of the effectiveness of the two techniques for "diagnosing" dream periods.

Wolpert (1960) recorded EEG, EOG, and (unspecified) arm and wrist EMG of subjects over a series of 20 experimental sleep sessions. His subjects were awakened for dream-narrative collections from Stage 1-REM periods following distinctive EMG patterns. He also awakened them during sleep Stages 2-4. Independent judges rated the dream narratives and EMG records and subsequently compared ratings of the decoded pairs. The results of this procedure indicated that wrist EMG was significantly greater during Stage 1-REM (dream) periods than during Stages 2, 3, and 4 ("nondreaming") periods of sleep. Additionally, significant associations between EMG activity and dream-narrative content were found for some subjects.

As one example, a subject was awakened when there was an isolated muscle action potential in his right arm, at which time he reported that as the dream was interrupted he was reaching for a jacket. In another instance, there was a combined bodily movement, following which the subject reported that at the end of the dream he jumped over a line of fish with sharp dorsal fins by extending his arms, legs, and trunk. Wolpert concluded that motor expression of dream content is greatly inhibited but not absent.

The tonic activity of the body musculature of six humans during natural sleep was studied systematically by Jacobson, Kales, Lehmann, and Hoedemaker (1964). EMG activity was measured in 29 muscle groups of the six subjects for a total of 24 subject-sleep sessions. There was also simultaneous recording of EEG and EOG. To emphasize the difference between tonic and phasic activity of skeletal muscle, tonic responding is sustained and continuous. Phasic muscle activity is rapidly changing, occurring in bursts. Hence, while it is common to find that tonus decreases during dreaming, there still is much rapid phasic activity. The distinction is especially important for us because we hypothesize that linguistic coding is carried in large part by phasic bursts of the skeletal musculature (rather than by tonic activity). During sleep, tonus of most head and neck muscles typically decreases at the onset of Stage 1-REM periods. As an example, hyoid EMG was found to decrease in 47 of the 61 REM periods observed. Muscle tonus of the trunk and limbs was found to remain unchanged in all of 487 REM periods observed, although frequent bursts of activity were noted. Jacobson *et al.* concluded that muscle tonus of the neck and head is related to EEG Stage 1-REM periods, while tonus of the trunk and limbs exhibits a relatively constant level.

It should be noted that there was little concentration on phasic activity in this study, yet phasic activity is the more important for studying mental content, whether awake or dreaming (e.g., McGuigan and Tanner, 1971; Sokolov, 1972). This point was also well made by Baldridge *et al.* (1965). In fact, Dement and Kleitman (1957) reported an increase in fine muscle movements during the dream phase that was essentially absent in nondream phases. They reported that these fine movements were observable directly but were not recorded with their EMG techniques, which were apparently not sufficiently sensitive for covert response research. The importance of the value of studying phasic muscle activity during dreaming should thus be underscored and kept independent from the often-made statement that EMG *decreases* during dreaming—while apparently tonic EMG *does* decrease, phasic activity does *not*. (See our mention of tonic versus phasic activity above in connection with the Jacobson *et al.*, 1964 study).

Baldridge, Whitman, and Kramer (1965) further examined Aserinsky and Kleitman's (1953) original report of an association between REMs and body movements during dreams of sleep. By the use of highly sensitive strain gauges, continuous measurements of eye, throat, hand, and foot movements were recorded during undisturbed sleep. The results indicated that movements appeared simultaneously from all locations and that this activity was significantly correlated with REMs. Body movement patterns correctly identified 32 of 41 peaks of eye movement activity, the typical criterion of when the subject was dreaming. Based on this and previous work, Baldridge *et al.* pointed out that the strain gauge method for detecting eye movement is "many times more sensitive than that recorded by means of the corneo-retinal potential" (p. 25). They emphasized that previous negative findings with regard to increased muscle activity during dreams have been based on very crude measurement techniques. Based on the previously reported association of REMs and dreams, Baldridge *et al.* concluded that fine muscle activity is associated with nocturnal dreams. They suggested three possible interpretations of the concurrence of fine body movements with dreaming: (1) that the dreamer is attempting to carry out the action of the dream as the dream unfolds; (2) that the covert responses provide increased proprioceptive input into the brain, which is then interpreted as a dream; or (3) that the dream and the muscle activity occur simultaneously as a result of some independent mechanism, such as heightened activity in the reticular formation.

Sassin and Johnson (1968) measured EEG, EOG, and arm, leg, and submental EMG while their five subjects slept in the laboratory for two consecutive nights. The object of the study was to specify the relationship between body motility (any "detectable" movement) and K-complex (i.e., sharp reversed-wave forms interspersed with slow components) of Stage 2 sleep, the latter often considered an indicator of arousal. The results showed that K-complexes preceded body movements (significantly) during Stage 2 sleep, the mean latency for 396 movements was 2.52 sec. The rate of body movements per minute was significantly lower in slow-wave (Stages 3 and 4) sleep than in Stages 1 and 2; rate of body movements was not significantly different in Stage 2 versus Stage 1–REM periods. Analysis of the type and duration of muscle movements indicated that 80% of Stage 3 and Stage 4 movements were global, involving the head, the extremities, and the trunk. Movements during Stages 1 and 2 were evenly divided between movements of the head, the face, or the mouth and global movements; a significant number of phasic limb movements occurred during Stage 1–REM periods. Sassin and Johnson concluded that body motility during sleep is not a random phenomenon and appears to be systematically related to the characteristic K-complex of Stage 2 sleep. Their finding of a significant number of *phasic* limb movements during dreaming is to be emphasized and related to our previous discussion of this point.

Larson and Foulkes (1969) examined the reported association between EMG suppression and passage from NREM sleep to REM sleep (cf. Berger, 1961; Jacobson *et al.*, 1964). They recorded nocturnal

EEG, EOG, and submental EMG from five subjects for a total of 42 nights. A total of 196 awakenings for the collection of dream narratives was classified among three awakening categories: NREM sleep preceding EMG suppression and REM onset; NREM sleep immediately following the EMG suppression, and early moments of REM sleep accompanied by EMG suppression. The researchers also recorded the time from calling the subject's name to the time at which he gave a coherent reply to the first questions following the awakening ("orientation time"). The results indicated that suppressed-EMG–NREM awakenings tended (not significantly) to be associated with lower dream recall frequency and lower Dreamlike Fantasy Scale ratings than were high-EMG–NREM awakenings. Two of five subjects showed significantly longer orientation times on suppressed-EMG–pre-REM awakenings than on high-EMG–pre-REM awakenings. Contrary to the traditional view of a monotonic transition from NREM sleep to REM sleep, Larson and Foulkes concluded that a momentary "deepening" of sleep (in terms of vivid mental content and decreased reactivity to the awakening stimulus) appears to accompany the pre-REM suppression of submental EMG potentials.

Experiments demonstrating an association between REMs and middle-ear muscle activity during sleep were described by Pessah and Roffwarg (1972). By use of acoustic impedance techniques, the authors continuously monitored the stapedius and tensor tympani muscles. The experimenters then observed whether or not REM periods followed middle-ear muscle activity (dream narratives were not called for). The results showed that middle ear activity typically precedes, and continues throughout, REM periods. Of all middle-ear muscle activity, 80% occurred within REM periods, and half of the remaining 20% occurred in 10-min intervals prior to REM-sleep onset. Pessah and Roffwarg concluded that this phenomenon requires further examination, with particular focus on the possible association of middle-ear muscle activity and auditory imagery.

Gardner, Grossman, Roffwarg, and Weiner (1973) studied the relation between fine limb movements and dream actions of REM sleep. The subjects, selected for good dream recall, were awakened for dream reports following EMG activity of the four extremities. They were awakened at four different times: (1) when there was no movement; (2) when there was upper limb activity with an absence of lower limb activation; (3) when there was lower limb activity with an absence of upper limb activation; and (4) when three was mixed upper and lower limb activation. The total of 209 dream reports and EMG records were coded, scored blindly, and then decoded for statistical analysis. The results indicated that a significant correlation existed in good dream recallers between the location of actual bodily movement and location and amount of dreamed action.

V. THE CURARE STRATEGY

One approach for ascertaining the role of skeletal muscle contraction (and afferent neural feedback resulting from such contraction) is to completely paralyze the skeletal musculature, usually attempted pharmacologically by the administration of neuromuscular blocking agents. The process of conditioning can thus be studied when the role of the skeletal musculature has presumably been eliminated. Some examples of reports of successful conditioning with curarized preparations are the works of Solomon and Turner (1962), Black, Carlson, and Solomon (1962), and DiCara and Miller (1968). Solomon and Turner, for example, concluded *"that certain types of transfer of training or problem solving can occur without the benefit of mediation by peripheral skeletal responses or their associated feedback mechanisms"* (p. 218, italics in original).

The assumptions upon which this strategy of paralysis is based are that the curare used (1) is actually effective in producing total paralysis of the skeletal musculature and (2) acts only at the myoneural junction and thus does not affect the central nervous system or peripheral sensory or autonomic mechanisms. The evidence for these assumptions, gained with the use of early impure forms of curare, is ambiguous (Solomon and Turner, 1962). D-Tubocurarine, a pure form of curare developed later, was first used in this context by Solomon and Turner (1962) and by Black, Carlson, and Solomon (1962) to conduct improved tests of the central versus the peripheral process interpretations of learning and transfer. These experiments necessarily relied heavily on the pharmacological research available at the time for information about the effects of D-tubocurarine on various bodily systems; we should, therefore, briefly review that pharmacological evidence. The three articles these authors cited still constitute the bulk of our information on curare derived from the study of humans: Smith *et al.* (1947), Unna and Pelikan (1951), and McIntyre, Bennett, and Hamilton (1951).

The pioneering work of Smith *et al.* (1947) is of special interest of psychologists because it resulted in a widely accepted (though unjustified) conclusion that individuals remain conscious and can "think" under total muscle paralysis due to curare; therefore, the notion is, muscle activity is not important in thought processes. Smith *et al.* (1947) administered D-tubocurarine, a neuromuscular blocking agent, to a healthy trained adult observer not undergoing an operation. The dosage was two and one-half times that necessary for respiratory paralysis and was therefore considered adequate for complete paralysis of the skeletal musculature. During the 54-min period of paralysis, it was reported that no changes occurred in the EEG, consciousness, or the sensory functions or in any aspect of the higher central nervous system (CNS), although objective tests of CNS functioning were not conducted. Smith *et al.* concluded that paralysis of the skeletal musculature did not affect central processes; this evidence has been used by others to disconfirm a motor theory of consciousness. While one must greatly admire this pioneering research, the experiment (using only one subject) must be realistically evaluated in light of its methodological inadequacies. Of six shortcomings cited by McGuigan (1966), the one most immediately relevant to the curare-conditioning studies is that the D-tubocurarine used may not have totally paralyzed the skeletal musculature, a point that could be easily decided through appropriate EMG monitoring. Hence, while there may well have been no *overt* responses in the curarized state, important minute (covert) responses still may have occurred (in addition, of course, to autonomic activity). Smith *et al.*'s experiment was repeated by Leuba, Birch, and Appleton (1968), but unfortunately it did not include the controls suggested by McGuigan (1966). Campbell, Sanderson, and Laverty (1964) also performed an experiment similar to that of Smith *et al.*, in which five human subjects were injected with succinylcholine chloride dihydrate. The authors stated that the drug breaks the connection between the motor neurons and the skeletal musculature and *very nearly* completely paralyzes the skeletal musculature, with no anesthetic effect. When subjects were asked after paralysis what they were aware of, they claimed that they were "aware of what was going on around them." They described their attempts to move during paralysis by saying that they were under the impression that their movements were very large, when in actuality they were small and poorly controlled. We should thus be admonished against the uncritical acceptance of subjects' reports. We should also be reluctant to reach broad conclusions about the status of a subject's awareness when there is a lack of *total* muscle paralysis.

Our criticism of the Smith *et al.* (1947) study is also pertinent to the second pharmacological study, by Unna and Pelikan (1951). In it, there was no EMG monitoring to establish that covert skeletal muscle responses were eliminated. In fact, an amazingly gross measure (viz., grip strength with the hand dynamometer) was used as the index of "muscular paralysis," and even that measure apparently did not decrease to zero under D-tubocurarine. An additional indication of lack of paralysis is that there was never any need for artificial respiration for their subjects. Illustrative of our concern here is Black's (1967) statement that "in experiments on the operant conditioning of heart rate under curare, it may very well be that electromyographic responses were actually conditioned and that these led to reflexive changes in heart rate" (p. 202). James Howard (personal communication, 1972) suggested a compatible physiological possibility: that the gamma-efferent system may have a significant role in conditioning since it is apparent that the gamma system of fibers has a higher threshold to the blocking effect of curare than the extrafusal muscle system (Buchwald, Standish, Eldred, and Halas, 1964). If Howard's reasoning is correct, successful conditioning of curarized preparations may have occurred because the covert behavior that remained was due to a still-functional gamma-efferent system and its feedback loop. The most sensitive method of determining whether or not the skeletal muscle system *is* actually paralyzed is to monitor it extensively with a sufficiently sensitive EMG apparatus. When one conducts a sufficiently stringent EMG test of the hypothesis that a neuromuscular blocking agent does effectively eliminate skeletal muscle activity, the subject should attempt to contract the skeletal musculature maximally. The subject could simply be instructed to contract certain muscles strongly, but a more satisfactory procedure would probably be to administer electric shock to him. Only when the procedures outlined herein are effected can we reach a firm conclusion as to whether or not curare (or whatever neuromuscular blocking agent is under test) can *totally* eliminate muscle action potentials, that is, produce EMG recordings of 0.0 μV throughout the body.

A few conditioning researchers did monitor EMGs when they used curare. EMGs were apparently recorded in only three of these autonomic conditioning studies, and in those the EMG sampling was limited and quite insensitive (the scales used were from 100 to 300 μV/cm; cf. McGuigan, 1973a). When one considers that important covert responses may be of the amplitude of less than a microvolt, it is apparent that more sensitive measurement techniques than those of ink-writing polygraphs are required. Even so, the sample EMGs offered by the experimenters cited in McGuigan (1973a) often do show variations in the curarized preparation; covert behavior of perhaps as much as 20 μV in amplitude may have been occurring in presumably paralyzed animals. Such covert behavior could have important consequences, such as the possibility considered in this context (though rejected) by Black (1965) that the "full occurrence of a response and its associated feedback is not necessary for the modification of that response by operant reinforcement" (p. 45). In this context, one may

recall the discussion above about the possibility that sufficient processing for conditioning may occur strictly through the high-threshold
gamma-efferent system, even though there is apparent "muscular
paralysis." In conclusion, it is hoped that future research in these
areas will include improved methodology, especially by employing
EMG monitoring control procedures.

The second assumption stated at the beginning of this section as
being necessary for successful application of the curare strategy is that
D-tubocurarine affects only the skeletal musculature. Unna and Pelikan
(1951) said that following administration of D-tubocurarine in six
subjects, "no evidence was obtained of any action other than on the
neuromuscular junction. . . . In particular no effects on autonomic
organs and also none on cerebral functions could be demonstrated"
(p. 480). That appears to be the totality of their offering in this
regard—Unna and Pelikan did not present any data (nor were any
cited) that substantiate that statement, nor did they further discuss the
matter of possible central or autonomic nervous system effects of D-
tubocurarine. (They did, though, indicate that Flaxedil affects blood
pressure and pulse rate.)

The third pharmacological study cited above was that by McIntyre
et al. (1951). In their consideration of this matter of possible brain
effects, McIntyre et al. first criticized the above-cited work of Smith et
al. (1947) on the grounds that the Smith et al. results came from
subjective observations. A second criticism was that Smith et al. did
not make sufficiently sensitive measurements of muscle activity.
McIntyre et al. concluded that "the balance of evidence establishes
beyond doubt that D-tubocurarine is capable of modifying central
nervous system activity independently of secondary effects due to
hypoxia" (p. 301). They did not elaborate, however, on the phrase
"balance of evidence."

Black et al. (1962) summarized evidence indicating that D-tubocurarine affects the brain, as indicated by EEG measures. Other considerable work is consonant with that conclusion. Estable (1959) concluded that curare produces an effect on all cholinergic synapses to
varying degrees. Okuma, Fujmori, and Hayashi (1965) reported elec-
trocrotical synchronization in animals as a function of the environmental temperature in which the animals received the curare. Amassian and Weiner (1966) and Brinley, Kandel, and Marshall (1958) found
an increase in the latency of evoked potentials in curarized animals.
And Hodes (1962) reported EEG effects from three different curare
compounds (D-tubocurarine, Flaxedil, and succinylcholine). Galindo
(1972) implicated both curare and pancuronium. In this same context, I
am grateful to James Howard for informing me that curare releases

histamine, which causes widespread bodily changes, including increased permeability and dilation of cerebral blood vessels (cf. Douglas, 1970; Koelle, 1960).

Apparently, then, D-tubocurarine does have CNS effects. Whether or not these effects are direct or whether they are produced indirectly by such peripheral mechanisms as inadequate artificial respiration parameters or reduction of necessary feedback of sensory, especially proprioceptive, impulses to the CNS is unclear. Unfortunately, we lack even primitive data here, since few conditioning researchers have monitored EEGs of their subjects. Consequently, we do not know whether or not brain activity of their subjects is, by an EEG index, affected (directly or indirectly) by the D-tubocurarine injected. Finally, with regard to the second assumption for using curare, while curare apparently affects the brain, other data indicate that curare has autonomic effects too (cf. Black, 1971; Grob, 1967; Koelle, 1960).

To summarize our discussion of the two assumptions for the curare strategy:

1. We simply lack sufficient data to decide on the validity of the assumption that the blocking agent produces total muscular paralysis. While under stringent conditions curare might completely eliminate the skeletal muscles as a source of mediation, we do not now possess empirical evidence sufficient to conclude that it does. Researchers who study autonomic and CNS activity by employing this strategy can add to our knowledge by (a) monitoring EMGs from *several* bodily sites using sensitive equipment and (b) monitoring EEGs, preferably from more than one location. In short, skeletal muscle responding has not been excluded by the "curare strategy" as a possible mediator in studies of brain and autonomic activity. Nor has it been shown that thought processes or awareness is or is not affected through the injection of curare.

2. With regard to the requirement that the muscular blocking agent not affect the brain, we should realize that it is methodologically very difficult to establish a *lack of relationship* (like attempting to "prove the null hypothesis"); this is particularly a problem with such complex variables as D-tubocurarine and CNS activity. The available evidence indicates that D-tubocurarine does (possibly indirectly) have CNS effects. Furthermore, curare apparently has autonomic effects in addition.

While it is not the major purpose here, it might be valuable to relate these conclusions to the question of autonomic conditioning. Successful autonomic conditioning of curarized animals has been reported, but there have been unsuccessful attempts that apparently defy explanation (e.g., Black, 1971; Ray, 1969). The situation seems to be that under curare, there is partial functioning and partial nonfunctioning of the autonomic system, of the skeletal musculature, and of the CNS. With this state of affairs, the logical possibilities are sufficiently numerous that one could argue for any of several interpretations. For one, the reported conditioning successes may have occurred because the autonomic system was still (incompletely) functioning, and the failures may have been due to the autonomic interference caused by the curare (cf. Black, 1971, p. 36–37). The same interpretation may be applied to the CNS, or even to the skeletal muscle system. One of the logical possibilities (unlikely as it might be) is that the reverse interpretation holds for the brain—that the successful instances of conditioning occurred *becasue* of the curare; that is, curare might directly or indirectly inhibit certain cortical functions so that the inhibition allows lower cerebral mechanisms concerned with autonomic funcitons to allow conditioning to occur.

In this section, we have concentrated on the classical approach, in which curare has been used. More recently, other neuromuscular blocking agents have replaced curare. Nevertheless, the lesson is the same: these other agents should not be uncritically employed, as curare has been. Whatever the neuromuscular blocking agent used, it should be subjected to the same stringent methodological evaluation discussed above. With regard to several other agents, Wilson and DiCara (1975) studied the effects of a single intraperitoneal injection of three neuromuscular blockers in rats: succinylcholine, dimethyl D-tubocurarine iodide, and D-tubocurarine chloride. They sampled EMG activity from two bodily regions and measured the EMG recovery time. They concluded that they had confirmed previous reports of the unpredictable consequences of paralysis induced by D-tubocurarine. In particular, their results confirmed the contention by Howard, Galosy, Gaebelein, and Obrist (1974) that D-tubocurarine chloride may be the least desirable choice of the neural blocking agents.

VI. STIMULATION, SURGICAL, AND CLINICAL STRATEGIES

It thus seems that the use of "the curare strategy" has not been adequate to isolate "*the* response of interest" from other bodily events that may themselves have been modified and controlled by that response. Other "strategies," such as electrical stimulation and surgical techniques, could conceivably be more successful in isolating relevant bodily systems (cf. McGuigan, 1966, p. 294). The work of Penfield (1958) illustrates the stimulation approach. Surgical techniques with animal subjects, like those in which Horridge (1965) successfully conditioned an insect without a brain or the peripheral nerve crushing and deafferentation procedures used by Light and Gantt (1936) and by Taub and Berman (1968), might yield valuable, unambiguous information.

In attempts to isolate bodily systems in order to ascertain their functions, limited data on pathological cases have sometimes been inappropriately used to negate broad theories. A criticism of Watson's theory of thinking is one example. It was argued that individuals with laryngectomies could still think, thus apparently disconfirming Watson's theory. Watson (1930) answered this criticism by saying that concerning "whether the man who cannot talk, cannot think . . . you will find that man thinks and talks with his whole body—just as he does everything else with his whole body" (p. 225). It is important to develop this point in greater detail, particularly because this long-standing methodological error of misusing otherwise valuable clinical data continues, despite advances in methodological sophistication and in our knowledge of neuromuscular systems since Watson's time. Shallice (1974), for example, opposed "a modified version of the motor theory of thought" because it holds "that one cannot think well without the involvement of the musculature, particularly that concerned with speech." Shallice continued, "It is unfortunate that no clinical neuropsychologist pointed out . . . that peripheral dysarthria, which prevents speech, leaves thought totally unaffected" (p. 1073).

The general conclusion from such reasoning is that the musculature does not have an essential function in cognitive activities. Let us consider six possible errors in this reasoning:

1. *Objective measures of thought under controlled conditions are wanting.* Reliable and valid measures are required to determine whether peripheral dysarthria (or any other pathological condition) in fact affects the thought process. Mere casual observation of a patient is not sufficient. Moreover, one can make valid inferences regarding *changes* in intellectual proficiency within individuals only if both pre- and postaccident measures have been taken. Ideally, too, the effect of the trauma that produced the pathology should be controlled, for any change in thought proficiency may have been produced by emotionality accompanying the trauma and not by the bodily damage *per se* (see also point 5 below).

2. *The extent of the insult to the neural and muscular systems is typically unknown.* Several clinical specialists (neurosurgeons, speech pathologists, etc.) have told me that in pathological cases in which the speech muscles or other linguistic apparatus is malfunctioning, the neuromuscular conditions are seldom (if ever) well defined—there is usually complex damage to muscles and also to associated neural

systems. With unknown or poorly determined muscular and neural damage, it is impossible to reach definitive conclusions about the influence of a single aspect of the complex speech system on cognitive functioning.

3. *Internal information-processing systems are redundant.* The entire body—not just a single system such as the speech musculature—is used in both verbal and nonverbal thought. Numerous other bodily activities and "parallel" processing systems occur during thought (cf. McGuigan and Schoonover, 1973); the value of such redundant circuits has been pointed out by Adams, McIntyre, and Thorsheim (1969) in other contexts. Hence, even if the *entire* speech musculature were nonfunctional (which seldom occurs), remaining neuromuscular channels could probably carry on thought. Usually, however, neuromuscular circuits involving portions of the chin, tongue, lips, throat, and jaw muscles remain operative, and these themselves might be sufficient to maintain cognitive proficiency.

4. *Neuromuscular conditions within a single syndrome are diverse.* Similarly classified individuals seldom exhibit identical symptoms. Shallice, for instance, stated that dysarthria "prevents speech"; however, this term is more commonly used to include a variety of speech disorders, some involving only lack of coordination of the speech act. Darley, Aronson, and Brown (1969a,b) distinguished five varieties of dysarthria. Such clinically diverse cases hardly form a sound, uniform basis for a generalized conclusion about thought.

5. *Causal variables are confounded.* Bodily damage, such as that to the speech musculature, is probably accompanied by emotionally traumatic events, such as an accident or surgery. The postshock state of the patient may thus be a function of the bodily damage, of the trauma that caused the injury, or of a complex interaction between these two variables. One can therefore not reach an unambiguous conclusion about the effects of a somatic-damage variable that is so confounded with other variables.

6. *Nonrepresentative sampling.* Finally, one should consider the extent to which generalizations can be made to a normal population from findings on pathological individuals. The lack of random selection of individuals to form a representative data base probably limits the extent to which one can generalize from a sample of unique clinical cases to information-processing systems in the normal individual or even to individuals with different pathologies.

Clinical observations are suggestive sources of hypotheses, but seldom can they furnish a firm foundation for definitive conclusions about the functioning of any single, limited bodily system. Suitable data on these issues might be acquired through rigorous research, but appropriate experiments are methodologically difficult (if not impossible) to conduct, given our present level of technical knowledge. The preceding discussion of how to adequately carry out the "curare strategy" in the laboratory illustrates how complex these issues can become. It is hoped that these considerations will help prevent the perpetuation of the methodological error of causal reasoning from clinical cases.

VII. CONCLUSIONS AND INTERPRETATION

On the basis of the preceding data and analyses, we may conclude that:

1. A variety of covert nonoral skeletal muscle responses *did* occur under a number of cognitive conditions, in that the response measure changed from baseline (Criterion 1).

2. To a large extent, those responses appear to have occurred because of the cognitive conditions studied by the researchers, since those responses often varied systematically as a function of the cognitive conditions (Criterion 2).

3. The most apparent conclusion with regard to Criterion 3 is that researchers generally did not make concurrent measures of other covert processes. The implication is obvious that researchers should apply this criterion more extensively. When this criterion *was* successfully applied, the nonoral response classes of interest (those specified in Column 1 of Table 1) about as frequently covaried with other response measures as they were independent of other covert reactions.

4. To a very large extent, the responses specified in Column 1 in some way specifically related to a cognitive condition. The various specific relationships are abstracted in the appendix.

In general, then, it seems clear that a variety of covert nonoral skeletal-muscle responses occur when individuals silently engage in a wide variety of cognitive activities. The specification of these numerous covert nonoral skeletal-muscle responses throughout the body is in conformity with the model presented in Figure 2. The problem now is to speculate about how these covert responses function during cognition.

Relative to our understanding of covert nonoral behavior, we possess a somewhat refined model for understanding the function of covert oral (speech) behavior (McGuigan, 1976). That model has been based to a large extent on the conclusions that (1) there is a discriminative relationship between class of covert oral behavior and the phonemic system and (2) that the speech musculature is physiologically capable of generating and transmitting such distinctive phonetic information to the linguistic regions of the brain. Because our model for the function of the speech musculature might facilitate our understanding of the cognitive functioning of nonspeech musculature, let us briefly review the bases for these two conclusions.

With regard to the first conclusion of a discriminative relationship between speech muscle behavior and the phonemic system, Blumenthal (1959) showed that tongue EMGs were of significantly greater magnitude when subjects thought of saying lingual–alveolar verbal materials (which would require major tongue movements during *overt* speech) than when they thought of saying bilabial materials (which engage the lips). In a series of experiments, Locke and Fehr (e.g., 1970) measured more covert lip activity during the subvocal rehearsal of labial words than during nonlabials. McGuigan and Winstead (1974) reported that covert responses in the tongue are relatively pronounced when the subject is reading, memorizing, and rehearsing prose that is heavily loaded with lingual–alveolar material, while covert lip behavior is especially pronounced when the subject is reading, memorizing, and rehearsing prose that is dominated by bilabial material. Of significance to speech perception, one extremely well-relaxed subject listened to sentences and words loaded with either labial or nonlabial verbal material. Lip EMGs significantly increased when this subject listened to labial material, but they did not while she was listening to comparable nonlabial material (McGuigan, 1973a). In short, it seems that the particular class of verbal material (bilabial, lingual–alveolar, etc.) silently processed evokes relatively heightened covert activity in the speech musculature that would be the focus of activity during the overt production of that class of verbal material.

Other data relevant to the first conclusion above are those that indicate that there is heightened tongue EMG during perceptual clarification of auditory linguistic input (the "Gilbert and Sullivan effect," as reported by Osgood and McGuigan, 1973, and by McGuigan, 1978). The general conclusion is that the speech musculature functions in the generation and transmission of a phonetic code to the brain. Such a phonetic code, while not itself meaningful, can cause differences in meaning. For instance, when the afferent neural volley of impulses generated by covert activity of the lips is transmitted to the language regions of the brain, a linguistic unit that includes bilabial components may be "retrieved" ("restructured," or whatever the central process might be). Hence, if one internally processes the externally impinging word *bad*, the afferent neural coding from the lips would retrieve /b/, which when followed by coding for [a] and [d], allows processing of *bad* versus, say, *dad*. In contrast, *dad* would be, in

part, centrally restructured because of an afferent neural volley generated by the tongue that carries a code for the lingual–alveolar verbal
unit of /d/, followed by [a] and [d].

With regard to the second conclusion about the refined physiological capability of the speech muscles for information processing, we
may note Sussman's (1972) summary of data relevant to the tongue,
the most important part of that musculature: "Not only can the higher
brain centers be kept informed as to the *initiation* of a high-speed
consonantal gesture of the tongue but also as to the *attainment* and
subsequent *release* of that gesture. . . . The neuromuscular system of
the tongue has been shown to be a built-in feedback system that can
signal the length and rate of movement of a muscle" (p. 266).
Consequently, "it is logical to assume that the *afferent discharge pattern
emanating from the tongue should contain high-level distinctive information*. Such discriminative information can be provided by the differential frequency discharge patterning of the muscle spindles due to the
orientation of the extrafusal fibers relative to the direction of movement" (p. 267, italics in the original).

The great versatility of verbal symbolism has led us to recognize a
priority for linguistic thought involving principally the speech musculature and the linguistic regions of the brain (McGuigan, 1966). Just as
clearly, however, nonoral behavior can also serve linguistic functions.
How often do we substitute gestures for spoken words, as in waving
good-bye to a friend of shrugging the shoulders? More refined nonoral
language functioning occurs when deaf individuals communicate with
dactylic language, when the blind read by braille, and when people
engage in cursive handwriting, and we may note in this context the
ability of the cutaneous senses to receive and process linguistic input
(cf. Geldard, 1966). (with speech we presume that there is commonal-
ity in production and perception processes [McGuigan, 1978]. We
make the same assumption here too.) No doubt the responding of the
nonoral musculature is involved in some way in processing information necessary for understanding the meaning of the stimulus input.
There is considerable precedent for this statement, as in Titchener's
context theory of meaning (1909), in which he held that the meaning
of words in part originates in bodily attitudes of the muscle systems.
Jacobson (1929) held that localized bodily tensions literally *mean* the
imagined act. When contractions in a given bodily region are recognized by a person who has been trained in progressive relaxation,
they are then qualitatively interpreted; for example, tension signals in
the right arm might mean to one individual that they are covertly
behaving (imagining) "as if" to overtly light a cigarette, or tensions in
the shoulders and back may be interpreted by a busy executive "as if"

hurrying to get the day's work done. Jacobson (1929) maintained the

> *working hypothesis that any report of the experience of muscular tenseness is incomplete until a function is stated.* The subject is simply asked, if necessary, "A tension to do what?" . . . Sherrington (1915) goes so far as to believe that tonus is always to be understood in the light of its aim or function. He states, "Every reflex can, therefore, be regarded from the point of view of what may be called its 'aim.' To glimpse at the aim of a reflex is to gain hints for future experimentation on it. Such a clue to purpose is often difficult to get." (pp. 78–79)

It has been previously argued that during linguistic processing (in which there are "thoughts" and the like), both oral and nonoral responses interact in some complex but supportive fashion (Figure 3). When one imagines lighting a cigarette with the right hand, for example, one covertly responds symbolically in the oral region (perhaps subvocally by saying "cigarette" or "fire") and almost simultaneously responds with the nonoral skeletal musculature with contractions of muscles in the right arm and hand (Jacobson, 1932). These oral and nonoral responses are hypothesized to interact in carrying information to the linguistic regions of the brain. (And we must not forget that there also follows an emotional component to thoughts through circuits that engage the autonomic system.)

Granting that the nonoral skeletal musculature has a linguistic capacity, whether or not it functions discriminatively in the generation and transmission of verbal coding—as the speech musculature apparently does—is still open to question. At first glance, one is inclined to answer this question in the negative. It is clear that the speech musculature—being an extremely complex and flexible system in which motor units of only several muscle fibers can be differentially activated—is physiologically capable of very precise discriminative reactions. In contrast, the nonoral skeletal musculature (with the exception of that in the eyes and the middle ears) is not as physiologically capable of precise differential responding (e.g., in the gastrocnemius muscle, there are typically some 2000 muscle fibers that must react in concert when each motor neuron is activated). Nevertheless, language *is* processed to at least some extent nonorally, often quite efficiently and in great detail. It may be that there exist discriminative relationships between linguistic categories and classes of nonoral responding. A specialized example of this would be a deaf individual proficient in dactylic language who, when silently processing a linguistic unit, exhibits heightened activity in exactly those fingers that would be engaged during overt communication of that particular linguistic unit.

Figure 3. An arbitrary behavioral unit that is commenced when an external language stimulus (S_{L_1}) evokes a covert oral (r_{o_1}) and a covert nonoral ($r_{\bar{o}_1}$) response. It is hypothesized that each covert oral and nonoral response results in an additional covert oral and nonoral response and that the sequence may continue indefinitely. The unit is arbitrarily said to be terminated when an overt language response (R_{L_1}) occurs; R_{L_1} may be the report of a solution to a problem posed by S_{L_1}, a tact of an internal event like a hallucination, etc. (From McGuigan, 1970.)

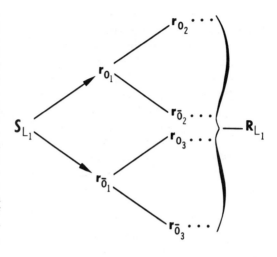

If the nonoral musculature does not function in the generation and transmission of a verbal code as complex and precise as the code carried by the oral musculature, what kind of code might reasonably be involved? We shall hypothesize two kinds of codes: first, a nonoral linguistic code, the nature of which is dependent upon the individual's verbal (but nonspeech) learning experiences, and second, a nonlinguistic code that has developed as a result of conditioning to various stimulus objects and events. The distinction is thus based on the difference between the learning of linguistic symbols versus nonlinguistic referents.

We shall designate the hypothesized linguistic code generated and transmitted by the nonoral skeletal musculature as an allographic code. The term *allogram* is analogous to *allophone* in that an allogram is a written linguistic unit, just as an allophone is a spoken linguistic unit. Similarly, an allogram is an instance of a grapheme class, as an allophone is an instance of a phoneme class. In the Latin alphabet, a grapheme would consist of many letters and letter combinations, each of which is an allogram (e.g., the *p* in *pin*, the *pp* in *hopping*, and the *gh* in *hiccough* are all allograms of the same grapheme).

What is the relationship between graphemes and phonemes? Certainly there is not a one-to-one relationship between spoken language and written language, but just as assuredly there is a considerable overlap. Osgood (personal communication) has suggested in effect that graphemes are more ambiguous than phonemes.[3] Such a difference might be related to the previous argument that the speech musculature is capable of more highly refined differential responding than most of the other muscles of the body, especially the writing arm and hand.

The notion, put forward here, is that activation of a pattern of nonoral skeletal-muscle responses generates afferent neural impulses that carry an allographic code, as we have hypothesized that the speech musculature generates and transmits a phonetic code. The allographic codes are transmitted through neuromuscular circuits to the linguistic regions of the brain. The particular linguistic units of the allographic code, as we said, would depend on the learning history of the individual. We would suppose that one who has learned cursive writing with the Latin alphabet might generate linguistic units consisting of letters or combinations of letters (syllables, etc.) from that alphabet. Those who have learned other languages (braille, Arabic, Chinese, symbolic logic, or the dactylic language of the deaf) might generate afferent neural volleys coded appropriately for that language by means of particular nonoral muscle patterns. In this way, then, we could have parallel linguistic information-processing involving the speech muscles and the nonspeech muscles. When one thinks "bicycle riding," for example, one covertly says the words, or some minute fractional component of the words (as suggested by heightened EMG speech muscle records), covertly writes the words (as suggested by increased EMG in the preferred arm), and also responds elsewhere in the body (particularly, in this instance, the legs). This last point brings us to the second kind of code that might be generated by the nonoral skeletal musculature.

The hypothesized nonlinguistic coding generated by the nonoral skeletal muscles involves a more primitive kind of symbolism than that needed for language—what may be called *referent coding*. It is feasible that referent coding also functions at the subhuman level. An animal who had had sufficient experience in responding to a given stimulus object may generate an afferent neural volley in the absence of that stimulus object by reinstating the conditional response pattern, as in dreaming, for example. The precise status of the skeletal muscle fibers during the evocation of the conditional response would then be representative of the conditional stimulus so that the resulting afferent neural volley would be coded for that stimulus. Referent coding would thus be a function of neuromuscular states that represent correspond-

---

[3] I am certainly grateful to Charles E. Osgood for his many contributions to my work that have grown out of our ongoing, friendly debate (cf. Osgood and McGuigan, 1973) and here especially for guiding me in the direction of the "grapheme concept."

ing external conditional stimuli. The view of a ball, for instance, would evoke complex muscle reactions throughout the body, but principally in the throwing arm. When those reactions generate neural impulses, coding for the object *ball* would be transmitted to the brain. This nonlinguistic coding may be directed through neural circuits to the minor (nonverbal) hemisphere. Such circuits for referent coding could help us to understand "nonverbal thought," a concept that Sperry (1973) found quite important in his split brain experimentation. Referent coding is relevant also to other considerations of nonverbal versus verbal thought, for example, Pavlov's first and second signal systems. The first (nonverbal) signal system may function through referent coding, while linguistic coding involving phonetic and allographic neuromuscular events may underlie the second signal system. Accordingly, while the nonoral skeletal musculature generates a verbal (allographic) code that might function with linguistic regions of the major hemisphere of the brain, additional circuits might function directly between the nonoral skeletal musculature and the minor hemisphere, principally for nonverbal thought.

In summary, as represented in Figure 4, during cognitive acts such as perception, imagery, thought, and dreams, we hypothesize for further consideration that the complex muscle response patterns include (1) those speech muscle components that function in the genera-

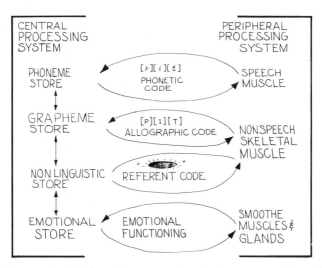

FIGURE 4. Neuromuscular information-processing circuits represented as a function of class of code generated and transmitted. We presume that the linguistic and nonlinguistic storage systems reside in the higher levels of the CNS, so that retrieval is possible through the interaction of the various peripheral–central circuits represented. There must be highly complex interactions among these classes of circuits, which, for simplicity, have not been represented here.

tion of a phonetic code; (2) those nonoral skeletal muscle components that function in the generation of an allographic code; (3) those nonoral skeletal muscle components that function in a nonlinguistic referent code; and (4) circuits involving the autonomic system for adding emotional tone. In conjunction, these various volleys are transmitted to their appropriate regions of the brain (the verbal coding to the linguistic regions for lexical–semantic processing, the nonverbal coding to nonverbal regions of the brain for nonlinguistic processing).

With Watson (1930) and many others, I here propose that there are critical nonoral muscular components of cognitive activity. A high-priority next step is to seek additional data relevant to nonoral coding systems. Our expectation is that further experimentation would specify highly differentiated covert responding in the nonoral musculature as a function of class of linguistic input. While it is unreasonable to expect covert nonoral responding (with the exception of eye activity) to be as differentiated as that of the oral musculature, we should expect to find some relationships between classes of bodily locations and linguistic input. Specification of those relationships should greatly contribute to our understanding of information processing in the nonoral musculature and hence of the functioning of the motor system during cognitive activities.

Appendix: Summary of Specific Relationships Identified in Column 4 of Table 1

Problem Solving

Golla (1921): Increases in forearm tonicity were positively related to the difficulty of the problem to be solved.

Tuttle (1924): Muscle tonus (patellar reflex) increased from relaxation to conversation to problem solving.

Freeman (1930): Leg tension increased during the first part of mental tasks directly as a function of task difficulty.

Clites (1936): Successful problem-solvers showed greater right forearm EMG and significantly less overt movement of that arm than did unsuccessful problem-solvers.

Davis (1937): Amount of right arm EMG was negatively related to amount of mental work accomplished.

Max (1937): The more intelligent and better-educated subjects gave smaller amplitude of manual arm responses to problem-solving situations.

Davis (1938): Right arm and neck EMG increased as the difficulty of the problem-solving task increased.

Davis (1939): There was a bodily focus of muscular activity for various psychological processes; for example, during multiplication the focus was in the right arm (relatively greater activity there than in the left arm, which, in turn, was greater than in the left leg). During learning of nonsense syllables, the focus was probably in the speech musculature. Response amplitude decreased as distance from the point of focus increased.

Ellson, Davis, Saltzman, and Burke (1952) (Experiment 7): Right arm EMG was greater during a conflict situation involving a right versus a left arm response than in the absence of conflict.

Ellson et al. (1952) (Experiment 8): Arm EMG response latencies were significantly shorter for critical lying responses than for critical nonlying responses.

Reuder (1956): Subjects under a task-oriented instruction exhibited higher EMG levels on the relatively difficult problems than they did on easy problems, whereas subjects who received ego-oriented instructions showed higher EMG levels for easy problems than they did for difficult problems.

Stennett (1957): As the subject's incentive was increased, there was an inverted-U relationship with integrated amplitude of EMGs from the left and right arms and also with palmar conductance.

Leshner (1961): During problem solving, EMGs decreased significantly for successful subjects and significantly increased for subjects who failed.

Pishkin (1964): Amplitude of EMG in the preferred arm significantly and positively increased with learning rate, and there was a negative correlation between preferred-arm EMG amplitude and time required per trial.

MacNeilage (1966): As difficulty of serial addition tasks increased, forehead and arm EMG significantly increased.

Pishkin and Shurley (1968): There was a positive correlation between number of errors made on a concept-identification task and forehead EMG; furthermore, that EMG activity increased significantly as a function of task complexity when the subjects were given both solvable and unsolvable sets.

Vaughn and McDaniel (1969): Amplitude of frontalis EMG during a match-to-sample visual discrimination task significantly increased when the subjects made correct responses and decreased following errors. Phasic responses were typically superimposed on a rising and falling EMG gradient.

McGuigan (1971): Amplitude of left arm and lip EMG significantly increased over baseline during problem solving, with the arm EMG being significantly greater than during a nonverbal control task. Integrated EEG from left motor area significantly decreased more during problem solving than during the control task.

Imagination

Jacobson (1927): Reduction in EMG tension prevented the subject from engaging in conscious processes like imagery, attention, reflection, and emotion.

Jacobson (1927, 1930a): Imagination of a right arm flexion produced heightened EMG in the right arm, whereas imagination of activity of other parts of the body did not produce right arm EMG increase. Jacobson's general conclusion was that imagination of voluntary movement is associated with neuromuscular activity in the locale of the imagined act. For his succeeding studies, we will maintain this general conclusion and cite only the specific findings.

Jacobson (1930b): Confirmed his (1930a) findings, except that he used a variety of specific imagination instructions such as "Imagine lifting a cigarette to your mouth," "Imagine throwing a ball," etc. The same relationship was found when the subjects were asked to recollect other muscular acts commonly performed with the right arm.

Jacobson (1930c): Imagining lifting a 10-pound weight produced EMG increases in the right biceps, but imagining lifting with the left did not. Furthermore, subjects could not simultaneously imagine lifting a weight and keep their arms relaxed; that is, they either had to disregard the relaxation instructions and imagine or disregard the imagination instructions in order to keep their arm relaxed.

Jacobson (1931a): Imagining lifting a weight with the right arm produced EMG increases in the right arm. On the other hand, *visually* imagining lifting the weight with the right arm typically increased EMG from the *ocular* region but did not typically increase biceps activity in the right arm.

Jacobson (1931b): Imagination of left hand flexion in an amputated arm was associated with a substitute reaction in the corresponding muscles of the right arm and in the remanent muscles of the upper left arm.

Shaw (1940): The magnitude of right arm EMG linearly increased as the magnitude of weights increased; the increase occurred while the subject actually lifted the weights and while he imagined lifting those weights.

Silent Reading

Jacobson and Kraft (1942): Right leg muscle EMG increased during a
30-min silent reading period, with the highest EMG level being
during the first and last several minutes of reading.

Strother (1949): EMG level in the forelimbs during the reading of
various kinds of emotional material was in order of descending
magnitude when the subjects were reading the following kinds of
prose: fear, hate-anger, happiness, tranquility-reverence.

Hardyck and Petrinovich (1970): Laryngeal, chin-lip, and right arm
EMG measures increased as a function of the difficulty of the
material read.

Speech Perception

Smith, Malmo, and Shagass (1954): EMG increased in the forearms
and chin while the subjects listened to a recording. During overtly
recalling, there were significant increases from the forehead, the
neck, both arms, and the chin.

Wallerstein (1954): Frontalis EMG significantly increased from baseline
while subjects listened to a detective story and to a philosophical
essay. Chin EMG increased significantly for the second and third
hearings of the story but not for the essay.

Bartoshuk (1956): Frontalis EMG was associated with interest in the
material listened to and was more closely associated with listening
than were forearm or chin EMGs.

Learning

Travis and Kennedy (1947): Rate and amplitude of super orbital EMGs
were inversely related to reaction time during an external feedback lookout task.

Berger, Irwin, and Frommer (1970): Right wrist EMG was higher while
subjects learned the manual alphabet for the deaf through observation than when they memorized word-number pairs visually
presented. The authors concluded that there was a relationship
between cognitive activity and localized muscle activity.

Beh and Hawkins (1973): Subjects with induced muscle tensions in the
arm learned significantly faster than significants who did not have
such induced tensions. Furthermore, delayed recall was significantly greater for those who learned under tension.

Petrinovich and Hardyck (1970): The mean number of generalized EMG responses from pictures to words was significantly higher than from words to pictures, suggesting that covert responses made during learning from pictures involved verbal coding of the names of the objects shown in the pictures.

Sleep-Dreams

Max (1935): Arm EMG increased during the dreams of deaf-mute subjects.

Stoyva (1965): In both deaf and hearing subjects, REM periods showed a consistently accelerated rate of finger EMG activity in comparison with other stages of sleep.

Wolpert and Trosman (1958): There was a strong relationship between frequency of recall of a dream if the dreamer was awakened during gross bodily movement.

Wolpert (1960): EMG was significantly greater during REM sleep than during Stages 2, 3, and 4. Additionally, there were significant associations between EMG activity and dream-narrative content for some subjects, but not for others.

Jacobson, et al. (1964): Muscle tonus of the neck and head is related to EEG stage 1-REM periods.

Baldridge, et al. (1965): Fine muscle activity in various parts of the body are associated with REM period.

Sassin and Johnson (1968): Phasic limb movements occur during Stage 1-REM.

Larson and Foulkes (1969): Momentary deepening of sleep is accompanied by pre-REM suppression of submental EMG.

Pessah and Roffwarg (1972): Middle ear muscle responses typically precede and continue throughout REM periods.

Gardner, et al. (1973): There is a significant correlation between location of actual bodily movement and locaton and amount of dreamed action.

References

ADAMS, J. A., McINTYRE, J. S., AND THORSHEIM, H. I. Response feedback and verbal retention. *Journal of Experimental Psychology*, 1969, *82*, 290–296.

AMASSIAN, V. E., AND WEINER, H. The effect of (+)-tubocurarine chloride and of acute hypotension on the electrical activity of the cat. *Journal of Physiology*, 1966, *184*, 1–15.

ASERINSKY, E., AND KLEITMAN, N. Regularly occurring periods of eye motility, and concomitant phenomena during sleep. *Science*, 1953, *118*, 273–274.

BALDRIDGE, B. J., WHITMAN, R. M., AND KRAMER, J. The concurrence of fine muscle activity and REMs during sleep. *Psychosomatic Medicine*, 1965, *27*,19–26.

BARTOSHUK, A. K. Electromyographic gradients and electroencephalographic amplitude during motivated listening. *Canadian Journal of Psychology*, 1956, *10*, 156–164.

BECHTEREV, V. M. *General foundations of human reflexology* (2d ed.). Moscow: Gosizdat, 1923.

BEH, H. C., AND HAWKINS, C. A. Effect of induced muscle tension on acquisition and retention of verbal material. *Journal of Experimental Psychology*, 1973, *98*, 206–208.

BERGER, R. J. Tonus of extrinsic laryngeal muscles during sleep and dreaming. *Science*, 1961, *134*, 840.

BERGER, S. M., IRWIN, D. S., AND FROMMER, G. P. Electromyographic activity during observational learning. *American Journal of Psychology*, 1970, *83*, 86–94.

BERRY, R. N., AND DAVIS, R. C. Muscle responses and their relation to rote learning. *Journal of Experimental Psychology*, 1958, *55*, 188–194.

BILLS, A. G. The influence of muscular tension on the efficiency of mental work. *American Journal of Psychology*, 1927, *38*, 227–251.

BLACK, A. H. Cardiac conditioning in curarized dogs: The relationship between heart rate and skeletal behavior. In W. F. Prokasy (Ed.), *Classical conditioning*. New York: Appleton-Century-Crofts, 1965.

BLACK, A. H. Transfer following operant conditioning in the curarized dog. *Science*, 1967, *155*, 201–203.

BLACK, A. H. Autonomic aversive conditioning in infrahuman subjects. In F. R. Brush (Ed.), *Aversive conditioning and learning*. New York: Academic Press, 1971. Pp. 3–104.

BLACK, A. H., CARLSON, N. J., AND SOLOMON, R. L. Exploratory studies of the conditioning of autonomic responses in curarized dogs. *Psychology Monographs*, 1962, *76*, 1–31.

BLUMENTHAL, J. Lingual myographic responses during directed thinking. Unpublished doctoral dissertation, University of Denver, 1959.

BRINLEY, F. J., JR., KANDEL, E. R., AND MARSHALL, W. H. The effect of intravenous D-tubocurarine on the electrical activity of the cat cerebral cortex. *Transactions of the American Neurological Association*, 1958, *83*, 53–58.

BUCHWALD, J. S., STANDISH, M., ELDRED, E., AND HALAS, E. S. Contribution of muscle spindle circuits to learning as suggested by training under Flaxedil. *Electroencephalography and Clinical Neurophysiology*, 1964, *16*, 582–594.

CAMPBELL, D., SANDERSON, R. E., AND LAVERTY, S. G. Characteristics of a conditioned response in human subjects during extinction trials following a simple traumatic conditioning trial. *Journal of Abnormal and Social Psychology*, 1964, *68*, 627–639.

CHASE, W. G. (Ed.). *Visual information processing*. New York: Academic Press, 1973.

CLITES, M. S. Certain somatic activities in relation to successful and unsuccessful problem solving, Part III. *Journal of Experimental Psychology*, 1936, *19*, 172–192.

DARLEY, F. L., ARONSON, A. E., AND BROWN, J. R. Differential diagnostic patterns of dysarthria. *Journal of Speech and Hearing Research*, 1969a, *12*, 246–269.

DARLEY, F. L., ARONSON, A. E., AND BROWN, J. R. Clusters of deviant speech dimensions in the dysarthrias. *Journal of Speech and Hearing Research*, 1969b, *12*, 462–496.

DASHIELL, J. F. *Fundamentals of general psychology* (3d. ed.). Boston: Houghton Mifflin, 1949.

DAVIS, R. C. The relation of certain muscle action potentials to "mental work." *Indiana University Publication, Science Series*, 1937, *5*, 5–29.

DAVIS, R. C. The relation of muscle action potentials to difficulty and frustration. *Journal of Experimental Psychology*, 1938, *23*, 141–158.

DAVIS, R. C. Patterns of muscular activity during "mental work" and their constancy. *Journal of Experimental Psychology*, 1939, *24*, 451–465.

DAVIS, R. C., GARAFOLOW, L., AND GAULT, F. P. An exploration of abdominal potentials. *Journal of Comparative and Physiological Psychology*, 1957, *50*, 519–523.

DELAFRESNAYE, J. F. (Ed.). *Brain mechanisms and consciousness.* Springfield, Ill.: Charles C Thomas, 1954.

DEMENT, W. C., AND KLEITMAN, N. The relation of eye movements during sleep to dream activity: An objective method for the study of dreaming. *Journal of Experimental Psychology*, 1957, *53*, 339–346.

DICARA, L. V., AND MILLER, N. E. Changes in heart rate instrumentally learned by curarized rats as avoidance responses. *Journal of Comparative and Physiological Psychology*, 1968, *65*, 8–12.

DOUGLAS, W. W. Autocoids. In L. S. Goodman AND A. Gillman (Eds.), *Pharmacological basis of therapeutics.* New York: Macmillan, 1970. Pp. 620–662.

DUNLAP, K. *Scientific psychology.* St. Louis: Mosby, 1922.

ECCLES, J. C. *Brain and conscious experience.* New York: Springer-Verlag, 1966.

ELLSON, D. G., DAVIS, R. C., SALTZMAN, I. J., AND BURKE, C. J. Report of research on the detection of deception. Contract N6onr-18011, ONR, 1952.

ESTABLE, C. Curare and synapse. In D. Bovet, F. Bovet-Nitti, and G. B. Marini-Bettolo (Eds.), *Curare and curare-like agents.* Amsterdam: Elsevier, 1959.

FREEMAN, G. L. Changes in tonus during completed and interrupted mental work. *Journal of General Psychology*, 1930, *4*, 309–334.

FREEMAN, G. L. The spread of neuro-muscular activity during mental work. *Journal of General Psychology*, 1931, *5*, 479–494.

GALINDO, A. Curare and pancuronium compared: Effects on previously undepressed mammalian myoneural junctions. *Science*, 1972, *178*, 753–755.

GALL, F. J., AND SPURZHEIM, G. *Recherches sur le systeme nerveux in général, et sur celui du cerveau en particulier.* Institut de France, 1809.

GAL'PERIN, P. YA. Razvitiye issledovaniy po formirovaniyu umstvennih deystviy/ Progress in the studies on formation of mental actions. In *Psychological science in the USSR*, Vol. 1. Moscow: APN RSFSR Press, 1959.

GARDNER, R., GROSSMAN, W. I., ROFFWARG, H. P., AND WEINER, H. Does sleep behavior appear in the dream? *Psychosomatic Medicine*, 1973, *35*, 450–451.

GELDARD, F. A. Cutaneous coding of optical signals: The optohapt. *Perception and Psychophysics*, 1966, *1*, 377–381.

GOLLA, F. The objective study of neurosis. *Lancet*, 1921, *2*, 115–122.

GOLLA, F. L., AND ANTONOVITCH, S. The relation of muscular tonus and the patellar reflex to mental work. *Journal of Mental Science*, 1929, *75*, 234–241.

GREENWALD, A. G. Sensory feedback mechanisms in performance control with special reference to the ideo-motor mechanism. *Psychological Review*, 1970, *77*, 73–99.

GRINGS, W. W. The role of consciousness and cognition in autonomic behavior change. In F. J. McGuigan and R. A. Schoonover (Eds.), *The psychophysiology of thinking.* New York: Academic Press, 1973.

GROB, D. Neuromuscular blocking drugs. In W. S. Root AND F. G. Hoffman (Eds.), *Physiological pharmacology*, Vol. 3: *The nervous system: Part C, autonomic nervous system drugs.* New York: Academic Press, 1967. Pp. 389–460.

HARDYCK, C. D., AND PETRINOVICH, L. F. Subvocal speech and comprehension level as a function of the difficulty level of reading material. *Journal of Verbal Learning and Verbal Behavior*, 1970, *9*, 647–652.

HEBB, D. O. *The organization of behavior.* New York: Wiley, 1949.

HEBB, D. O. Concerning imagery. *Psychological Review*, 1968, *75*, 466-477.

HODES, R. Electrocortical synchronization resulting from reduced proprioceptive drive caused by neuromuscular blocking agents. *Electroencephalography and Clinical Neurophysiology*, 1962, *14*, 220-232.

HORRIDGE, G. A. The electrophysiological approach to learning in isolatable ganglia. *Animal Behavior*, 1965, Suppl. 1, 163-182.

HOWARD, J. L., GALOSY, R. A., GAEBELEIN, C. J., AND OBRIST, P. A. Some problems in the use of neuromuscular blockage. In P. A. Obrist, A. H. Black, J. Brener, and L. V. DiCara (Eds.) *Cardiovascular psychophysiology: Current issues in response mechanisms, biofeedback and methodology.* Chicago: Adline Publishing Co., 1974.

HUNTER, W. S. The problem of consciousness. *Psychological Review*, 1924, *31*, 1-37.

JACOBSON, E. Action currents from muscular contractions during conscious processes. *Science*, 1927, *66*, 403.

JACOBSON, E. *Progressive relaxation.* Chicago: University of Chicago Press, 1929.

JACOBSON, E. Electrical measurements of neuromuscular states during mental activities, I: Imagination of movement involving skeletal muscle. *American Journal of Physiology*, 1930a, *91*, 567-608.

JACOBSON, E. Electrical measurements of neuromuscular states during mental activities, II: Imagination and recollection of various muscular acts. *American Journal of Physiology*, 1930b, *94*, 22-34.

JACOBSON, E. Electrical measurements of neuromuscular states during mental activities, IV: Evidence of contraction of specific muscles during imagination. *American Journal of Physiology*, 1930c, *95*, 703-712.

JACOBSON, E. Electrical measurements of neuromuscular states during mental activities. V. Variation of specific muscles contracting during imagination. *American Journal of Physiology*, 1931a, *96*, 115-121.

JACOBSON, E. Electrical measurements of neuromuscular states during mental activities, VI: A note on mental activities concerning an amputated limb. *American journal of Physiology*, 1931b, *96*, 122-125.

JACOBSON, E. Electrophysiology of mental activities. *American Journal of Psychology*, 1932, *44*, 677-694.

JACOBSON, E. *Biology of emotions.* Springfield, Ill.: Charles C Thomas, 1967.

JACOBSON, E. Electrophysiology of mental activities AND introduction to the psychological process of thinking. In F. J. McGuigan and R. A. Schoonover (Eds.), *The psychophysiology of thinking.* New York: Academic Press, 1973.

JACOBSON, E., AND KRAFT, F. L. Contraction potentials (right quadriceps femoris) in man during reading. *American Journal of Physiology*, 1942, *137*, 1-5.

JACOBSON, A., KALES, A., LEHMANN, D., AND HOEDEMAKER, F. S. Muscle tonus in human subjects during sleep and dreaming. *Experimental Neurology*, 1964, *10*, 418-424.

KOELLE, G. B. Neuromuscular blocking agents. In L. S. Goodman and A. Gillman (Eds.), *Pharmacological basis of therapeutics.* New York: Macmillan, 1960. Pp. 601-619.

LACEY, B. C., AND LACEY, J. I. Studies of heart rate and other bodily processes in sensorimotor behavior. In P. A. Obrist, A. H. Black, J. Brener, and L. V. DiCara (Eds.), *Cardiovascular psychophysiology: Current issues in response mechanism, biofeedback, and methodology.* Chicago: Aldine Publishing Co., 1974. Pp. 538-564.

LANGFELD, H. S. The historical development of response psychology. *Science*, 1933, *77*, 243-250.

LARSON, J. D., AND FOULKES, D. Electromyogram suppression during sleep, dream recall, and orientation time. *Psychophysiology*, 1969, *5*, 548-555.

Lashley, K. S. The brain and human behavior. *Proceedings of the Association for Research in Nervous and Mental Disease*, 1958, *39*, 1-18.

Leont'ev, A. N. *Problems for psychic development*. Moscow: APN RSFSR Press, 1959.

Leshner, S. Effects of aspiration and achievement on muscular tensions. *Journal of Experimental Psychology*, 1961, *61*, 133-137.

Leuba, C., Birch, L., and Appleton, J. Human problem solving during complete paralysis of the voluntary musculature. *Psychological Reports*, 1968, *22*, 849-855.

Light, J. S., and Gantt, W. H. Essential part of reflex arc for establishment of conditioned reflex: Formation of conditioned reflex after exclusion of motor peripheral end. *Journal of Comparative Psychology*, 1936, *21*, 19-36.

Locke, J. L., and Fehr, F. S. Subvocal rehearsal as a form of speech. *Journal of Verbal Learning and Verbal Behavior*, 1970, *9*, 495-498.

MacNeilage, P. F. Changes in electroencephalogram and other physiological measures during serial mental performance. *Psychophysiology*, 1966, *2*, 344-353.

Max, L. W. An experimental study of the motor theory of consciousness. *Psychological Bulletin*, 1933, *30*, 714.

Max, L. W. An experimental study of the motor theory of consciousness, III: Action current responses in deaf mutes during sleep, sensory stimulation and dreams. *Journal of Comparative Psychology*, 1935, *19*, 469-486.

Max, L. W. An experimental study of the motor theory of consciousness, IV: Action-current responses in the deaf during awakening, kinaesthetic imagery and abstract thinking. *Journal of Comparative Psychology*, 1937, *24*, 301-344.

McGuigan, F. J. *Thinking: Studies of covert language processes*. New York: Appleton-Century-Crofts, 1966.

McGuigan, F. J. Covert oral behavior during the silent performance of language tasks. *Psychological Bulletin*, 1970, *74*, 309-326.

McGuigan, F. J. Covert linguistic behavior in deaf subjects during thinking. *Journal of Comparative and Physiological Psychology*, 1971, *75*, 417-420.

McGuigan, F. J. Conditioning of covert behavior—Some problems and some hopes. In F. J. McGuigan and D. B. Lumsden (Eds.), *Contemporary approaches to conditioning and learning*. Washington: Winston, 1973a.

McGuigan, F. J. Electrical measurement of covert processes as an explication of "higher mental events." In F. J. McGuigan and R. A. Schoonover (Eds.), *The psychophysiology of thinking*. New York: Academic Press, 1973b.

McGuigan, F. J. The function of covert oral behavior in linguistic coding and internal information processing. Kurt Salzinger (Ed.), *Small Annals of the New York Academy of Sciences*, 1976.

McGuigan, F. J. *Cognitive psychophysiology—Principles of covert behavior*. Englewood cliffs, N.J.: Prentice-Hall, 1978.

McGuigan, F. J., and Pavek, G. V. On the psychophysiological identification of covert nonoral language processes. *Journal of Experimental Psychology*, 1972, *92*, 237-245.

McGuigan, F. J., and Rodier, W. I., III. Effects of auditory stimulation on covert oral behavior during silent reading. *Journal of Experimental Psychology*, 1968, *76*, 649-655.

McGuigan, F. J., and Schoonover, R. A. (Eds.), *The psychophysiology of thinking*. New York: Academic Press, 1973.

McGuigan, F. J., and Tanner, R. G. Covert oral behavior during conversation and visual dreams. *Psychonomic Science*, 1971, *23*, 263-264.

McGuigan, F. J., and Winstead, C. L., Jr. Discriminative relationship between covert oral behavior and the phonemic system in internal information processing. *Journal of Experimental Psychology*, 1974, *103*, 885-890.

McIntyre, A. R., Bennett, A. L., and Hamilton, C. Recent advances in the pharmacology of curare. In A. R. McIntyre (Ed.), *Curare and anticurare agents, Annals of the New York Academy of Sciences*, 1951, *54*, 297–530.

Novikova, L. A. Electrophysiological investigation of speech. In N. O'Connor (Ed.), *Recent Soviet psychology*. New York: Liveright, 1961.

Okuma, T., Fujmori, M., and Hayashi, A. The effect of environmental temperature on the electrocortical activity of cats immobilized by neuromuscular blocking agents. *Electroencephalography and Clinical Neurophysiology*, 1965, *18*, 392–400.

Osgood, C. E. Motivational dynamics of language behavior. In M. R. Jones (Ed.), *Nebraska symposium on motivation*. Lincoln: University of Nebraska Press, 1957.

Osgood, C. E., and McGuigan, F. J. Psychophysiological correlates of meaning: Essences or tracers? In F. J. McGuigan and R. A. Schoonover (Eds.), *The psychophysiology of thinking*. New York: Academic Press, 1973.

Pavlov, I. P. *Lectures on conditioned reflexes*, Vol. 2: *Conditioned reflexes and psychiatry*. Translated and edited by W. H. Gantt. New York: International Publishers, 1941.

Penfield, W. Some mechanisms of consciousness discovered during electrical stimulation of the brain. *Proceedings of the National Academy of Sciences*, 1958, *44*, 51–66.

Pessah, M. A., and Roffwarg, H. P. Spontaneous middle ear muscle activity in man: A rapid eye movement sleep phenomenon. *Science*, 1972, *178*, 773–776.

Petrinovich, L. F., and Hardyck, C. D. Generalization of an instrumental response between words and pictures. *Psychonomic Science*, 1970, *18*, 239–241.

Pishkin, V. Electromyographic variation concomitant with concept identification parameters. *Perceptual and Motor Skills*, 1964, *18*,649–652.

Pishkin, V., and Shurley, J. T. Electrodermal and electromyographic parameters in concept identification. *Psychophysiology*, 1968, *5*, 112–118.

Ray, R. Classical conditioning of heart rate in restrained and curarized rats. Unpublished doctoral dissertation, University of Tennessee, 1969.

Reuder, M. E. The effect of ego orientation and problem difficulty on muscle action potentials. *Journal of Experimental Psychology*, 1956, *51*, 142–148.

Sassin, J. F., and Johnson, L. C. Body motility during sleep and its relation to the K-complex. *Experimental Neurology*, 1968, *22*, 133–144.

Sechenov, I. M. *Refleksy golovnogo mozqa* (St. Petersburg, 1863). Translated as *Reflexes of the Brain*, by A. A. Subkov. In *I. M. Sechenov, Selected works*. Moscow and Leningrad: State Publishing House for Biological and Medical Literature, 1935. Pp. 264–322. In R. J. Herrnstein and E. G. Boring (Eds.), *A source book in the history of psychology*. Cambridge, Mass.: Harvard University Press, 1965.

Shallice, T. Mental states and processes. *Science*, 1974, *183*, 1072–1073.

Shaw, W. A. The distribution of muscular action potentials during imaging. *Psychological Record*, 1938, *2*, 195–216.

Shaw, W. A. The relation of muscular action potentials to imaginal weight lifting. *Archives of Psychology, New York*, 1940, *247*, 1–50.

Sherrington, C. S. Postural activity of muscle and nerve. *Brain*, 1915, *38*, 191–234.

Skinner, B. F. *Verbal Behavior*. New York: Appleton-Century, 1957.

Skinner, B. F. Verbal behavior. In F. J. McGuigan (Ed.), *Thinking: Studies of covert language processes*. New York: Appleton-Century-Crofts, 1966.

Smith, A. A., Malmo, R. B., and Shagass, C. An electromyographic study of listening and talking. *Canadian Journal of Psychology*, 1954, *8*, 219–227.

Smith, M. O. History of the motor theories of attention. *The Journal of General Psychology*, 1969, *80*, 243–257.

Smith, S. M., Brown, H. O., Toman, J. E. P., and Goodman, L. S. The lack of cerebral effects of D-tubocurarine. *Anesthesiology*, 1947, *8*, 1–14.

Sokolov, A. N. *Perception and the conditioned reflex.* New York: Macmillan, 1963.

Sokolov, A. N. *Inner speech and thought.* New York: Plenum, 1972.

Solomon, R. E., and Turner, L. H. Discriminative classical conditioning in dogs paralyzed by curare can later control discriminative avoidance responses in the normal state. *Psychological Review,* 1962, *69,* 202-219.

Sperry, R. W. Lateral specialization of cerebral function in the surgically separated hemispheres. In F. J. McGuigan and R. A. Schoonover (Eds.), *The psychophysiology of thinking.* New York: Academic Press, 1973.

Stennett, R. G. The relationship of performance level to level of arousal. *Journal of Experimental Psychology,* 1957, *54,* 54-61.

Stoyva, J. M. Finger electromyographic activity during sleep: Its relation to dreaming in deaf and normal subjects. *Journal of Abnormal Psychology,* 1965, *70,* 343-349.

Strother, G. B. The role of muscle action in interpretative reading. *Journal of General Psychology,* 1949, *41,* 3-20.

Sussman, H. M. What the tongue tells the brain. *Psychological Bulletin,* 1972, *77,* 262-272.

Taub, E., and Berman, A. J. Movement and learning in the absence of sensory feedback. In S. J. Freedman (Ed.), *The neurophysiology of spatially oriented behavior.* Homewood, ILL.: Dorsey, 1968.

Titchener, E. B. *Lectures on the experimental psychology of the thought-processes.* New York: Macmillan, 1909.

Travis, R. C., and Kennedy, J. L. Prediction and automatic control of alertness, I: Control of lookout alertness. *Journal of Comparative and Physiological Psychology,* 1947, *40,* 457-461.

Tuttle, W. W. The effect of attention or mental activity on the patellar tendon reflex. *Journal of Experimental Psychology,* 1924, *7,* 401-419.

Unna, K. R., and Pelikan, E. W. Evaluation of curarizing drugs in man, VI: Critique of experiments on unanesthetized subjects. In A. R. McIntyre (Ed.), *Curare and anti-curare agents, Annals of the New York Academy of Sciences,* 1951, *54,* 297-530.

Vaughn, A. O., and McDaniel, J. W. Electromyographic gradients during complex visual discrimination learning. *Psychonomic Science,* 1969, *16,* 203-204.

Vigotsky, L. S. *Thought and language.* New York: Wiley, 1962.

Wallerstein, H. An electromyographic study of attentive listening. *Canadian Journal of Psychology,* 1954, *8,* 228-238.

Washburn, M. F. *Movement and mental imagery.* Boston: Houghton-Mifflin, 1916.

Watson, J. B. *Behaviorism.* Chicago: University of Chicago Press, 1930.

Wilson, J. R., and DiCara, L. V. Influence of neuromuscular blocking drugs on recovery of skeletal electromyographic activity in the rat. *Psychophysiology,* 1975, *12,* 249-253.

Wolpert, E. A. Studies in psychophysiology, II: An electromyographic study of dreaming. *AMA Archives of General Psychiatry,* 1960, *2,* 231-241.

Wolpert, E. A., and Trosman, H. Studies in psychophysiology of dreams, I: Experimental evocation of sequential dream episodes. *AMA Archives of Neurology and Psychiatry,* 1958, *79,* 603-606.

Young, R. M. *Mind, brain, and adaptation in the nineteenth century.* New York: Clarendon (Oxford University Press), 1970.

3 Regulation of the Stream of Consciousness: Toward a Theory of Ongoing Thought

KENNETH S. POPE AND JEROME L. SINGER

Consciousness—that familiar constellation of memories, sensations, plans, fantasies, fleeting images, and sometimes unrecognizable forms that constitutes our awareness from moment to moment—has received rough treatment at the hands of 20th-century American psychology. Neither the elaborate Titchnerian method of introspection nor the stirring, graceful prose of William James managed to extend the life of consciousness as a legitimate area for psychological investigation much past the turn of the century. As Roger Brown (1958) wrote, "In 1913 John Watson mercifully closed the bloodshot inner eye of American psychology. With great relief the profession trained its exteroceptors on the laboratory animal" (p. 93). Even the impact of Freudian thought and psychoanalysis, with its great interest in and respect for the inner life of the individual, failed to generate a renewed study of consciousness because it emphasized the overwhelming power of the unconscious and portrayed man's life as determined by a hydracliclike system of drives of which the individual was generally unaware. More recently, careful, creative, rigorously executed scientific work (Holt, 1964; Paivio, 1971; Segal, 1971; Sheehan, 1972; Singer, 1974a,b) has managed to open the door a bit toward a systematic study of consciousness, though psychology is still occasionally chastised for its "diverting preoccupation with a supposed or real inner life" (Skinner, 1975, p. 46).

KENNETH S. POPE · Department of Psychiatry, University of California, San Francisco, California.   JEROME L. SINGER · Department of Psychology, Yale University, New Haven, Connecticut.

I. THE STREAM OF CONSCIOUSNESS AS A PSYCHOLOGICAL PROBLEM: ARTS AND SCIENCES

To anyone but a psychologist, it would seem incredible that textbooks on thinking (Bourne, Ekstrand, and Duminowski, 1971; Johnson, 1955) can ignore or say little about the stream of consciousness and imagination, that books on personality (Mischel, 1971) or on adolescence (Seidman, 1960) can say so little about daydreaming or fantasy. Insofar as we are aware of this phenomenon of ongoing thought in our day-to-day lives and of its virtual absence within psychological research and theory, we may feel a discontent similar to that voiced by Virginia Woolf (1925/1953) in discussing its absence from a certain kind of novel: "But sometimes, more and more often as time goes by, we suspect a momentary doubt, a spasm of rebellion, as the pages fill themselves in the customary way. Is life like this?" (p. 154). Though ongoing thought remains to this day a relatively neglected concern of formal psychology, the fine arts showed little hesitation in responding to the challenge William James (1890/1950) posed in his famous chapter "The Stream of Thought."

The excitement engendered in the first two decades of this century by the efforts of James Joyce to produce what Edmund Wilson (1922) called "perhaps the most faithful x-ray ever taken of the ordinary human consciousness" (p. 64) reflected the seriousness with which writers responded to James's insights. Writing in 1919, Virginia Woolf (1925/1953) expressed the concern of many writers lest this aspect of human life be denied or ignored:

> Examine for a moment an ordinary mind on an ordinary day. The mind receives a myriad impressions—trivial, fantastic, evanescent, or engraved with the sharpness of steel. From all sides they come, an incessant shower of innumerable atoms; and as they fall, as they shape themselves into the life of Monday or Tuesday, the accent falls differently from of old. . . . Life is not a series of gig lamps symmetrically arranged; but a luminous halo, a semi-transparent envelope surrounding us from the beginning of consciousness to the end. . . . Let us record the atoms as they fall upon the mind in the order in which they fall, let us trace the pattern, however disconnected and incoherent in appearance, which each sight or incident scores upon the consciousness. (pp. 154–155)

This literary effort was not brief and faddish. Poets and novelists have continued to represent man's stream of consciousness as well as the stream of behavior and events. The works of Theodore Roethke (the stream of consciousness of a developing child in *Praise to the End*), Erica Jong (Isadora's wildly vivid sexual fantasies in *Fear of Flying*), Saul Bellow (the aged man's reflections in *Mr. Sammler's Planet*), and Hubert Selby, Jr. (Georgette's jumble of words and images, fantasies, and physical sensations as he makes homosexual love in *Last Exit to Brooklyn*) render an aspect of human experience that is relatively inaccessible if we attend only to overt behavior, social conversation, and "gig lamp" descriptions of events.

While James Joyce, Virginia Woolf, and T. S. Eliot (1950) in his 1919 discussion of the "objective correlative" were forming the basis for the use of the stream of consciousness as a literary and poetic medium, filmmakers like Sergei Eisenstein perceived an opportunity in moving pictures to capture even more effectively the ongoing thought stream. By developing the "montage" and the technique of "partial representations," Eisenstein (1942) sought to create films that would evoke for the viewer the same ongoing thought experience occurring in the mind of the artist or of one of the film's characters.

Recent films illustrate cinema's dramatic effectiveness in capturing the characteristics of normal thought. In Sidney Lumet's *The Pawnbroker*, Sol Nazzerman makes his way into a crowded New York City subway train and we see in briefest flash a cattle car crowded with Jews en route to a concentration camp, a memory from the pawnbroker's own experience. In Eric Rohmer's *Chloe in the Afternoon*, a young man spends an afternoon desirously admiring the women he sees but never approaching them. We then see through his mind's eye his walk through the streets, during which, because he is wearing a "magic" stone around his neck, every woman he sees comes up to ask him to her bed. In Woody Allen's *Play It Again, Sam*, Alan Felix prepares his apartment in anticipation of his best friend's wife's joining him alone for dinner and to watch TV. As he sets the table, we see brief images of him calling her "darling" and leaning over to kiss her. This imaginary preview plays itself over and over again in his mind, each time growing a little longer and a little more elaborate. When he pictures himself pulling her over to him, we see her begin to struggle and yell, "RAPE!!!" As the daydream reaches its horrifying conclusion, Alan feverously sweeps the table settings off the table into the wastebasket, deciding that they should safely go out to dinner and to a movie instead.

Unlike writers, filmmakers, and other artists, the behavioral scientists must work within the framework of the scientific method. This constraint pulls for experiments that are easy to set up and control, generally focusing on outcome products of specific directed thinking tasks or on the study of isolated features of thought (e.g., the time it takes to rotate mentally a geometric form; the effectiveness of imagery in paired-associate learning; comparing the size of real or imagined wooden balls). Only very recently have researchers addressed such problems as the ethical thinking of the individual or the

private estimations and evaluations we make about human relationships. Yet even these studies are typically cast within the format of
problem solution in a structured fashion. The emergent picture of
thought process, therefore, often possesses a quality of organization
and rationality that is hard to reconcile with the nature of ongoing
thought as it is presented by artists or with our own stream of
consciousness if we take the trouble to observe it in its natural course.

II. PSYCHOANALYTIC APPROACHES AND THE NOTION OF REGRESSION

Drawing upon his interactions with patients rather than upon
clean laboratory studies, Freud was able to observe and write about
the complexities of thought, the irrational, wishful, self-preoccupied
aspect of private experience. His work is difficult to evaluate; various
structural characteristics of the theory—*id, ego, superego, unconscious,
conscious, preconscious, primary,* and *secondary processes*—were conceptualized and discussed at different times and were never finally
brought into correspondence (Gill, 1963). And yet, the overall impression is that the irrational, wish-laden, idiosyncratic mode of thinking
characterized as "primary process" belongs to childhood, mental
illness, and dreams. The well-analyzed adult has developed an ability
and facility at secondary process thought. True, even the most mature
mind falls prey to those irritating memory blanks, mental lapses, and
misleading associations known as the psychopathologies of everyday
life—yet these are simply false steps from which the well-analyzed,
mature mind can recover to resume its purposeful, directed thinking.
It is difficult, however, to agree with the notion that the numerous
phenomena characterized as primary process should, as a whole, be
considered merely immature or failed secondary process thinking.
Suzanne Langer (1964) argued the case persuasively when she discussed dreams:

> There are several theories of dreams, notably, of course, the Freudian
> interpretation. But those which—like Freud's—regard it more as excess
> mental energy or visceral disturbance do not fit the scientific picture of the
> mind's growth and function at all. A mind whose semantic powers are
> evolved from the functioning of the motor arc should *only think:* any
> vagaries are "mistakes." If our viscera made as many mistakes in sleep as
> the brain, we should all die of indigestion after our first nursing. It may be
> replied that the mistakes of dreams are harmless, since they have no motor
> terminals, though they enter into waking life as memories, and we have to
> learn to discount them. But why does the central switchboard not rest
> when there is no need of making connections? (p. 43)

Some analysts have tried to modify or open up this characterization of the normal, mature mind in terms of rational processes. Ernst Kris (1951), for instance, introduced the concept "regression in the service of the ego" to explain some of the mind's more creative activities. And yet the term *regression* brings along with it that heavy emphasis on the directed, rational, "secondary process" quality of normal, mature ongoing thought. It seems inadequate to maintain that a poet who can vividly recapture early memories and also create dramatic combinations from current experiences relies on a more childlike mode of thought. Similarly, consider the minds of Beethoven or Bach, teeming with melody, with novel and striking combinations of themes, instrumental coloration and interweaving lines of music, or the minds of Ingmar Bergman or Robert Altman, constantly rearranging, coordinating, and juxtaposing the actors, the dialog, the pauses, images, and perspectives of the scenes that comprise their movies. Should we describe these minds as representing a somehow more primitive style of thought than that of a mathematician mentally solving a math problem or a logician solving a riddle? The problems with this sort of conceptualization are many. The overemphasis on verbal or language processes as being of a higher order than auditory or visual imagery content in adult thinking may reflect a prejudice pervasive among professionals who are so dependent on the ultimate verbal, logical expression of material in print. More importantly, the recent heightened awareness we have of the differential processing capacities of the brain and its functional asymmetry for verbal-quantitative and imagery-spatial representational capacities suggests that the process of effective thought, particularly in complex situations, is far more complex than previously recognized. If we can step away from the hydraulic energy models that have been so much a part of our thinking about thinking during most of this century, then we may be able to develop more adequate notions than the oversimplified primary-secondary process or regression views that have been a part of that model.

III. Toward a Formulation of Ongoing Thought

A. Overview and Outline

Building a model of our stream of consciousness calls to mind the minister who stepped up into the pulpit and announced that he was going to preach on "God, the Universe, and Other Things." However, in this section, we attempt to identify and discuss very briefly some of those fundamental factors that regulate our moment-to-moment awareness, that bring us toward certain thoughts at a particular time or mood or place, that make it likely that we will think of one thing rather than another.

Table 1 presents our organization of this section and these factors.

In searching for an adequate account of the regulation of the stream of consciousness, we found the first step to be a realization that the mind itself is not static, not a large storage bin nor a passive blank slate; it is an organ of activity, process, and ongoing work. To a great extent, this active organ concerns itself with the processing of sensory input. The sense organs, then, exert considerable influence over what material will be ultimately available to consciousness. The material that reaches consciousness from immediate sensory input may be conceptualized as at one pole of a continuum of awareness that runs from a public pole (physical stimuli from the environment, clearly measurable or capable of consensual description by other people as well as by the individual) through internal bodily stimuli (not so readily accessible to the public but still on the whole traceable to physically measurable characteristics) to the "private" pole of the continuum (images, associations, and other material related to short- and long-term memory).

Attention is the process by which the material available is screened and selected for introduction into the stream of consciousness. There appears to be a distinct bias toward attending to sensory material, a characteristic of obvious survival and adaptational value. When the environment becomes predictable, dull, or barren, however, the tendency is for the consciousness to move toward the more private end of the continuum, for memories, associations, and imaginary

TABLE 1
Determinants of the Stream of Consciousness

1. The mind as activity
2. Sensory input
3. A continuum of awareness
4. Attention: the ability to screen and select
5. A bias favoring sensory input
6. Predictable, dull, or barren environments: an opportunity for private processing
7. The matching function: judging environmental input as predictable, dull, and barren OR as surprising, exciting, and rich
8. Affect
9. Current concerns, unfinished business, and unresolved stress
10. The set toward internal processing
11. Structural characteristics of the stimuli

materials to flow into the stream of consciousness. The quality of being "predictable," "dull," or "barren" does not inhere solely in the environment but depends to a great extent on the individual's image or scheme of incoming stimuli and on how well these representations are able to "match" or anticipate the environmental stimulation.

At this point, we turn to the theoretical framework of Silvan Tomkins (1962–1963) concerning the affects or emotions as primary sources of motivation. The affects, then, are used to explain in greater detail the workings of the factors described thus far in regulating the stream of consciousness. The basic set of affects operates with telling effectiveness to bring to consciousness material from the body, from the environment, and from entirely private sources (memories, dreams, fantasies, etc.).

The wealth of private material each of us constantly carries around is enormous. To specify which parts or aspects of this material gain admission to consciousness, we introduce the notions of current concerns, unfinished business, and unresolved stress.

Two additional factors seem to regulate the stream of consciousness. One is the "set" adopted toward the processing of "private" material. This "set" can be longstanding and habitual or it can be situation-specific. The other factor is the structural characteristics of the stimulus, though very little empirical work has been done relating this variable systematically to ongoing thought.

1. The Mind as Activity

As Luria (1973) stressed in the title of his book, the physiological basis for our mind is *The Working Brain*. Our minds handle tremendous amounts of information. The sheer enormity of the storage capacity, convincingly demonstrated in numerous recent experiments on the effectiveness of recognition memory (Kagan and Kogan, 1970), is not as significant as the techniques by which the material is stored. Apparently, the storage process involves not only sensory content but also presumably some degree of organization of material. Bartlett (1975) demonstrated that environmental sounds that cannot be easily identified or labeled may still be stored as organizations rather than as purely sensory components for later recognition. Such studies lead us away from thinking of the mind's storage capacity as a mere binful of discrete contents. We must consider the processing and organizing activities, the "working":

> The mind does not seem much like a place anymore. Instead we think
> of it as an organ, analogous to a bodily organ, with a specific function.
> That function is the processing of information. A staggering wealth of

information reaches the sense organs of the body, but only certain aspects
of it are truly informative about crucial aspects of the environment. Hence,
the input must be analyzed, abstracted, coded, and reworked if the
organism is to survive; in many cases it must also be stored for later
retrieval and use. . . . There are not simply "sensations," supplemented by
"association" to form "perceptions" which are stored and recovered.
Instead there is a vast array of stages, activities, and processes at every
level. (Neisser, 1972, p. 237)

The work of the mind—carried on through the "vast array of
stages, activities, and processes at every level"—may be continuous,
not only while we are awake but also while we sleep. Night dream
research has generated substantial amounts of content report from
people interrupted during all stages of sleep, although the REM
periods of Stage 1 EEG cycles seem to be correlated with the most
vivid and "dreamlike" descriptions.

2. Sensory Input

Having considered the brain as a continually active working
organ, we now turn our attention to the material available to it for
processing. A large amount of this material is delivered, of course,
through the sense organs. Among those factors that regulate our
stream of consciousness, the network of sense organs exert enormous
influence:

All our purposeful behavior, all our awareness of physical "reality," all
our ideas about the universe ultimately derive from data which our sense
organs alone can provide: "Nihil est in intellectu, quid non est in sensibus."
Thus for the biologist and the philosopher alike the study of the structure
and function of the sense organs is of outstanding importance.
    No two animals or people live in exactly the same world, for no two
are precisely identical in sense perception. (Kalmus, 1952, p. 64)

Thus, such factors as our location on the continuum from acute
auditory sensitivity to total deafness or the degree of night blindness
we experience powerfully affect the material that will immediately or
ultimately find its way into our stream of consciousness.

Even when sense organs function "normally" or without defect,
research suggests numerous individual differences in the impact that
sensory data exert on the perceptual systems. The work of Schachter
and Rodin (1974) and Rodin and Singer (1976), for instance, suggests
that overweight people are much more acutely sensitive to external
cues generally as well as those relating to food and eating. Petrie (1967)
has explored in detail what she calls each person's "perceptual
reactance" (p. 2). In regard to a person's modulation of sensory

experience, Petrie and her colleagues have

> identified three kinds of persons—the reducer, the augmenter, and the
> moderate—who differ from one another in their ways of processing their
> experience of the sensory environment. The reducer tends subjectively to
> *decrease* what is perceived; the augmenter to *increase* what is perceived; the
> moderate neither to reduce nor to augment what is perceived. In general
> these perceptual types occupy adjoining positions on a continuous scale.
> (Petrie, 1967, pp. 1-2)

3. A Continuum of Consciousness

Various amounts of sensory data enter into the continuous activity of the mind. But not all of the mind's activity finds its way into the stream of consciousness. Some aspects, in fact, remain stubbornly hidden. If someone asks us to name the smallest state in the United States or to add three plus six, the answers probably pop into the consciousness without our being aware of what our minds were doing to produce those answers. Posner and Boies (1971) have cited research indicating that "conscious awareness is itself rather late in the sequence of mental processing" (p. 407).

Other aspects of this continuous mental work, however, are certainly available to our awareness. When Shepard (1975) asked people to judge whether two abstract geometrical forms, presented from different perspectives, were isomorphic, the subjects were able to describe with some precision the subjective experience of arriving at an answer. Most subjects looked at the two stimulus figures, formed mental images of the two figures, then mentally rotated one of the figures around to see if it would "fit" within the other.

As an example more characteristic of everyday life, imagine yourself deeply involved in a conversation with a close friend as the two of you stroll through an unfamiliar neighborhood. Although you are totally absorbed in the conversation, your mind is constantly processing information about the environment necessary to enable safe, effective movement. Somehow you take into account the curbs, the steps, the potential obstacles in your path, and you manage to avoid tripping, bumping into people, or wandering out into the street into the path of an oncoming car. The conversation may be so engrossing that the process of navigating through the physical environment simply does not register in your stream of consciousness. Yet this process is available to our consciousness should we choose to attend to it; if the conversation lags, for instance, you may suddenly realize the beauty of the surroundings or perhaps that the two of you have lost your way.

The continuous workings of the brain present varieties of stimuli available to our consciousness, but it seems likely that we acquire a selective inattention toward much of its working, just as we learn not to notice the many gurglings of our stomachs, twitchings of our toes, and spontaneous firings of various nerve endings that are occurring all the time as we go about our day-to-day activities. However, it is important to note that certain aspects of the mind's workings themselves constitute fields of stimuli (much like those delivered through the perceptual systems) and can furnish novel or unique material that may itself be processed or "worked on."

To clarify this concept, let us postulate a continuum of stimulation that is capable of engaging the workings of the mind. The continuum runs from the public to the private. At the public pole are physical stimuli from the surrounding environment, clearly measurable or capable of consensual description by other people as well as by the individual. Slightly closer to the private pole are interoceptive stimuli generated mostly from the circulatory, digestive, and respiratory systems, and proprioceptive stimuli generated by the position and movement of parts of the body in space and in relation to each other. The stimuli available from these sources are not so readily accessible to the public but are still traceable on the whole to physically measurable characteristics. Further along the internal dimension is the more complex matching of exteroceptive, interoceptive, and proprioceptive stimuli to relatively recent stimulation held in short-term memory and some degree of organizational or coding activities. Still further along the internal dimension, one might find rehearsal and replay activities from long-term memory, some of them set off by external stimuli as in the famous case of Marcel Proust's taste of the Madelaine cookie crumbs in his tea that brought flooding back a whole series of vivid images of the town of Combrai.

Perhaps most interior on this dimension would be the associations related primarily to the most private material drawn from long-term memory, as in the case of associations several steps removed from the initial taste of the tea to sets of associations generated primarily by material drawn almost completely from long-term memory. For the most part, as best we can ascertain, our dreams, except those clearly referable to an outside noise such as the alarm clock going off, are responses to such private stimuli. A little introspection will demonstrate how often many of our ongoing thoughts while performing other tasks represent a series of chained associations of varied degrees of vividness related only to other material drawn from long-term memory. The material that arises in this regard may, of course, be other than carbon copy reproductions of former thoughts or experiences; the material may have been considerably altered (e.g., condensed, incorporated into long-term plans or current concerns, altered in light of new experiences) through further mental processing, whether conscious or unconscious.

Erdelyi and Becker (1974) have shown that pictorial stimuli actually show an increase in recall functions over time, while verbal stimuli, in keeping with Ebbinghaus's findings, show decay. It seems likely from this research (Erdelyi and Kleinbard, 1977) that private rehearsal and reminiscence of visual imagery are more extensive and ongoing than for verbal material. Very likely such processes may also account for the patterns of intrusive imagery or peremptory ideation (Horowitz, 1975; Klein, 1967) or the phenomena of the so-called "day residue" in dreams.

It is somewhere near to that last point that we must probably place the "private" pole of the continuum of stimuli available for consciousness. Beyond that pole are those mental activities that are not only unobservable by the public but also obscured from the direct awareness of the individual as well. It is this class of mental activities to which Lashley referred in maintaining that it was the products of thought rather than the process of thinking that were available to the consciousness of the individual (Lashley, 1958).

4. Attention: The Ability to Screen and Select

The ways in which we distribute our attention among these different sources of available stimulation is an important factor in the regulation of the stream of consciousness. Hernandez-Peon *et al.* (1956) demonstrated the astounding power of attention to regulate which of the available stimuli in the external environment will be processed. Using a metronome, he presented a rhythmic series of clicks to cats. He was able to measure a strong, steady series of impulses from the auditory nerve of the cat. However, if the cat saw a mouse or smelled a fish, the auditory nerve impulse that corresponded to the metronome's stimuli dropped almost to zero. More than the cat's simply failing to pay attention to what he was hearing, it was almost as if his hearing of the metronome itself was completely nonexistent.

If the human individual, in a similar manner, finds the stimuli from one pole of the continuum (say, that of external stimulation) worth his attention to the exclusion of the other pole, it has implications not only for what material will appear in his consciousness at present but also for the material that will pass into short- and long-term memory (against which future incoming stimuli will be matched) and that will shape subsequent mental activities.

> All the things that a man can call to mind, and all the skills a man can use, were established with materials that once formed a part of his awareness, that appeared in the stream of consciousness. There is no evidence, so far as I am aware, that any of the things he ignored are stored away—at least not in any available form—in the central nervous system. Thus, a man, in selecting what he will attend to, selects what is to be preserved not only in the sequential record of experience but in the numerous mechanisms of the brain. (Penfield, 1969, p. 166)

Attention's ability to screen and select among the available material of the moment not only regulates the moment-to-moment awareness of the individual but also, through doing so, influences what passes into the memory and into that "vast array of stages, activities, and processes at every level."

In summary of the discussion so far, we can say that, in general, attention regulates the stream of consciousness, drawing material from a mind continuously active, always at work. The material available for consciousness falls along a continuum running from a public pole, drawn mainly from immediate sensory input, to a private pole, drawn mainly from associations, toward transformations of very private material from long-term memory. To what extent can we specify more precisely how this process operates?

5. A Bias Favoring Sensory Input

The normal, adult human mind seems generally to assign priority in processing to salient or important material from the external, public segments of the continuum. Rapaport (1960) proposed that there may be a "permanent gradient towards external cathexis" serving man's adaptive purposes. Clearly, it appears most adaptive to attend to external cues while we are awake. There are numerous potential hazards involved in our navigating through the environment; failing to take notice of sharp instruments, of windows opening onto a drop many stories to the street below, or of oncoming traffic may have fatal consequences. And, at least in man's early history, alertness to the external environment was necessary for the procuring of food as well.

A view of a limited-channel capacity within an information-processing model is perhaps more appropriate to describe the demand character of external stimulation. To the extent that we are indeed awake and moving around in an environment, the amount of feedback we get from external sources is likely to limit available channel space for processing internal material. There is considerable evidence that the same pathways appear to be used for processing private visual imagery as for processing externally derived visual stimulation (Antrobus, Singer, Goldstein, and Fortgang, 1970; Segal and Fusella, 1970). Thus, the active processing organs of a waking person are likely to overload and limit internal processing. Moreover, we undoubtedly train ourselves not to attend to private stimuli much as we learn not to notice the nose on our face or the hundreds of twitches and gurglings of our active body machinery. Clinical observations of severely disturbed schizophrenic patients suggest that long-standing difficulties they have in body representation, associational control, and some of the withdrawal from attempts either to involve themselves in social situations or to think about significant social situations all lead to their tendency to confuse these private bodily sensations with external stimulation (Angyal, 1944; Blatt, 1974; Singer, 1975).

6. Predictable, Dull, or Barren Environments: An Opportunity for Private Processing

Salient, informative stimulation from the external surroundings, then, can monopolize channel space and severely attenuate, if not interrupt entirely, the processing of private material. But the natural tug of our attention toward the immediate public end of the continuum loses its urgency in an environment that fails to present difficult or valuable material. We expect material from the private side of the continuum increasingly to find its way into the stream of consciousness when the environment is relatively barren of novel or complex stimulation. This appears to be the general case both in normal sleeping (the dream research discussed earlier) and waking (e.g., the private material that preoccupies our thoughts during periods spent in uninteresting waiting rooms or while we lie in bed waiting for sleep to come) and in more extreme situations (the wealth of vivid private material, sometimes accompanied by quasi hallucinations, in sensory deprivation studies). West (1962) illustrates the principle:

> An oversimplified but perhaps helpful model of these conditions pictures a man in his study, standing at a closed glass window opposite the fireplace, looking out at his garden in the sunset. He is absorbed by the view of the outside world. He does not visualize the interior of the room in which he stands. As it becomes darker outside, however, images of the objects in the room behind him can be seen reflected dimly in the window glass. For a time he may see either the garden (if he gazes into the distance) or the reflection of the room's interior (if he focuses on the glass a few inches from his face). Night falls, but the fire still burns brightly in the fireplace and illuminates the room. The watcher now sees in the glass a vivid reflection of the interior of the room behind him, which appears outside the window. This illusion becomes dimmer as the fire dies down,

and finally, when it is dark both outside and within, nothing more is seen. If the fire flares up from time to time, the visions in the glass reappear.

In perceptual release, the daylight (sensory input) is reduced while the interior illumination (general level of arousal) remains bright, and images originating within the rooms of our brains may be perceived as though they came from outside the windows of our senses.

The theory thus holds that a sustained level and variety of sensory input normally is required to inhibit the emergence of percepts or memory traces from within the brain itself. When effective (attention-commanding) sensory input decreases below a certain threshold, there may be a release into awareness of previously recorded perceptions through a disinhibition of the brain circuits that represent them. (p. 275)

Antrobus, Singer, and Greenberg (1966) studied this principle in a controlled laboratory setting by manipulating the amount and complexity of external stimulation presented to the subject. Subjects sat alone in the laboratory processing (detecting) auditory tones. At random moments during this task, the subjects were interrupted and asked to signify (indicate yes or no) whether, immediately prior to the interruption, they were thinking of the task at hand (i.e., were processing stimuli from the external environment) or whether they were aware of unrelated ("stimulus-independent") thoughts or images. Increasing both the complexity of the task and the penalty for inaccurate detections did indeed significantly reduce the frequency of stimulus-independent thoughts. Yet the intrusion of private material into the stream of consciousness of the subjects persisted at all levels of complexity within this experiment.

Drucker (1969), however, found that he could more completely inhibit the occurrence of stimulus-independent thoughts within a similar paradigm by presenting the signals at an uneven rate, thus making it difficult for subjects to pace themselves as they could when signals came at regular intervals. More recent laboratory studies have indicated that the ability of external stimuli to suppress the processing rate of private material is somewhat modality-specific. That is to say, if a person is processing visual stimulation from the environment, he or she is likely to show some reduction in general level of stimulus-independent thought of a visual nature. There is, however, no apparent change in his level of auditory fantasy activity (Antrobus *et al.*, 1970).

Csikszentimihalyi's (1974) studies of the flow of behavior generally and especially of what he termed "autotelic behaviors" (those actions that are not in themselves clearly directed toward satisfaction of the more basic drives or the economic motives of the human condition) furnish illuminating evidence drawn from more normal everyday life and not so constrained by laboratory conventions. His findings indicate that private material (what Antrobus and Singer termed "stimulus-independent" thought) normally and naturally appears in the stream of consciousness but that it may be attenuated and sometimes suppressed altogether through the immediate stimulus demands of the environment. Csikszentimihalyi and his colleagues asked various groups of people (dancers, surgeons, rock climbers, chess players) to report their ongoing behavior, including mental activity, through both questionnaires and personal interviews. Two-thirds of a group of 21 surgeons interviewed reported frequent, often elaborate daydreaming, even while performing surgery. These daydreams ranged widely in content, touching on music, wine, food, and particular individuals of the opposite sex. But the processing of private material during surgery was confined to the dull and routine aspects, such as sewing up the incision, in which the environment offered no surprises. When the external stimulation was more complex and less predictable, as when the surgeon cut into the patient's tissues toward a directed goal, private material seemed to vanish from the stream of consciousness. The following representative statements are by four of the surgeons:

> You are not aware of your body except your hands . . . not aware of yourself or your personal problems.
> If involved, you are not aware of aching feet, not aware of self.
> Just concentrate on what you are doing.
> Totally enmeshed in what I am doing and I forget fatigue and forget the night before. (Csikszentimihalyi, Holcomb, and Csikszentimihalyi, 1974, p. 211)

7. The Matching Function: Judging Environmental Input as Predictable, Dull, and Barren OR as Surprising, Exciting, and Rich

If the stream of consciousness is more likely to flow near the public end of the continuum when the environment offers surprising, exciting, and rich input and is more likely to flow near the private end of the continuum when the environment is predictable, dull, or barren, our task becomes to specify more precisely what determines or constitutes the salience or importance of external stimuli. Whereas an accomplished surgeon may allow unrelated private thoughts to fill his or her consciousness while sewing up a fellow human being during a life-or-death operation (with no resulting loss of skill or efficiency), others of us with less skill, nerve, or practice may find ourselves totally preoccupied with sewing a button onto an old coat. Even the signal detection tasks in scientific laboratories, with their precise measurements of exactly how much "information" is being presented to the subject at any one time, are of limited use for an understanding of what sorts of environmental events offer "priority information" (with accompanying demands for processing) to the individual as he goes about a normal, everyday life. Here it is useful to develop the notion of a central executive function and optimal levels of stimulation (Hebb, 1955).

The elaborate and varied works of Anokhin (1969), Rescorla (1969), Shepard (1975), Sokolov (1963), and others suggest that an important function of the mind is the making of images or schemes. That is, the human organism steers itself through its environment by schematizing its experiences into at least some relatively simple categories or rubrics, then elaborating further on these through encoding processes that allow not only an image (not necessarily visual) of the status quo but also anticipations of future patterns of stimulation. Each new set of environmental stimuli must be encoded and matched against stored material. The notion of a central matching process based in part on anticipatory images or plans is a key feature of current cognitive systems (Miller, Galanter, and Pribram, 1960; Neisser, 1967, 1972; Pribram, 1971; Tomkins, 1962–1963). The notion of a central matching concept has great significance for the problems of cognition and attention. Obviously, some selective process is necessary to allow man to function effectively and to avoid being overwhelmed by the immense range of external stimulation constantly available. To some extent, issues such as degree of structure or gestaltlike qualities of inherent goodness (Garner, 1974) may make certain external cues "important" or salient, but these in turn are already in part prepared for by the sets of plans or expectations that we bring into each new environmental situation.

As Fiske and Maddi (1961) pointed out in their work on the functions of varied experiences, many environments provide ample external inputs and yet because of their redundancy or limited complexity do not demand attention. Optimal stimulation really means something more than some simple quantitative measure of input, and we must look beyond such concepts for an adequate notion of what makes external stimuli "important" or salient. Having laid the groundwork for an approach to this problem in the concepts of a central executor, the generation of schemes, and the matching function, we will focus on the role of affect as a critical regulator of this process.

8. Affect

Perhaps the most sophisticated and well-developed theory of the interrelationship of affect with the central executor, the generation of schemes, and the matching function has been set forth by Tomkins (1962-1963). We will outline this theory here to sharpen our understanding of what material appears in the stream of consciousness. The discussion will deal first with the appearance of material from within the physical body (stimuli not readily apparent to the public but still traceable on the whole to physically measurable characteristics), second with the appearance in consciousness of material at the most public end of the continuum (physical stimuli from the surrounding environment, clearly measurable or capable of consensual description by other people as well as the individual), and third with the appearance of material from the private end of the continuum (long- and short-term memories, etc.).

According to Tomkins, the affects or emotions are one of five fundamental systems that regulate man's behavior: homeostatic (the autonomic regulatory system), the drive system, the affect system, cognition, and the motor system. The primary role of the drives, in terms of human motivation, is to signal the presence of deprivation states within the physical body. It is this task of bringing deprivation states to consciousness and to conscious control that distinguishes the drive system from the more general homeostatic mechanisms of the body:

> We know that the majority of biological processes within the body of man and the rat are silent. They have no conscious representation but are nonetheless capable of running the complex machinery so that the animal remains alive. These processes do not "need" conscious representation because they "know" what they need to know, to do what they have to do. If the finger is cut, the blood knows how to clot, unless this information is missing, as it is in the genes of bleeders. The body employs a "drive" only when it lacks the information necessary to maintain the body. Then it beats on the door of consciousness until the person is goaded into some activity which will meet the body's needs. The need for air is, ordinarily, no more a drive than is the need for blood in the various organs of the body. The human being is born with the information which enables him to circulate his blood and to breathe to supply that blood with oxygen. He may spend most of his life unaware of both processes. . . . At this point you may argue that breathing is a consummatory response to a drive signal whether the latter is conscious or not. If the breathing rate varies as a function of signals from the carotid sinus, which in turn varies its response as a function of the carbon dioxide content of the blood, is this not a drive signal system? We would say no more than the blood clotting mechanism is a drive signal system. The breathing rate comes under drive governance rather than homeostatic control when the awareness of breathing and suffocation mobilizes the individual to breathe more rapidly or more slowly and more deeply, or less so, *or* to take immediate action to remedy whatever is threatening his air supply, or both. What of the case when the drive signal is "sent" but not "received"? Since there is competition between channels for transformation of messages into conscious form, some drive signals may be sent but never transmuted into reports. Is an

unconscious hunger signal a drive? We would say it is no more a drive than an unperceived sensory message is a percept. The drive mechanism includes in its design favored entry into consciousness. (Tomkins, 1962, pp. 31–32)

The affect system, however, serves in Tomkins's theory as the major motivating system. Affects may amplify drive signals, or they may in their own right provide rewarding or punishing experiences to the individual. The affects themselves, however, are subject to the information-processing activities of the brain (cognitive system) and particularly the rate and complexity with which new material has to be processed.

In Section 7 above, we touched briefly on a "matching" function: a central executor processes incoming stimuli; schemes, representations, or "neural models" are constructed from this stimulation (and, in turn, more elaborate anticipatory schemes or plans may be generated from these models); future incoming stimuli are then matched against these schemes or models. According to Tomkins, there is a limited number of differentiated affects that may be triggered by fairly specific differences in this information-processing task that man continually faces. For example, massive inputs of novel or unassimilable information produces startle or fear responses; moderate rates of new information generate interest or excitement, which are both rewarding affects; and the sudden reduction of high levels of seemingly unassimilable information (as in delayed recognition of an old friend, seeing the point of joke, or gaining a sudden insight into a riddle) leads to the rewarding experiences of joy or laughter. High rates of unassimilable or complex information persisting over long periods of time lead to the punishing affects of anger, despair, and sadness. Thus, the flow of information, the readiness of the individual based upon his past experience, his cognitive style, his anticipation of a situation, or his planning for the situation—all these serve to determine whether punishing, negative affects emerge or whether the rewarding, positive affects of interest (a moderately rising gradient of new information), joy (a moderately declining gradient from a high level of novelty), or laughter (a sharp decline from a high level of novelty) are experienced.

Inspection of Figure 1 will help the reader grasp what has been presented in an extremely condensed, outline form here. Tomkins employed the term "density of neural firing," which conveys the degree to which there is a massive involvement of neural activity from various brain areas. This variable is not easily measured, however, and we have chosen to translate it into "assimilability of information."

Picture yourself taking a stroll through a quiet neighborhood,

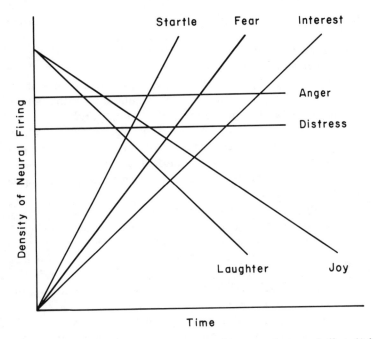

FIGURE 1.   Graphical representation of a theory of innate activators of affect. (Adapted from Tomkins, 1962, Vol. 1.)

totally preoccupied with your own thoughts. Someone walks up behind you without your noticing. Suddenly the person says, "Hey." Had you been expecting a friend to join you and had you heard him or her approaching, this stimulus would easily have been "matched"; it would have offered no unassimilable information. As it is, however, you are momentarily startled. You turn around and it is a tall, muscular stranger. He refuses to speak for a few seconds. Unable to assimilate or "figure out" what is happening, your primary affect may be fear. You might then recognize the man as the postman who usually delivers your mail, someone you did not recognize out of uniform and "out of context." This sudden "putting together" of the man before you with information available from memory may cause you to break out in a smile or even a laugh of recognition.

The momentarily startled silence and then breaking into laughter or joyful applause of many audiences viewing *The Sting* or *Sleuth*, movies with elaborate turns of plot leading to sudden recognition of "what is really going on," exemplifies the pleasurable affects resulting from such sudden assimilations of seemingly unassimilable material. The chances of negative affect's occurring are much greater, of course, if high levels of unassimilable material continue for long periods of time, as happens, for instance, in Kafka's *The Trial*.

The innate triggering of affects, thus, is closely related to the information-processing load and patterning of environmental stimulation. As a primary component of the human motivational system, the affects contribute significantly to the regulation of the stream of consciousness: the ability of the mind to "match" and further assimilate environmental input into schemes or plans serves, in part, to shape our affects, which in turn cue our attention toward priority information from the environment (and, more precisely, toward specific aspects of the constant flood of sensory input) or signals a generally predictable, dull, or barren environment.

Let us here add the notion that the information-processing or matching functions serving as innate activators of the affects are not restricted to stimulus input from the immediate, present environment. Demands for matching or processing may also be made by difficult-to-assimilate material from the "vast array of stages, activities, and processes at every level" that is the mind itself. That is to say, private material (such as memories, plans, dreams, or associations) can constitute a stimulus field that can compete with the external stimulus input for processing. As discussed in Section 6 above, the priority of this private material increases as the availability of priority material from the immediate environment decreases.

As an example of how the processing of private material can activate the affects, imagine Mr. and Mrs. Archer driving toward the fanciest restaurant in town. In the car with them are their guests: Mr. Archer's employer (Mrs. Arnold) and the employer's husband (Mr. Arnold). Mr. Archer is well on his way to convincing the Arnolds that he is not only a very competent and responsible worker but also a witty, sophisticated, and thoroughly delightful social companion. He figures that this will not harm his chances for the big promotion that he feels he is due. In the midst of one of Mrs. Arnold's oft-told witty anecdotes, Mr. Archer's eyes turn glassy. He has suddenly realized that when changing clothes he forgot to put his wallet in the pocket of the pants he is now wearing. He will be unable to pay for the dinner, unless he turns the car around and goes to his house to pick up the wallet with his credit cards or else, equally humiliating, asks his guests to loan him the money. He sees in his mind's eye the shocked, unbelieving faces of his guests when he is forced to tell them of his foolish mistake. He sees the promotion fade away. If he can't handle a simple dinner arrangement, could he really be that responsible an employee? He sees himself collecting unemployment as he looks for another job. The horrifying expressions passing across his face, though unseen by the people in the back seat, are still noticeable to his wife, who is thoroughly puzzled. (Mrs. Arnold's stories, though dull and virtually interminable, have never been cause for alarm.) In effect, then, a private event and the unrolling of a memory sequence elaborating itself into vivid anticipations may have much the same psychological impact and capacity to trigger affect as complex, externally derived information may.

A similar example may be used to point out how positive affect can be aroused on the basis of a sequence of private events. Having suffered in silence for several minutes, Mr. Archer suddenly recalls that his wife also has a set of credit cards, which she carries with her in her purse. It will be an easy matter to charge the dinner on her account. He may suddenly feel a dramatic drop in the persisting level of unassimilable material and break into a grin or chuckle. He is now showing strong positive affect, which, fortunately, coincides with the witty ending of Mrs. Arnold's humorous story, and all is right with the world once again.

The affect system, then, exerts great influence in regulating the stream of consciousness, in identifying "priority" information, in distributing attention among the most public events (incoming sensory data from the immediate surroundings), less public events (bodily states and processes, often signaled by the drive system), and private events (memories, fantasies, dreams, etc.). The public range of stimuli is, by definition, fairly identifiable. If we walk into a room where music plays loudly, we will very likely become conscious, if only briefly, of the music. It is easy to point to the music, to its loudness and momentary novelty, as "cause" for our attending to it at that moment; our environment presents it saliently, and until it is processed, it demands some immediate channel space in consciousness. Similarly, a drive-activated body state can "beat on the door of consciousness"; having dived deeply into the water, we can become aware of little else than our acute need to breathe until we once again reach the surface and can take air into our lungs. The temporary lack of new oxygen demands channel space in consciousness. But what of the vast amount of private material that is always with us in that "vast array of stages, activities, and processes at every level"? Each of us has an astounding number of memories, for instance. Though we have developed the principle that such private material is more likely to appear in the stream of consciousness when there are lessened demands for processing of material from the immediate surroundings or from the drive system, can we specify any more precisely which or what sorts of private material are likely to assert themselves in consciousness? If we become bored in a particular environment, what memory or fantasy themes might pop into consciousness?

9. Current Concerns, Unfinished Business, and Unresolved Stress

The principle of matching and its connection with the arousal of surprise and interest as well as joy when the final match is made to somewhat established schemes may also be related to the increasing indications that recurring thoughts or dream contents are related to current unfinished business or current concerns and unresolved immediate stresses (Breger, Hunter, and Lane, 1971; Klinger, 1971; Lewin, 1916; Singer, 1975). A great deal of our conscious experience can be characterized by the recurrence of thoughts about tasks initiated but as yet uncompleted, plans set in motion but as yet far from execution, actions taken quite recently that one realizes were inadequate to a task or incorrect, deadlines in work assignments still to be met, promises in relationship to others still to be kept. This process is adaptive in a variety of ways: "Since fantasy content is normally adrift, it provides continuous reminders of concerns other than those [one] is working on which [one] needs to bear in mind" (Klinger, 1971, p. 356). In this manner, fantasy helps maintain the hierarchical structure of plans and routines generated to guide man's behavior. A plan or intention that we are not able to execute or complete immediately is not lost forever; nor must we make an active, exhaustive search through every shred of material in our long-term memory to find out if there is still something we need to do. The uncompleted plan maintains itself and increases its likelihood of completion by entering the stream of consciousness when we are less than totally occupied with the present external environment or bodily processes. Plans not only maintain themselves but are capable of being changed and elaborated upon as we anticipate situations and imagine the consequences of our actions: "Fantasy thus serves as a channel for performing preparatory work fortuitously between emergencies" (Klinger, 1971, p. 356).

Unfinished business and uncompleted plans denote, of course, not only our intentions of physically doing something (such as mailing a letter or buying groceries) but also incomplete mental activity (novel perceptions, for example, that we were not able to assimilate or match sufficiently to material from long-term memory). The relevant material is maintained in "rehearsal" or "buffer" storage (Broadbent, 1971) and tends to repeat itself in our consciousness until it is adequately processed.

The phenomenon is a familiar one in everyday life. An innovative movie presenting striking scenes may be literally "thought provoking" and lead us to dwell on its images for days afterward. The sudden, unexpected death of a neighbor, someone whom we may know only casually but who is part of our day-to-day life, may constitute a considerably stressful event, and we may find ourselves unintentionally dwelling on it for some time. Antrobus, Singer, and Greenberg (1966) have found that subjects overhearing a news report about a serious escalation of the Vietnam war prior to entering a signal detection experiment showed a considerable increase in reports of stimulus-independent thought, with the content of such thought relating to fantasies about the implications of this bad news. This finding suggests that particular events or perceptions may be recognized as of such importance to the organism or of such salience that they may generate strong demands for processing. If we are not able to complete the processing very quickly, we may find further processing of the events occupying our stream of consciousness even as we try to turn our attention to other tasks or material. If while reading a magazine article to pass the time in the waiting room before our appointment we hear a loud scream of pain from the dentist's office, we may have great difficulty directing our attention back to the magazine article. Horowitz and Becker (1971) found a most powerful experimental source of such intrusive thoughts during a signal detection task by showing the subjects, prior to their entering the booth, the harrowingly explicit film *Subincision*. Subsequent work directed by Horowitz (1975) extends this result to other emotional inputs from films.

10. The Set toward Internal Processing

A further notion seems important and worth developing as it relates to the stream of consciousness. On one hand, material from the current public stimulus field can make demands upon the continuous processing activities of the mind and find its way into the stream of consciousness. The types of external stimulation most likely to make strong demands are those occupying a central position in our plans or anticipations (see Miller, Galanter, and Pribram, 1960) and those novel or unexpected aspects that we have some degree of difficulty assimilating or "matching" either to our plans or to material from long-term memory. Physical stimulation relating to internal body states is most likely to gain admission to consciousness when deprivation states are signaled by the drive system.

On the other hand, when material from the current "public" stimulus field is insufficient to fill up our consciousness, private material can gain our awareness. As we have seen, the types of material most likely to gain admittance to our stream of consciousness are current concerns, unfinished business, incompleted plans, and particular events or perceptions that have not been sufficiently assimilated, matched, or processed. In a sense, such private material competes with current external stimulation for channel space and, if sufficiently strong, may divert our attention from that external stimulation (as in the Horowitz and Becker study). Another notion important to an understanding of the stream of consciousness is the set of plans or anticipations with which we approach the stream itself and the material available from both internal and external sources. There seem to be striking individual differences in the extent to which we set up expectations for recalling our ongoing fantasy activity. A good deal of the time during any day we simply fail to label our passing thoughts for recurrence, just as we may fail to label where we parked the car or the name of a person we have just been introduced to. That is to say, we do not assign them sufficient basis for recurrence within the other complex material being processed. By failing to set up formal labeling or retrieval routines, we may often be surprised when such thoughts do surge up into awareness in periods of preparation for sleep, when there are fewer competing stimuli, or during our dreams.

Some people, however, are practiced daydreamers. That is, they adopt a conscious attitude of attention to their stream of consciousness, and therefore the accessibility of symbolic materials, novel combinations, and unique private representations is much greater for them. Such people may gain relatively quick insights into the transformations from conventional English sentences that may occur in their dreams or reveries. Psychoanalysis often encourages a person to adopt just such an attitude. It encourages him to notice dreams, momentary images, slips of the tongue, and novel associations, to replay this material mentally several times, even sometimes to write it down. Psychoanalysis also furnishes him with a classifying, labeling, or coding system that will increase the likelihood of recall. Needless to say, various schools of psychoanalysis use different classifying, labeling, and coding systems, and the range of terms, interpretations, and associations is astronomically increased if we consider the wide range of psychological, philosophical, artistic, or religious approaches that emphasize attending to private material. The particular set of terms, interpretations, and associations used will naturally influence what is noticed, how it is interpreted, its likelihood of later recall, and the associations it evokes. Under such circumstances, it is unlikely that we can recapture, without distortion, the veridical content of a dream or establish the true and absolute interpretation of a thought fragment, and we may glumly have to agree with a paraphrase of conservative economics: there is no such thing as a free association.

There is convincing evidence suggesting that people learn or acquire a fairly consistent, habitual, and long-term set of plans with which to approach, attend to, and process their ongoing conscious experience. Insofar as we have learned as children to enjoy make-believe and games of imagination, we may also become comfortable and feel some degree of control over our own ongoing thought activities, particularly those concerning private material (Singer, 1973).

The work of a number of investigators (Giambra, 1974; Huba, Segal, and Singer, 1977a,b; Segal and Singer, 1976; Singer and Antrobus, 1963, 1972; Starker, 1974) using factor-analytic methods suggests three fairly general and stable patterns of daydreaming. One is a guilty-dysphoric style characterized by an abundance of fantasies involving guilt and self-recrimination, others involving hostile, aggressive wishes, and some involving fears of failure mingled with striving for achievement. Another pattern is characterized more by fleeting, uncontrollable fantasies, generally full of anxiety. There is considerable distractibility and mind wandering, which includes inability to pursue or to hold fast to thoughts and difficulty in inhibiting attention to current external events. A third factor seems to be more associated with positive contents in fantasy, vivid visual and auditory imagery, and future-oriented and planful fantasies. In general, people who are associated with this pattern tend to affirm daydreaming as a worthwhile, enjoyable activity. Insofar as an individual is given to one or another of these patterns of thought, he has in a sense become habituated to approaching his search of internal material with a view to organizing it in relation to these patterns.

To the idea of a fairly consistent, long-standing, habitual approach to processing private and external material, let us add the notion of temporary, situation-specific strategies or plans. As an example, imagine a person who has set aside two hours for reading each evening. During one of the hours, he reads a book of mathematics. As he reads, memories of the busy day pop into his mind, but he quickly pushes them from consciousness because they draw his mind from the text and keep him from concentrating on the material. At one point, the book becomes dull and the man's mind drifts off to a chain of memories about an old friend he hasn't seen for years. Again he becomes aware of the book in front of him and, with effort, immediately begins to resume his learning, irritated that this brief daydream has interrupted his learning. During the other hour, however, the man reads a book of poems. The lines call up vivid images in his mind's eye. The words evoke memories and feelings. The man pauses in his reading to let this material play itself out. Another poem sets off a responsive chain of associations, which is not so much an interruption in the reading of the poem as it is part of the process. Obviously, the man has adopted one set of "plans" toward private material and the stream of consciousness for reading the math book and quite another for reading the book of poems. Two investigators have explored the nature of such plans on the basis of careful, creative experimental work.

In a very complex experiment, Miller (1972) asked subjects to adopt one of two strategies while listening to a brief poetry or prose passage. One strategy corresponded to that of the imaginary man described above as he reads the math book: the subject was asked to be "listening in a problem-solving way . . . with a rational, logical, and scientific orientation to the material." The other strategy corresponded to that of the man as he reads poetry: "In essence, you listen so as to let whatever ideas, images, thoughts, and feelings which happen, happen. The purpose of this kind of listening is just to *experience*, rather than to be able to repeat or summarize or even to give some verbal response to what you hear." Miller then obtained data not on responses to the passages to which the subjects were asked to attend but rather on the subject's recognition rate to other verbally presented (and ostensibly, to the subject, irrelevant) material occurring in the experimental situation. Among his findings is that the "scientific" listener has a significantly greater rate of recognition for low-imagery, abstract relational words than the "just experiencing" listeners and vice versa. We are able, then, to adopt temporary, situation-specific "plans" for mental processing, and these plans have definite, measurable effects.

Klinger (1974) studied people who reported their thoughts aloud during each of four situations: solving a manual puzzle, solving a logic problem, reverie, and quasi-hypnogogic thought. Klinger termed the strategy appropriate for the first two (problem-solving) situations "operant thought." The strategy appropriate for the other two (non-problem-solving) situations he termed "respondent thought." He was able to distinguish operant from respondent thought on the basis of characteristic utterances: "During the manual puzzle and logic problem activity, they produced significantly more utterances in which they evaluated their previous problem-solving thoughts or acts and in which they indicated that they were controlling their attention than during reverie and hypnogogic thought" (p. 44). The findings seem to offer more support for the notion that we are capable of adopting temporary plans for reacting to ("evaluated their previous problem-solving thought") or controlling ("controlling their attention") the material that appears in our stream of consciousness.

11. Structural Characteristics of the Stimuli

Another possible influence upon the stream of consciousness is the form of the material. The flow of long- and short-term memories, current concerns, unassimilated fragments, novel material, background noises, odd associations—certain of these may reflect particular properties of structure or of "good gestalten" that will attract attention and lead to further rehearsal of the material.

The stream-of-consciousness material in Joyce's *Ulysses* (1922/1961) includes numerous examples of well-turned or interestingly structured phrases that recur. Often the sounds as well as the meanings of the phrases are important, as in "loudlatinlaughing" (p. 42) or "It flows purling, widely flowing, floating foampool, flower unfurling" (p. 49). Alliterative phrases that may not have any personal significance may remain in the attention longer or recur more frequently in one's interior monologue. Other properties, such as consonance, assonance, or rhyme, may likewise call attention to themselves and to the material that embodies them. Possibly there is a certain goodness of fit about particular structures, such as well-known songs or snatches of melody and rhythm, that lead them, once noticed, to be replayed regularly, sometimes to the point of annoyance at the recurrence of the material. Many of us may have had the maddening experience of unintentionally humming all day a song we don't like or bits of a TV commercial jingle we despise. As Mark Twain noted in a humorous story, a catchy rhyme may in effect take possession of one's consciousness. In this case, one person after another is plagued by the little phrase "Punch, brothers, punch with care; punch in the presence of the passenjare!"—a jingle about trolley car conductors; each person who heard it could not get rid of it until he had finally told someone else about it.

Salience of what might be termed "naturally occurring structures" is of course hard to demonstrate in respect to private conscious experience and in any case may play a much less significant role than the other influences discussed thus far.

IV. OPTIMAL LEVELS OF STIMULATION: A COGNITIVE–AFFECTIVE VIEW

We wish to conclude this extremely brief outline of a theory of what regulates the stream of consciousness with an emphasis on the extreme interrelatedness of the cognitive and affective processes. The stream of consciousness does not flow epiphenomenally or without great efficacy in our day-to-day affairs. Among a number of influences, not only the mental work, the information processing of a wealth of stimuli, but also our feelings, in their own right or serving to amplify other systems, regulate the flow of the stream of consciousness. And this continuous flow, in turn, helps regulate our thoughts, feelings, and behavior.

An understanding of the stream of consciousness, then, has significance for approaches to psychotherapy as well as for a general understanding of the human organism. Various behavior-modification techniques, such as systematic desensitization, work with conscious images produced by the client to produce behavior change. Other psychotherapeutic techniques may seek to impart certain cognitive or behavioral skills through focusing on conscious techniques of problem solving, self-assertiveness, etc. The point is that the successful use of such techniques dealing with the conscious processes may not only increase the autonomous, successful behavior and cognitive skills of the client and thus have an indirectly beneficial effect on his mood or feelings about himself but may *directly* influence the affects. The consciousness regulates and is regulated by affective as well as cognitive components. And the affective dimension is significant. Thus, in an extremely dull and predictable external environment, the person who has (or can learn to have) a willingness to explore internal activities, to entertain herself or himself with fantasies, recollections, and recombinations of experiences, may tune into stimulation leading to the same pleasurable affects of surprise, joy, and interest that Tomkins outlined for the processing of external stimuli. There are indications, for instance, from studies of sensory deprivation that suggest that those persons already comfortable with private fantasy activity are less likely to report either gross discomfort with sensory deprivation or being susceptible to hallucinatory experiences. Similarly, people who are accepting of and positive toward their inner experience report much less discomfort while sitting in barren "waiting" rooms or in performing dull signal detection tasks (Singer, 1974b). When Csikszentimihalyi asked his subjects to deprive themselves of daydreams and other "autotelic behaviors," those who were practiced daydreamers reported extremely negative affective reactions.

V. SOME RESEARCH PROSPECTS

We have attempted to touch on some of those influences that shape and interact with the stream of consciousness. Our inability to

speak with greater precision or certainty about the stream of consciousness is due in part to the fact that our research tools and
techniques are primitive and not yet perfected. The great difficulty in
developing sound, reliable methods to study the ongoing stream of
thought that is so much a part of our day-to-day activities and is
captured with dramatic effectiveness by the arts may have been a
prime factor in American psychology's willingness to deny the stream
of consciousness, to treat it as an epiphenomenon, or to downplay its
inherent interest and importance during most of the first half of this
century. In closing, then, let us look briefly at some of the innovative
methods—each, of course, with its own problems and limitations—
being developed to learn about the naturally occurring stream of
consciousness.

Of major importance are questionnaire studies such as Singer and
Antrobus's Imaginal Processes Inventory. The great advantage is that
subjects attempt to report accurately and with some precision about
their stream of consciousness as it has occurred in their everyday
lives. The conceptions of private experience that emerge from these
studies, therefore, are less artificial, less the result of laboratory
pokings, proddings, and manipulations uncharacteristic of everyday
life. A similar technique with the same advantage is interviewing
people, asking them to report on their stream of consciousness as they
have experienced it (Hariton and Singer, 1974). Whereas questionnaires are much easier to administer to a large number of people, the
interview technique offers greater opportunities to follow up the
idiosyncrasies and unique material of each person in greater detail.
Both methods, however, are limited in that they obtain retrospective
reports and thus depend upon the individual's memory. A person
who does not, for instance, attend closely to the bits and pieces of
fantasy, memory fragments, and imagined conversations running
through his mind, who does not rehearse them or "ticket" them for
further recall, may not remember them at the end of the day and may
not report that such material is highly characteristic of his stream of
consciousness.

Asking people to "think aloud," to verbalize their thoughts as
they occur (Antrobus and Singer, 1964; DeGroot, 1965; Klinger, 1971,
1974; Rychlak, 1973) is a method not so dependent on the reporter's
memory. The question arises, of course, what do the subjects do while
they report, how are they engaged while in the laboratory or reporting
room? The answers so far range from the highly artificial signal-
detection tasks (Antrobus and Singer, 1964) to tasks not uncharacteristic of everyday life, such as chess playing (DeGroot, 1965) or manual
puzzles and logic problems (Klinger, 1974), to giving the subject no

activity or task but simply asking the subject to sit or lie comfortably and report (Klinger, 1971, 1974; Pope, 1977; Rychlak, 1973).

The "thinking-aloud" procedure, however, has its difficulties. It asks people to perform what is in some cases a demanding task: putting their thoughts into words and doing so quickly enough so that they neither slow down (nor further distort) their thoughts nor leave out parts of a description because they are in a hurry or because they can't find the right words. It is a problem faced by the early stream-of-consciousness writers. Wyndham Lewis (1926) had this to say about *Ulysses* soon after its publication: "Joyce had to pretend that we were really surprising the private thought of a real and average human creature, Mr. Bloom. But the fact is that Mr. Bloom was abnormally *wordy*. He *thought in words*, not images, for our benefit, in a fashion as unreal, from the point of view of the strictest naturalist dogma, as a Hamlet soliloquy" (pp. 413–414).

A study by Pope (1977) offers support for this basic insight and suggests that verbalization may indeed slow down or otherwise influence the report of the stream of consciousness. Of importance to the study was the occurrence of "shifts" in thought (changes of content or the direction of thought). Subjects who kept track of their stream of thought nonverbally (momentarily releasing a key each time a shift of consciousness occurred) indicated a significantly higher shifting rate than subjects who reported by "thinking aloud" (both when the shifts were supplied by the subjects themselves and when the shifts were reliably judged from transcripts by independent raters). Data were obtained from a variety of physical situations (subjects reporting while lying down, while seated, while walking around) and from differing social conditions (subjects alone or with other people present). In this study, subjects reporting their flow of consciousness nonverbally reported a shift of thought on the average of every 5 or 6 seconds, while subjects thinking aloud reported shifts only on the average of about every 30 seconds. The data suggest that explorations relying solely on a thinking-aloud procedure may present a distinctly biased picture of the stream of consciousness. One useful tactic, then, may be to have subjects convey only a limited amount of information about their stream of thought (e.g., whether their thought at the moment is preoccupied with the environment or with processing other material) through simple key-press devices (Pope, 1977). Although it delivers only limited information about the ongoing thought (and lacks the richness of language), the method may be less intrusive, less inhibiting of the natural flow of the stream of consciousness. Another useful method is "thought sampling" (Klinger, 1971), in which a subject is interrupted at irregular intervals and asked to describe his thoughts just prior to the interruption. This method gives the subject time to make his description as phenomenologically accurate and fully communicative as his vocabulary allows, but it does sacrifice the moment-to-moment movement of the stream.

In closing, we would like to advocate three aspects or strategies of research that we feel would be most fruitful. First, we must continue to move beyond the laboratory in exploring the stream of consciousness. The material obtained from people whose customary surroundings, familiar patterns of behavior, and day-to-day routines have been minimally altered or disturbed is invaluable in supplementing, guiding, verifying, and furnishing a meaningful touchstone for the frequently more artificial or contrived research carried on within the constraints of the more traditional laboratory. Hurleburt (1976), for instance, equipped people serving as subjects with mechanical "beepers." The subjects then went about their normal, everyday life. At random, generally at infrequent intervals, the small device (carried within a pocket or purse) emitted a brief tone. The subject then jotted down whatever contents were flowing through his or her stream of consciousness at the time of the tone. Such research may lead us to a more accurate picture of the thoughts and feelings people experience during the course of their normal, daily routines. A recent unpublished study by Catherine McDonald, using this method, indicated that subjects averaged 43% of reports of stimulus-independent or daydreamlike thought during a given day.

Second, if we are to increase our knowledge of the subtle movements and nuances of the stream of consciousness, we must devote more time to the individual subject, taking into account the personal complexities and idiosyncratic factors characteristic of that particular person. A little introspection by the reader of the fleeting thoughts passing through his mind while reading this paper should turn up considerable material unrelated or related only distantly to the manuscript at hand: memories, awareness of particular room noises, daydreaming perhaps, mental notes to perform a particular task when the reading is done, fragmentary images. The variation in material from reader to reader is probably quite large. Though we can spell out certain general principles governing the occurrence of this material, the determinants regulating the appearance of particular material for a particular reader are probably quite personal, intimately related to the unique history, states, traits, and other characteristics of that individual. If we are to construct theories of ongoing thought that are meaningful, precise, and capable of verification or disconfirmation, we must take the time to learn something of these characteristics and how they, as supposed determinants, relate to the ongoing consciousness of the individual. Such work will add the necessary precision to (and serve as a check on) the general principles obtainable through studies involving large numbers of people.

Third, we must begin to incorporate more than one level of factors at a time into our research designs. Almost without exception, the research on which this paper was based explored only single aspects of the workings of the stream of consciousness. A number of influences have been outlined here as serving to regulate the flow of thought. Current concerns, drive states, sets toward particular processing styles, amount and complexity of incoming sensory stimulation, etc., have each separately served as the subject of research. What is lacking is an attempt to see, within a research paradigm, how they interrelate: Is the influence they contribute additive? Do they interact in unforeseen ways? Can we specify which ones will be effective in a given situation?

A given experimental situation viewed as an analogue of many network-occurring situations can be analyzed into a combination of interacting factors, for example, the environmental determinants, including physical characteristics of the stimuli and their meaningfulness or abstraction; the situational demands, such as the request made by the experimenter or the social meaning of the situation; and finally, personal determinants brought to the situation by the subject, the emotions aroused before he comes into the room, perhaps, and a long-standing personality predisposition, such as introversion–extroversion or cognitive style (Singer, 1952). An experiment by Rodin and Singer (1976) introduced many of these intersecting variables into a situation in which the focus was upon the relation of private cognitive activity to the way a person's eyes moved about during a two- or three-person interview. The interviewer, seated facing the subject, asked a series of questions that required different degrees or types of reflective thought. Some questions called for overlearned reactions, for example, "What is your mother's name?" Others called for more reflective verbal or arithmetical sequential processing, for example, number series or "How many r's are there in 'around the ragged rock the ragged rascal ran'?" Other questions called for reflective visual-imagery processing, for example, "What did your first-grade teacher look like?" or "What way does John F. Kennedy face on the half-dollar coin?" There were thus very different kinds of cognitive inner activity required, presumably governed by different portions of the brain (bilateral asymmetry hypothesis) and reflected by differential degrees and directions of lateral eye movement.

To ascertain whether eye shifts could be influenced not only by the nature of the cognitive operations required but also by the social and physical stimuli of the setting, the experiment varied the presence or absence of an additional person, seated sometimes to the left and sometimes to the right of the interviewer. Since the face of another person is a compelling stimulus, it was felt that subjects would have to avert their gaze from the interviewer if they were developing an elaborate private image in order to avoid overloading the visual channel (Meskin and Singer, 1974). The presence of still another person to the interviewer's left or right should compel a shift of gaze toward the blank third of the subject's forward plane of regard while he is reflecting on a visual image.

The predispositional variables in the experiment included the cognitive style of the subjects, their predilection, and, finally, the *weight* of the subject. As suggested earlier, overweight persons have been shown to be excessively dependent upon external cues. One would expect that overweight subjects would have special difficulty in processing visual-imagery material while facing another person and so would be forced to shift gaze more.

The results, as might be anticipated, were complex, but they do point up the subtle interactions of these factors. Overweight subjects reported less visual imagery in their daydreams or ongoing thought. They were also much more likely to shut their eyes while processing complex materials in the face-to-face situation or to shift their gaze toward the blank area if faced by two persons. These effects were even more striking when the material to be processed emphasized visual spatial imagery rather than verbal materials. And, finally, when compared to the other subjects, overweights who were also field-dependent in their cognitive style were particularly likely to shift their gaze toward the blank area. These results do suggest that (1) style differences in how much emphasis is habitually placed on verbal versus visual interior monologue, (2) demands for attention to the inner versus the external pole, and (3) the nature of the social and physical setting all interact in fairly predictable ways to determine the flow of ongoing thought.

The work that remains to be done whets the appetite. The stream of consciousness, so much a part of our day-to-day lives and intimate experience, is once again a legitimate subject for research in American psychology. It provokes research and some exciting, vital, scientific thinking and writing. Psychology is coming to life in this area—responding to the challenge posed by William James 85 years ago.

REFERENCES

ANGYAL, A. Disturbances of thinking in schizophrenia. In J. S. Kasanin (Ed.), *Language and thought in schizophrenia*. Berkeley: University of California Press, 1944.

ANOKHIN, P. K. Cybernetics and the integrative activity of the brain. In M. Cole and I. Maltzman (Eds.), *Handbook of contemporary Soviet psychology*. New York: Basic Books, 1969.

ANTROBUS, J. S., AND SINGER, J. L. Visual signal detection as a function of sequential variability of simultaneous speech. *Journal of Experimental Psychology*, 1964, *68*, 603–610.

ANTROBUS, J. S., SINGER, J. L., GOLDSTEIN, S., AND FORTGANG, M. Mind-wandering and cognitive structure. *Transactions of the New York Academy of Sciences*, 1970, *32*, 242–252.

ANTROBUS, J. S., SINGER, J. L., AND GREENBERG, S. Studies in the stream of consciousness: Experimental enhancement and suppression of spontaneous cognitive processes. *Perceptual and Motor Skills*, 1966, *23*(2), 399–517.

BARTLETT, J. C. *The coding of naturalistic sounds*. Unpublished doctoral dissertation, Yale University, 1975.

BLATT, S. J. Levels of object representation in anaclitic and introspective depression. *Psychoanalytic Study of the Child*, 1974, *29*, 107–157.

BOURNE, L. E., EKSTRAND, B. R., AND DUMINOWSKI, R. L. *The psychology of thinking*. Englewood Cliffs, N.J.: Prentice-Hall, 1971.

BREGER, L., HUNTER, I., AND LANE, R. W. *The effect of stress on dreams*. New York: International Universities Press, 1971.

BROADBENT, D. E. *Decision and stress*. London: Academic Press, 1971.

BROWN, R. *Words and things*. Glencoe, Ill.: The Free Press, 1958.

CSIKSZENTIMIHALYI, M. *Flow: Studies of enjoyment*. PHS Grant Report N. R01 HM 22883-02, 1974.

CSIKSZENTIMIHALYI, M., HOLCOMB, J. H., AND CSIKSZENTIMIHALYI, I. The rewards of surgery. In M. Csikszentimihalyi (Ed.), *Flow: Studies of enjoyment*. PHS Grant Report N. R01 HM 22883-02, 1974.

DEGROOT, A. *Thought and choice in chess*. The Hague: Mouton, 1965.

DRUCKER, E. *Studies of the role of temporal uncertainty in the deployment of attention*. Unpublished doctoral dissertation, City University of New York, 1969.

EISENSTEIN, S. *The film sense*. New York: Harcourt & Brace, 1942.

ELIOT, T. S. Hamlet and his problems. In *Selected essays*. New York: Harcourt & Brace, 1950.

ERDELYI, M. H., AND BECKER, J. Hypermnesia for pictures: Incremental memory for pictures but not words in multiple recall trials. *Cognitive Psychology*, 1974, *6*, 159–171.

ERDELYI, M. H., AND KLEINBARD, J. Has Ebbinghaus decayed over time? The growth or recall (hypermnesia) over days. *Cognitive Psychology*, in press.

FISKE, D. W., AND MADDI, S. R. *Functions of varied experience*. Homewood, Ill.: Dorsey, 1961.

GARNER, W. R. *The processing of information and structure*. Potomac, Md.: Erlbaum, 1974.

GIAMBRA, L. Daydreaming across the life span: Late adolescent to senior citizen. *Aging and Human Development*, 1974, *5*, 116–135.

GILL , M. Topography and systems in psychoanalytic theory. *Psychological Issues*, Monograph 10. New York: International Universities Press, 1963.

HARITON, E. B., AND SINGER, J. L. Women's fantasies during sexual intercourse: Normative and theoretical implications. *Journal of Consulting and Clinical Psychology*, 1974, *42*, 313–322.

HEBB, D. O. Drives and the central nervous system. *Psychological Review*, 1955, *62*, 243–253.

HERNANDEZ-PEON, R., SCHERRER, H., AND JOUVET, M. Modification of electrical activity in the cochlear nucleus during "attention" in unanesthetized cats. *Science,* 1956, *123,* 331–332.

HOLT, R. Imagery: The return of the ostracized. *American Psychologist,* 1964, *19,* 254–264.

HOROWITZ, M. Intrusive and repetitive thought after experimental stress. *Archives of General Psychiatry,* 1975, *32,* 1457–1463.

HOROWITZ, M. J., AND BECKER, S. The compulsion to repeat trauma. *Journal of Nervous and Mental Diseases,* 1971, *153,* 32–40.

HUBA, G. J., SEGAL, B., AND SINGER, J. L. Consistency of daydreaming styles across samples of college male and female drug and alcohol users. *Journal of Abnormal Psychology,* 1977a, *86*(1), 99–102.

HUBA, G. J., SEGAL, B., AND SINGER, J. L. Organization of needs in male and female drug and alcohol users. *Journal of Consulting and Clinical Psychology,* 1977b, *45*(1), 34–44.

HURLEBURT, R. *Self-observation and self-control.* Unpublished doctoral dissertation, University of South Dakota, 1976.

JAMES, W. *The principles of psychology,* Vol. 1. New York: Dover, 1890/1950.

JOHNSON, D. M. *The psychology of thought and judgment.* New York: Harper, 1955.

JOYCE, J. *Ulysses.* New York: Random House, 1961. (Originally published in 1922.)

KAGAN, J., AND KOGAN, N. Individual variation in cognitive processes. In P. Mussen (Ed.), *Carmichael's manual of child psychology,* Vol. 1. New York: Wiley, 1970.

KALMUS, H. Inherited sense defects. *Scientific American,* 1952, *186,* 64–70.

KAMIN, L. J. Predictability, surprise, attention, and conditioning. In B. A. Campbell and R. M. Church (Eds.), *Punishment and aversive behavior.* New York: Appleton-Century-Crofts, 1969.

KLEIN, G. S. Peremptory ideation: Structure and force in motivated ideas. In R. Holt (Ed.), *Motives and thought. Psychological Issues,* 1967, *5,* 80–128.

KLINGER, E. *Structure and functions of fantasy.* New York: Wiley, 1971.

KLINGER, E. Utterances to evaluate steps and control attention distinguish operant from respondent thought while thinking out loud. *Bulletin of the Psychonomic Society,* 1974, *4*(1), 44–45.

KRIS, E. On preconscious mental processes. In D. Rapaport (Ed.), *Organization and pathology of thought.* New York: Columbia University Press, 1951. Pp. 474–493.

LANGER, S. K. *Philosophy in a new key.* New York: Mentor Books, 1964.

LASHLEY, K. S. Cerebral organization and behavior. In *The brain and human behavior, proceedings of the Association for Research on Nervous and Mental Disease.* Baltimore: Williams & Wilkins, 1958.

LEWIN, K. Die psychische Tatigkeit bei der Hemmong von Willensvorgangen und das Grundgesetz der Assoziation. *Zeitschrift für Psychologie,* 1916, *77,* 212–247.

LEWIS, W. *The art of being ruled.* New York: Harper, 1926.

LURIA, A. R. *The working brain.* New York: Basic Books, 1973.

MESKIN, B., AND SINGER, J. L. Daydreaming, reflective thought and laterality of eye movements. *Journal of Personal and Social Psychology,* 1974, *30*(1), 64–71.

MILLER, G., A., GALANTER, E., AND PRIBRAM, K. *Plans and the structure of behavior.* New York: Holt, 1960.

MILLER, T. *Some characteristics of two different ways of listening.* Unpublished doctoral dissertation, New York University, 1972.

MISCHEL, W. *Introduction to personality.* New York: Holt, Rinehart, & Winston, 1971.

NEISSER, U. *Cognitive psychology.* New York: Appleton-Century-Crofts, 1967.

NEISSER, U. Changing conceptions of imagery. In P. W. Sheehan (Ed.), *The function and nature of imagery.* New York: Academic Press, 1972. Pp. 223–251.

PAIVIO, A. *Imagery and verbal processes.* New York: Holt, Rinehart, & Winston, 1971.

PENFIELD, W. Consciousness, memory, and man's conditioned reflexes. In K. H. Pribram (Ed.), *On the biology of learning.* New York: Harcourt & Brace, 1969. Pp. 129–168.

PETRIE, A. *Individuality in pain and suffering.* Chicago: The University of Chicago Press, 1967.

POPE, K. S. *The stream of consciousness.* Unpublished doctoral dissertation, Yale University, 1977.

POSNER, M. I., AND BOIES, S. J. Components of attention. *Psychological Review,* 1971, *78,* 391–408.

PRIBRAM, K. H. *Languages of the brain.* Englewood Cliffs, N.J.: Prentice-Hall, 1971.

RAPAPORT, D. The psychoanalytic theory of motivation. In M. R. Jones (Ed.), *Nebraska Symposium on Motivation.* Lincoln: University of Nebraska Press, 1960.

RESCORLA, R. A. Conditioned inhibition of fear. In N. J. Mackintosh and W. K. Honig (Eds.), *Fundamental issues in associative learning.* Halifax: Dalhousie University Press, 1969.

RODIN, J., AND SINGER, J. L. Eye-shift, thought and obesity. *Journal of Personality,* 1976, *44,* 594–610.

RYCHLAK, J. F. Time orientation in the positive and negative free fantasies of mildly abnormal vs. normal high school males. *Journal of Consulting and Clinical Psychology,* 1973, *41,* 175–180.

SCHACHTER, S., AND RODIN, J. *Obese humans and rats.* Washington, D.C.: Erlbaum/Wiley, 1974.

SEGAL, B., AND SINGER, J. L. Daydreaming, drug and alcohol use in college students: A factor analytic study. In *Addictive Behaviors,* Vol. 1, Pergamon Press, 1976. Pp. 227–235.

SEGAL, S. J. *Imagery: Current cognitive approaches.* New York: Academic Press, 1971.

SEGAL, S. J., AND FUSELLA, V. Influence of imaged pictures and sounds on detection of auditory and visual signals. *Journal of Experimental Psychology,* 1970, *83,* 458–464.

SEIDMAN, J. M. *The adolescent, a book of readings, revised.* New York: Holt, Rinehart, & Winston, 1960.

SHEEHAN, P. *The function and nature of imagery.* New York: Academic Press, 1972.

SHEPARD, R. N. Form, formation, and transformation of internal representation. In R. Solso (Ed.), *Information processing and cognition: The Loyola Symposium.* Hillsdale, N.J.: Erlbaum, 1975.

SINGER, J. L. Personal and environmental determinants of perception in a size constancy experiment. *Journal of Experimental Psychology,* 1952, *43,* 420–427.

SINGER, J. L. *The child's world of make believe: Experimental studies of imaginative play.* New York: Academic Press, 1973.

SINGER, J. L. *Imagery and daydream methods in psychotherapy and behavior modification.* New York: Academic Press, 1974a.

SINGER, J. L. Navigating the stream of consciousness: Research in daydreaming and related inner experiences. *American Psychologist,* 1974b, *30,* 727–738.

SINGER, J. L. *The inner world of daydreaming.* New York: Harper & Row, 1975.

SINGER, J. L., AND ANTROBUS, J. S. A factor analysis of daydreaming and conceptually related cognitive and personality variables. *Perceptual and Motor Skills,* 1963, Monograph supplement 3-V17.

SINGER, J. L., AND ANTROBUS, J. S. Daydreaming, imaginal process, and personality: A normative study. In P. Sheehan (Ed.), *The function and nature of imagery.* New York: Academic Press, 1972.

SKINNER, B. F. The steep and thorny way to a science of behavior. *American Psychologist,* 1975, *30,* 42–49.

SOKOLOV, E. N. *Perception and the conditioned reflex.* New York: MacMillan, 1963.

SOKOLOV, E. N. The modeling properties of the nervous system. In M. Cole and I. Maltzman (Eds.), *Handbook of contemporary Soviet psychology.* New York: Basic Books, 1969.

STARKER, S. Daydreaming styles and nocturnal dreaming. *Journal of Abnormal Psychology,* 1974, *83,* 52–55.

TOMKINS, S. *Affect, imagery, and consciousness,* Vols. 1 and 2. New York: Springer, 1962–1963.

WEST, L. J. A general theory of hallucinations and dreams. In L. J. West (Ed.), *Hallucinations.* New York: Grune & Stratton, 1962.

WILSON, E. Ulysses. *New Republic,* 1922, *31,* 164.

WOOLF, V. Modern fiction. In V. Woolf, *The common reader.* New York: Harcourt & Brace, 1953. (Originally published, 1925.)

4   *Self-Deception, Self-Confrontation, and Consciousness*

Harold A. Sackeim and Ruben C. Gur

I. Introduction

> Our position is like that of a puppy who sees himself in a mirror; after sniffing at his reflection he walks behind and sees only strips of wood and tacks. We too tend to see one side or the other of our problem: the physiological and behavioral side on one hand and on the other the side of experience and sensations. Our difficulty is to see the problem and to see it whole, to see both the mirror and our reflection, and to understand their unity. (Cherry, 1957, p. 299)

These comments were made by Colin Cherry in a discussion of the mind–body question. However, the significance of Cherry's remarks may be more general. A peculiar characteristic of the study of mind and, therefore, the discipline of psychology is that the study is necessarily self-reflective. Whether one examines observable behavior or develops theoretical models of contents of the "black box," consciousness is employed to investigate the products of consciousness. In this sense, like the puppy, the psychologist is self-confronted; the mind observes and attempts to understand the mind.

In any science, what can be determined is limited, in part, by the methodologies that are available to the scientist. Schools of psychology have been criticized for equating what can be determined with all that there is. Behaviorists have been taken to assert not only that we must limit ourselves to the study of observable influences on behavior but

Harold A. Sackeim · Department of Psychology, Columbia University, New York, New York. Ruben C. Gur · Department of Psychology, University of Pennsylvania, Philadelphia, Pennsylvania. Preparation of this chapter was aided in part by a National Science Foundation grant #BNS 75-23061.

also that only observable events do influence behavior. Similarly, in the study of the nature of consciousness, we are limited for the most part to what we can become aware of. If we were to equate consciousness with awareness, then we would be led to the claim that consciousness is unitary and transparent. When one asserts that consciousness is unitary, one claims that consciousness is not divided into separate and independent functional structures or control systems. Rather, one claims that there is one structure, or one "mind," regardless of organization. When one asserts that consciousness is transparent, one claims that all contents of consciousness are capable of reaching awareness. Identifying awareness of the contents of consciousness with the nature of consciousness is an example of equating what our methodologies enable us to investigate with what there is. William James (1890/1950) termed this logical error "the psychologist's fallacy par excellence": "We must avoid substituting what we know the consciousness *is*, for what it is a consciousness *of*" (p. 197).

There have been long-standing debates in both philosophy and psychology concerning views of consciousness as unitary and/or transparent. Descartes's (1641/1967) position was that consciousness is both unitary and transparent, a core assumption also held by Wundt (1912/1973). Psychologists, in criticizing experimental research on the nature of consciousness, often have implicitly assumed that consciousness is characterized by these properties. For instance, as Erdelyi (1974) pointed out, Bruner and Postman (1949), Howie (1952), Luchins (1950), and others held that the phenomenon of perceptual defense is a conceptual impossibility because it entails the logical paradox of claiming that an individual may perceive and not perceive at the same time. Howie (1952) wrote, "To speak of perceptual defense is to use a mode of discourse which must make any precise or even intelligible meaning of perceptual defense impossible, for it is to speak of a perceptual process as somehow being both a process of knowing and a process of avoiding knowing" (p. 311). On the other hand, some philosophers and psychologists have argued that consciousness is neither unitary nor transparent. Plato (circa 359 B.C./1953) claimed that if one can assert that individuals may be self-deceived—that is, that individuals may lie to themselves—then consciousness must be viewed as nonunitary and/or nontransparent. James (1902) stated:

> I cannot but think that the most important step forward that has occurred in psychology since I have been a student of that science is the discovery, first made in 1886, that, in certain subjects at least, there is not only the consciousness of the ordinary field, with its usual centre and margin, but an addition thereto in the shape of a set of memories,

> thoughts, and feelings which are extra-marginal and outside the primary
> consciousness altogether, but yet must be classed as conscious facts of
> some sort, able to reveal their presence by unmistakable signs. (p. 233)

Freud's most radical claim and perhaps his most important contribution to psychology is the idea that not only is consciousness nonunitary and nontransparent but also that, at times, selective awareness and nonawareness of the contents of consciousness are, in part, motivated. This view of the nature of consciousness underlies Freud's concept of repression. Concerning the significance of this concept, Freud (1914/1957) states that repression is "the cornerstone on which the whole structure of psychoanalysis rests" (p. 16). Since this statement, scores of experimental investigations have been interpreted as either propping up or as tearing down this cornerstone. In evaluating the results of such endeavors as they bear on the utility of concepts like repression, it is important to keep in mind that the evidence must be relevant to considerations concerning the nature of consciousness, not specifically its contents.

Investigators in this area have rarely attempted to outline necessary and sufficient criteria for ascribing the concept of repression. Freud himself offered several differing formulations of what is meant by *repression* and discussed this concept in reference to topological, economic, and dynamic perspectives of consciousness. Clearly, without a statement of the necessary and sufficient criteria for ascribing the concept, it is difficult to see how one can determine the extent to which any evidence bears on the ontological status of the concept. Recently, Holmes (1974) presented three criteria that he felt must be met for any given phenomenon to be viewed as an instance of repression. He argued that repression is an instance of motivated selective forgetting. Furthermore, repression is not under conscious control. Finally, the material that is repressed is not lost but rather stored in the unconscious. Holmes and others (e.g. Hilgard, 1973) who have reviewed investigations that attempt to demonstrate the existence of repression have concluded that the evidence is at best equivocal and that "there is no consistent research evidence to support the hypothesis derived from the theory of repression" (Holmes, 1974, p. 649). Our purpose here is not to review the evidence that forms the basis of this conclusion. Rather, we wish to point out some conceptual difficulties in the arguments used both by protagonists and by antagonists in the debate concerning the existence of repression.

Holmes (1972, 1974) and Eysenck and Wilson (1973) have made the argument that if the phenomena that the repression literature has attributed to the influences of repression can instead be explained from biochemical, response competition, or interference perspectives, then, *ipso facto,* the phenomena cannot be asserted to be consequences or examples of repression. This perspective turns the concept of repression into a type of explanation of or mechanistic influence on behavior rather than a descriptive term used to state that a phenomenon is characterized as meeting a specific set of criteria. Certainly, finding that the reputed consequences of repression are explainable from an interference or biochemical view may rule out the ascription of repression, if the criteria for the ascription are such that they are contradicted by such explanations. However, in the absence of such contradictions, it could be the case that repression or its consequences comes about through biochemical, interference, or response-competitive influences. Discussions of the "how" questions of processes and mechanisms only indirectly bear on the issues related to the ontological status of a given class of concepts.

On the other hand, investigators who have attempted to demonstrate the existence of repression may be criticized for employing methodologies that were inherently inadequate for that purpose. The concept of repression requires that consciousness be shown to be nonunitary and nontransparent and, in particular, that cognitions that are not subject to awareness be stored in an unconscious. Studies of repression have concentrated, in the main, on examining instances of momentary forgetting. Demonstrations that items in memory may be forgotten or retrieved depending on motivational considerations should not be taken as a demonstration that there are separate and independent control systems that influence behavior directly. Indeed, it is difficult to imagine how one might go about demonstrating the existence of an unconscious and what sorts of evidence would be relevant to such a conclusion. The results of studies on repression do bear on the lesser claim that consciousness is nontransparent and that selective awareness and nonawareness may be motivated. However, even in this respect, the evidence to date has not been compelling.

The concept of repression may be viewed as a special instance of the more general category of self-deception. If self-deception does not exist, it is unlikely that repression exists. Failure to demonstrate the existence of self-deception would cast strong doubts on the likelihood that repression could be demonstrated to exist. It would seem, therefore, that conceptual analysis and experimental investigation of the concept of self-deception are of paramount importance in the attempt to come to an understanding of the nature of consciousness.

The concept of self-deception has received much attention in philosophical and literary writings (e.g., Camus, 1956; Fingarette, 1969; Gide, 1955; Sartre, 1958). A number of psychologists have also discussed self-deception as a possible explanation for a wide range of behavior. Meehl and Hathaway (1946) and Anastasi (1961) have stressed the importance of self-deception in producing non-content-based responding to self-report personality inventories. In discussing the significance of lie scales, Meehl and Hathaway wrote, "What is much more important, they [lie scales] are mainly directed at the sort of *conscious* falsehood which most writers have stressed, while ignoring the more subtle tendencies to self-deception which are probably of even greater importance in affecting scores" (p. 528). In the area of motivation and personality, Hilgard (1949) presented two formulations by which to conceptualize defense mechanisms or mechanisms of adjustment. These mechanisms may be perceived as defenses against anxiety or "It is entirely appropriate to consider self-deception as one of the defining characteristics of a mechanism" (p. 376). Murphy (1970) related the concept of self-deception to possible interpretations of the experimental findings on perceptual defense. In fact, Mischel (1974) has viewed all neurotic behavior as instances of self-deceptive acts. In the area of problem-solving behavior, Wason and Johnson-Laird (1972) invoked the concept of self-deception as a possible explanation of the persistence of subjects in maintaining hypotheses in the face of disconfirmation. Furthermore, the concept of self-deception may also be relevant to accounts of behavioral and attitudinal change based on cognitive dissonance (Festinger, 1957) and reactance (Brehm, 1966) theories. For example, a question for investigation may be whether the subject who initially states that an experiment is dull and then, after dissonance manipulations, avers that the experiment was interesting can be said to be self-deceived.

Considering the role given to self-deception in several areas of study, it is surprising that psychologists have not attempted to define what is meant by this term. Furthermore, there have been no previous experimental investigations that have examined the appropriateness of characterizing individuals as self-deceived. Rather, self-deception has served as an explanatory construct whose conceptual boundaries and construct validity or ontological status are undetermined.

In this chapter, we discuss our attempts to come to grips with the concept of self-deception on both conceptual and empirical levels. Recent discussions of self-deception in the philosophical literature have centered on whether the logic of self-deception should be viewed as similar to the logic of other-deception. We outline here a logicolinguistic analysis of the concept of self-deception that argues that when consciousness is claimed to be nontransparent, the assimilation of self-deception with other-deception is justified (cf. Sackeim and Gur, 1976). On the basis of this analysis, we present four criteria as necessary and sufficient for the ascription of self-deception. Furthermore, it is argued here that the criteria for ascribing self-deception are necessary but are not sufficient for the ascription of repression. As a result, acts of repression may be viewed as specific instances of the broader category of self-deceptive behaviors.

Once we have established conceptual boundaries for the concept of self-deception, it is necessary to demonstrate that the criteria for the ascription of the concept are operationable. It is necessary that investigations of defensive behavior employ methodologies that are sensitive to motivational factors. Freud (1915/1957) argued that the contents of consciousness that are repressed are highly individual and that repression itself is mobile, varying with the motivational concerns of the individual. In our experimental studies of self-deception, we have examined the behavior of subjects when they recognize and fail to recognize audio stimuli of the self. A number of psychologists have studied the reactions of people when their attention is directed inward through the use of mirrors, audio- and videotape playbacks, and audience effects. It has been found that when individuals are self-confronted and their attention is directed inward, psychophysiological, cognitive, affective, and behavioral responses differ markedly from responses of individuals whose attention is directed outward to the environment. We briefly review here the results of studies on self-confrontation. This review not only forms a basis both for the operationalization of the criteria for ascribing self-deception and for the hypotheses to be tested in the experiments on self-deception that we report but also presents a set of arguments pertaining to the relationship between awareness of the self and the nature of consciousness. It is argued here that consciousness of the self produces an inherently different state of awareness than consciousness of others or of events in the environment. Furthermore, it is claimed that self-consciousness is aversive for many individuals and that they avoid it. Evidence is presented for the view that the greater the cognitive discrepancy within an individual—that is, the greater the dissatisfaction with aspects of self—the more intense is the aversiveness of the state of self-confrontation. In sum, it is argued that differences in states of awareness, in terms of their properties and consequences, may be a function, in part, of the contents of the awareness.

After reviewing studies of self-confrontation, we present an operationalization of the criteria for ascribing self-deception that applies our knowledge of the effects of self-confrontation. We discuss how one might go about demonstrating that individuals hold contradictory beliefs and that individuals may hold beliefs that are not subject to awareness. The criterion of nonawareness has proved to be particularly intractable to demonstration without the use of highly obtrusive measures in areas of investigation such as learning without awareness (Martin, Hawryluk, and Guse, 1974) and selective attention (Moray, 1972). We propose that it is possible to devise unobtrusive measures of awareness and nonawareness, and we hypothesize that awareness or nonawareness of particular beliefs leads to differential behavioral outcomes in our experimental setting. We discuss alternative methods for demonstrating that the awareness or nonawareness of beliefs or cognitions may be motivated. New data are presented from an experiment that tested the proposed operationalization of the criteria for ascribing self-deception. We argue that these results indicate that self-deception is "an experimentally real phenomenon." It is concluded that much processing of information occurs outside of awareness and that the products of this processing may not be subject to awareness. Furthermore, we argue that our data support the contention that the awareness and nonawareness of cognitions or beliefs may be motivated. In this respect, there is evidence for the assertion that consciousness is nontransparent and that selectivity of awareness is determined, in part, by the motivational concerns of the individual.

We view our work in this area as providing only initial steps in coming to an understanding of self-deception and of the implications of this concept for theories concerning the nature of consciousness. Establishing that self-deception does occur brings many questions to the fore. In the final section, we present a number of speculations concerning the generality of self-deception as a mode of defense against threatening stimuli, and we raise the issue of individual differences in tendencies to engage in self-deceptive behaviors. Fingarette (1969) originally raised the possibility that differences between the two cerebral hemispheres in the processing of information may be involved in the mechanisms that underlie self-deception. We review here evidence from studies of hemisphericity and functional brain asymmetry and argue that Fingarette's hypothesis deserves serious experimental attention. We conclude with an overview of the work that has been presented here and a discussion of the implications of our methods of investigation for the study of consciousness.

II. CRITERIA NECESSARY AND SUFFICIENT FOR ASCRIBING SELF-DECEPTION

"There is nothing worse than self-deception—when the deceiver is always at home and always with you" (Plato, circa 386 B.C./1953).

Recent philosophical discussions of self-deception have centered on the question of whether the logic of self-deception can be assimilated to that of other-deception, for example, lying to others. When Jones lies to Smith, Jones makes Smith hold a belief, p. Jones does not believe that p. In fact, Jones believes that not-p. If Jones is successful in the deception, then Smith will believe that p at the same time that Jones believes that not-p. Furthermore, Smith will not be aware that Jones believes that not-p. Assimilating other- to self-deception, when the deceiver and the deceived are one and the same individual, entails that the individual hold two contradictory beliefs at the same time. When consciousness is viewed as unitary and transparent, this assimilation produces a paradox:

> The one to whom the lie is told and the one who lies are one and the same person, which means that I must know in my capacity as deceiver the truth which is hidden from me in my capacity as the one deceived. Better yet, I must know the truth very exactly in order to conceal it more carefully—and this not at two different moments, which at a pinch would allow us to re-establish a semblance of duality—but in the unitary structure of a single project. How then can the lie subsist if the duality which conditions it is suppressed? (Sartre, 1958, p. 49).

Note the similarity between the formulation of the paradox proposed by Sartre and the conceptual difficulties offered by Howie (1952) and others in reference to the concept of perceptual defense.

There appear to be two methods of dealing with this situation. The paradox can be avoided by a rejection of the assimilation of self-deception with other-deception. This route requires that an alternative framework be provided by which to analyze self-deception. On the other hand, the paradox is problematic only if it is maintained that self-deception takes place "in the unitary structure of a single project." When it is not claimed that consciousness is necessarily unitary and transparent, it may be possible to maintain the assimilation and yet avoid contradiction.

Philosophers who have rejected the assimilation thesis have focused their accounts of self-deception on the relationship between a belief and the circumstances in which it is held. Canfield and Gustafson (1962) proposed that to be self-deceived, an individual must hold a belief in adverse circumstances; that is, the evidence does not support the belief. Penelhum (1966) recognized that Canfield and Gustafson's formulation is insufficient in that it does not provide criteria by which instances of self-deception can be discriminated from instances of ignorance. He argued that not only must an individual hold a belief in the face of countervailing evidence but also, to be considered self-deceived, the individual must be aware of the evidence and its import. Penelhum did not view this position as a simple restatement of the original paradox because he concluded that the self-deceiver is in a "conflict state," half believing in both contradictory propositions.

Both formulations provide criteria that are neither necessary nor sufficient for ascribing self-deception.

They do not provide necessary criteria because it can be shown that there are instances, in which people are considered self-deceived, that do not meet these criteria. Individuals may hold, at times, beliefs that are not supported by the objective evidence. Because of their fear, surprise, pleasure, whatever, they may deny these beliefs. These instances are often considered to be examples of self-deception. However, in such cases, the new beliefs are supported by objective circumstances, and the circumstances are favorable. In other words, the belief that the individual professes and about which the individual is said to be self-deceived happens, in some instances, to be true (as in the case of denial of superstitions).

The criteria provided by these positions are not sufficient because it can be shown that there are instances in which the criteria are fulfilled and self-deception is not ascribed. As Gardiner (1970) has pointed out, in blind faith, individuals may hold, at times, firm beliefs that are contrary to the prevailing evidence and be fully aware of the evidence and its import. However, the beliefs that are supported by the evidence are not entertained even as possibilities. Such may be the case in firm religious convictions or, as in Gardiner's example, in cases such as Hitler's unshaken belief in eventual victory in the face of disaster.

That these positions have not provided criteria necessary and sufficient for the ascription of self-deception is an indication that the status of evidence in relation to beliefs is not germane to consideration of the logical constituents of self-deception. The formulations that are criticized above have structured their analyses of self-deception in beliefs, partially, in terms of the truth conditions of those beliefs. A distinction must be drawn between the issues involved in how we come to know that given individuals are self-deceived (an epistemological question) and what constitutes self-deception (a logical question). Statements about the objective evidence that reflects on beliefs may provide some clues as to whether it is likely that given individuals are self-deceived. However, statements about evidence are no more related to logical accounts of the properties of holding a belief in general than they are to the logical properties of being self-deceived.

If these arguments are successful in countering the formulations that have rejected the assimilation of self-deception and other-deception, one is left with the original paradox. Arriving at this position by default does not particularly convince one that there is substantial justification for the assimilation. However, it can be argued that the public language use of the concept of self-deception and related concepts indicates that there are positive grounds supporting the assimilation.

When individuals claim that a given person is self-deceived, they often state that although the person believes that p, in that person's "heart" or "deep inside" the person believes that not-p. Likewise, individuals, upon recognizing that they are self-deceived—that is, when self-deception is broken—often use such phrases as "I knew all along that . . . not-p." Therefore, it appears that individuals use language to discuss instances of self-deception in a manner that, at face value, conforms to the assimilation thesis.

Another approach to the formulation of criteria necessary and sufficient for ascribing self-deception has centered on denying that consciousness is unitary and/or transparent. Starting with Plato (circa 359 B.C./1953), a number of philosophers have attempted to resolve the conceptual difficulties of attributing contradictory beliefs to the same individual by positing that consciousness is nonunitary and/or nontransparent. When it is denied that consciousness is unitary, self-deception becomes almost a duplicate of other-deception. Two, at the least, autonomous agencies (within the same individual) each hold separate and contradictory beliefs. Since the assimilation with other-deception also requires that "Jones is not aware that Smith actually believes that not-p," such a formulation of nonunitary nature of consciousness also entails a nontransparent nature. The self-deceived individual, who expresses belief in p, is not aware that not-p is also believed. On the other hand, a view that denies the assumption of a transparent nature of consciousness does not entail ¯a nonunitary nature. Individuals may be said to fail "to notice that they have a belief" or to be unaware of or unable to notice that they have a belief, without an implication of any assumptions about autonomous structures (Demos, 1960). If an adequate account of self-deception can be formulated on the basis of assuming a nontransparent nature of consciousness, for reasons of parsimony there is little need to consider the nonunitary view, as this perspective entails the first assumption along with another, more drastic one.

On the basis of the assimilation thesis, it is argued that to be self-deceived, an individual must hold two contradictory beliefs at the same time. Furthermore, the assimilation thesis requires that the individual who holds these beliefs be unaware that he holds one of them. If a nontransparent view of consciousness is assumed, then there is no longer a paradox. The issue that remains, however, is whether these criteria are both necessary and sufficient for ascribing self-deception.

There are reasons for claiming that these criteria are not sufficient. If Jones believes that the morning star is very large and Jones also believes that the evening star is very small, Jones believes in two contradictory propositions at the same time. However, Jones does not realize that the morning star and the evening star are the same star, that is, Venus. In situations such as this, one is more likely to attribute ignorance or error to Jones rather than self-deception.

The illustration points to one aspect of the insufficiency of the criteria currently offered. The notion of self-deception implies an active as opposed to a passive organization of beliefs on the part of the self-deceived individual. The term *self-deception* has meaning only when it is claimed that the failure to notice or to be aware of one of the beliefs is motivated and not happenstance.

> The role of motives in self-deception has been to some extent ignored or played down in recent discussions of the topic, yet it is surely crucial. It is, for example, not clear what could be meant by, or what justification there could be for, speaking of somebody as deceiving himself if it were at the same time contended that what he was said to be deceiving himself about was a matter of total indifference to him, in no way related to his wants, fears, hopes and so forth: could we, e.g., intelligibly talk about "disinterested" or "'gratuitous" self-deception? (Gardiner, 1970, p. 242)

The tie between "motivation" and self-deception complicates the issue considerably. One can not simply assert that self-deception involves motivated behavior. One must attempt to specify the role of motives.

The account we wish to advance here claims that in instances of self-deception, individuals are motivated in their denial of holding one belief as opposed to another. The act of not noticing a particular belief is a motivated act and leads to differential outcomes for the individual (Irwin, 1971). As Fingarette (1969) has pointed out, when purposefulness is attributed to an act of forgetting or not noticing in the self-deception situation, it must also be claimed that the very act is not retrievable or noticed. An individual who holds two contradictory beliefs, denies to the self or fails to notice one of these beliefs, and yet is aware of having made such a denial or failure to notice would be a queer individual and an unlikely candidate for a self-deception ascription. It must be claimed, therefore, that the acts of deciding between which beliefs to endorse or which beliefs not to notice are not themselves reflected upon. Just as one cannot go to sleep while reflecting upon going to sleep, one can not determine between beliefs to be denied while reflecting upon the determination. The assumption of a nontransparent nature to consciousness further contributes to the viability of such a view.

Although the terms used to discuss the motivational aspects of self-deception have been words like *deny, determination, notice,* etc., we do not claim that the "motivated act" is intentional. Between formulations like that of Demos (1960), who failed to attribute purposefulness to the act of not noticing, and that of Fingarette (1969), who attributed full-blown intentionality, there is room for a less extreme position. The act of noticing a belief or of originally deciding between beliefs may be motivated in the sense that such acts lead to differential outcomes for the individual. However, it is not necessarily claimed to be a type of act that is planned, considered, or expected by an individual.

Aside from being less extreme than either of the other positions, there are positive grounds for asserting this view. One of the differences between lying and deception expression statements is that intentionality is necessarily associated with lying but not with deception. Smith can not intelligibly say, "I unintentionally lied to Jones." Smith has made a meaningful statement, however, when he says, "I unintentionally deceived Jones." Since statements of this sort can be made, it is apparent that intentionality is not a necessary condition for acts of other-deception. In line with the assimilation thesis, intentionality is not considered a necessary criterion for ascribing self-deception. By the same type of analysis, it can be shown that motives are necessary constituents of self-deception. Just as Smith cannot intelligibly claim, "There was no reason or cause for my lying to you," he also cannot claim, "There was no reason or cause for my deceiving you." This is not to argue that individuals, while self-deceived, are aware of their motives for self-deception. Rather, this demonstrates that self-deceptive acts are motivated and that when individuals break through self-deception, they will attribute motivational accounts to their behavior.

In summary, there are four criteria necessary and sufficient for ascribing self-deception:

1. The individual holds two contradictory beliefs (p and not-p).
2. These two contradictory beliefs are held simultaneously.
3. The individual is not aware of holding one of the beliefs (p or not-p).
4. The act that determines which belief is and which belief is not subject to awareness is a motivated act.

These four criteria are necessary but are not sufficient for ascribing repression. It has been argued (Holmes, 1974) that repression involves motivated selective forgetting. The belief (p) that is "forgotten" is not lost but is stored in the unconscious. Psychoanalytic theory has elaborated on the types of defense mechanisms that individuals employ to assert various forms of the belief that not-p on a conscious level. Thus, the concept of repression entails that an individual simultaneously hold two contradictory beliefs. The fact that the belief p is not subject to awareness and that its "forgetting" is motivated satisfies the third and fourth criteria for ascribing self-deception. However, the ascription of repression requires the additional claim that the belief that is not subject to awareness is stored in an unconscious. The unconscious is a functionally independent control system, capable of intentional influence on behavior. In this respect, the concept of repression entails that consciousness is not only nontransparent but also nonunitary. It is for these reasons that we believe that the demonstration of the existence of self-deception is logically prior to a demonstration of the existence of repression and, further, that such a demonstration in the case of repression is likely to involve a more arduous adventure.

An obvious candidate for providing instances of self-deception is the situation in which, like our puppy, individuals are confronted with aspects of themselves that they find difficult to accept. We will presently review the effects of self-confrontation in order to provide a foundation for our operationalization of the criteria for ascribing self-deception.

III. EMPIRICAL INVESTIGATIONS OF SELF-CONFRONTATION

In recent years, there has been a growing interest in the self-confrontation experience. One group of researchers has investigated the implications of self-confrontation for areas associated with social psychology. The effects of manipulations that either direct attention inward, to the self, or outward, to the environment, have been studied in relation to conformity, social facilitation, cognitive dissonance, communication sets, and attribution phenomena (e.g. Carver, 1974; Duval and Wicklund, 1972, 1973; Ickes, Wicklund and Ferris, 1973; Insko, Worshel, Songer, and Arnold, 1973; Martens, 1969; Storms, 1973; Wicklund and Duval, 1971; Wicklund and Ickes, 1972). Other investigators have been concerned with the psychophysiological, affective, and cognitive correlates of the self-confrontation experience (Holzman and Rousey, 1966; Holzman, Rousey, and Snyder, 1966;

Olivos, 1967; Rousey and Holzman, 1967; Sackeim, 1974). Self-confrontation outside of conscious awareness (Castaldo and Holzman, 1967, 1969; Huntley, 1940; Wolff, 1943) and the connection between voice playback and vocal masking (Holmes and Holzman, 1966; Holzman and Rousey, 1970; Klein, 1965; Klein and Wolitzky, 1970) have also been investigated. Finally, the effects of self-confrontation on therapeutic outcome in clinical settings has been reported in case studies and in experimental investigations (e.g. Alkire and Brunse, 1974; Bailey and Sowder, 1970; Boyd and Sisney, 1967; Danet, 1968; Fryrear, Nuell, and Ridley, 1974; Paden, Himelstein, and Paul, 1974). In this section, we review many of these findings and the interpretations that they have sparked.

A. Psychophysiological and Psychological Correlates

There is a good deal of evidence that indicates that self-confrontation leads to increased autonomic arousal. Most of this work has involved auditory feedback of subjects' own voices. Holzman, Rousey, and Snyder (1966) had male subjects listen to a tape of 20 different male voices, each repeating the same neutral 20-word sentence. The individual subjects' own voices were dubbed into the 12th position, and the psychophysiological measures included galvanic skin responses (GSR), frontalis muscle electromyograms (EMG), and finger plethysmograms. The results indicated that subjects showed significantly greater physiological reactivity to their own voices than to the voices of others, despite the fact that in a postexperimental interview, only 8 out of 20 subjects reported that they had recognized their own voices.

Olivos (1967) replicated the Holzman et al. (1966) experiment with a larger sample. A 1–2 sec recording (the first three words in Holzman et al.'s 20-word sentence) was made for 110 subjects. Each subject listened to 20 recordings, with their own voice recorded in the 12th position. Olivos took five measures of psychophysiological reactivity: response time between the beginning of the response and response maximum for GSR and galvanic skin potential (GSP), response amplitude of the maximum response to a stimulus as compared to prestimulus level for GSR and GSP, and electroencephalographic (EEG) alpha wave blocking. For all five measures, there was greater psychophysiological reactivity following the tape of the subjects' own voices than after the tape of the voices of the others, regardless of whether the subjects recognized their own voices. The Olivos experiment was an improvement over the Holzman et al. (1966) experiment in that the subjects were required to state 15 seconds after every playback whether the recording was of themselves or not, rather than in a postexperimental interview. Under these conditions 55% of the subjects correctly identified their own voices.

Gur and Sackeim (1976) presented subjects with 30 stimulus voices ranging in temporal duration from 2 to 24 sec. The voice of the self appeared five times, and the subjects' task was to make self–other identifications as soon as possible after stimulus onset. Under these conditions, GSR reactivity to voice of the self was greater than reactivity to voices of others, regardless of the correctness of identifications (Figure 1). Sackeim (1974) presented subjects with videotapes of innocuous interviews of themselves and a stranger. In this study as well, stimuli of the self were associated with greater GSR reactivity.

In every study that we are aware of (cf. Dickinson and Ray, 1965; Murray, 1963; Verwoerdt, Nowlin and Agnello, 1965) using a variety of psychophysiological measures, arousal levels were higher after

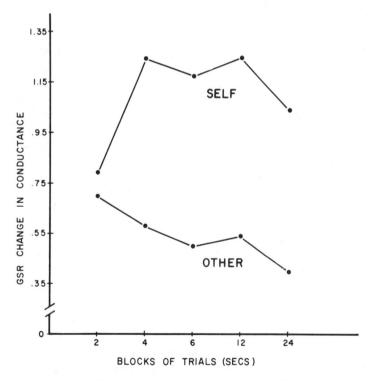

FIGURE 1. Levels of psychophysiological reactivity (in micromhos) for audio stimuli of self and other, as a function of block of trials.

presentation of the self. Stating that the self-confrontation experience leads to increased autonomic activity is of little value unless the type of emotional arousal that is produced can be specified.

Although it has been argued that on the basis of psychophysiological data alone specific emotional reactions cannot be specified (e.g., Lader and Marks, 1971), recent work on the patterning of psychophysiological indices suggests that this claim may be unwarranted (Schwartz, Fair, Salt, Mandel, and Klerman, 1976). The findings that the experience of self-confrontation results in gross changes in activity levels in several response systems should provide an impetus for the examination of patterns of psychophysiological changes, and with such research, we should expect a clearer understanding of the psychological changes that are produced by confrontation situations.

There have been several experiments employing self-confrontation methodology that have investigated the psychological changes within subjects that occur during the confrontation. Although these studies have, in the main, used double-blind procedures to determine loadings on the dependent measures, only relative confidence is justified in the interpretation of individual experiments because of the unknown validity of the dependent measures employed. However, taken as a whole, these studies have produced consistent results.

Holzman et al. (1966) had subjects free-associate before and after listening to their own voices. The task was to produce as many words as possible, as quickly as they came to mind. The results indicated that after listening to their own voices, subjects produced fewer words than before the playback and fewer than a group that had free-associated after listening to a stranger's voice. Self-confronted subjects tended to associate in safe, mechanical ways. The words produced referred to objects in the room or to neutral topics. Emotional words became significantly less frequent.

Holzman and Rousey (1966) used an interview technique to elicit verbal responses after self-confrontation; 32 subjects heard their own voice playback and 14 subjects comprised a control group, which heard a recording of a stranger's voice. Subjects in the experimental group listened to their own voices until they evidenced an emotive response, generally within 5 sec of playback onset. The tape was then turned off, and an experimenter elicited a verbal report by repeating the remarks made by the subject or by pointing out that the subject had made some facial expression. With the control group, in whom affective reactions were rare, the experimenter stopped the tape after 5 sec and initiated a response by inquiring, "What occurs to you?"

Transcripts of subjects' responses were coded by the use of two scoring schemes, voice confrontation responses (VCR) and Mahl's

(1959) speech disturbance categories (SDC). The results indicated that the experimental group showed more affective reaction, primarily oriented to voice qualities and not syntax or grammar. Experimental subjects also significantly noted more discrepancies between what they expected to hear and what they heard, and they reacted with more negative words.

To guard against the effects of experimenter bias, the static nature of the scoring tests, and the fact that the disruptive influence of the self-confrontation experience may be too transitory to be measured in an interview, Holzman and Rousey (1966) did an additional study with one experimental and two control groups. All groups filled in three equivalent forms of Osgood, Suci, and Tannenbaum's (1957) semantic differential, rating the concept "my voice" (Coyne and Holzman, 1966). The exmperimental group filled in one form before hearing a tape of their own voices, directly after hearing a 5-sec playback, and again 5 min later. One control group recorded their own voices but heard a stranger's voice, and the second control group simply filled in the three forms, without recording or hearing any tapes. The results indicated that on the three factors measured by the semantic differential (evaluative, potency, and activity factors), the experimental group differed from the control groups only on Form 2 (filled in directly after hearing their own voices) and only on the evaluative and activity factors. The experimental group moved significantly toward the negative end of the evaluation factor and the passive end of the activity factor.

From these experiments and others like them (e.g., Rousey and Holzman, 1968; Holzman, Berger, and Rousey, 1967), the view had been advanced that verbal behavior, aside from its expressive functions in communication, also has a monitoring or editing function. When self-confronted, the individual consciously perceives aspects of self that have not been completely censored.

> The voice-confrontation experience suggests that when we are given the opportunity to hear ourselves as others do, to regard the voice as a percept rather than as a mediator of expression, we may hear not only the results of the censoring but what it is that we are attempting to censor. We are assuming then that part of the disturbance that people experience when they hear their own voices is accounted for by the unsuccessful or incomplete editing of aspects of themselves which they did not consciously intend to express and which they now hear in the recording. (Holzman and Rousey, 1966, p. 85)

Obviously, these assertions are a major jump from the evidence so far examined. One might argue that there is a far more simple explanation to account for the physiological and psychological correlates of the self-confrontation. When one hears one's voice from a tape-recording playback, one does not hear the same thing as when one listens directly to one's voice. When one listens directly to one's voice, the sound is equally mediated by bone and air conduction (Bekesy, 1949). When one is listening to a tape recording, bone mediation is largely eliminated and voice quality alters. However, some reasons have been offered that suggest a rejection of this alternative explanation.

Holzman, Berger, and Rousey (1967) had subjects whose first language was Spanish and who were also fluent in English but who had first learned English after age 16 record tapes of their voices in both languages. The interview technique described above, with VCR and SDC scoring schemes, was again employed. The results followed the predictions of the experimenters in that subjects responded with more affective and defensive reactions to tapes of their Spanish-speaking voices than to the tape of their voices in their second language.

Rousey and Holzman (1968) replicated their earlier study (Holzman and Rousey, 1966), using scores on the semantic differential as the dependent variables, but had experimental and control subjects listen to either their own or others' voices under five degrees of distortion. Distortion was accomplished by the filtering out of selected frequencies. The responses of the male portion of the sample were unreliable. The results for female subjects, however, indicated that consistent disruption and discrepancy effects to their own voices as opposed to the voices of others were maintained regardless of the degree of distortion.

These two experiments were interpreted as ruling out any explanation of the self-confrontation experience that rests purely on the differences in the physical properties of recorded and natural speech. That the results do rule out such an interpretation is not apparent. The fact that female subjects do not show differential reactions to degrees of distortion is not in itself proof that distortion *per se* is not a significant element in determining responses. Likewise, the fact that Holzman *et al.* (1967) predicted that subjects would show greater affective reactions to speech in their native language does not demonstrate with certainty that it was not the distortion of that speech that was the significant variable, particularly when subjects were more practiced in hearing recorded feedback in their acquired language (Holzman *et al.*, 1967, p. 427). Since there is no positive evidence that the psychophysiological and psychological correlates of self-confrontation are a function of the distortion in recorded voices, the issue is not resolved.

If it could be shown that the "distortion" explanation should be rejected, this would not provide any direct support for Holzman and Rousey's interpretation of emotional reactions to self-confrontation. The significance of the experiments discussed above is limited by their reliance on dependent measures that may have only limited validity. Dibner (1958) found only suggestive evidence linking the SDC and anxiety. Rousey and Holzman (1968) argued that the semantic differential may not be appropriate for men. In addition, before a view that verbal behavior serves a monitoring and editing function can be accepted, it is necessary to provide evidence that without the availability of verbal feedback, the monitoring function is inhibited.

B. Vocal Masking Experiments

The standard methodology of vocal occluding studies is to fit subjects with earphones that give off white noise, which prevents them from hearing their own voices. An obvious constraint on this technique is that it cannot be firmly established whether any changes in behavior are due to the occluding of the voice or the activating and/ or aversive effects of the white noise. This issue is particularly significant since in the experiments to be discussed below, Klein and Wolitzky (1970) and Holzman and Rousey (1970), white noise masking (WNM) was set at levels of 100 db and 98 db, respectively. However, there is no apparent or ethically justifiable technique now available to occlude an individual's voice except under noise conditions.

Granting this drawback, it can still be ascertained whether denying vocal feedback with noise leads to a decrease in the editing function of overt speech. Experiments in self-confrontation have indicated that when the voice becomes a percept there are increases in negative evaluations and defensive reactions and a constriction of emotional content. One would expect that for Holzman and Rousey's (1966) claims to be supported, the opposite trends should occur under vocal occluding.

Klein (1965) and Klein and Wolitzky (1970) have provided evidence for this position. In the latter experiment, subjects were given an imagery task under WNM and normal conditions. The task consisted of the presentation of slides of two de Chirico surrealist paintings, each for 10 sec. After each slide presentation, there was a 3-min response period during which subjects were asked to describe what they saw and anything else that came to mind. They were not required to stay with the initial picture. The scoring of the responses was in several categories of content and formal speech characteristics.

The content categories were adapted from Holt and Havel's (1960) method of content analysis, with the major two categories being unweighted drive (all ideational themes expressing appetitive and aggressive states) and weighted drive (with greater emphasis on blatant, unsocial drive expressions). A number of subsidiary content categories were also examined. The formal speech characteristics were measured by an adaptation of Mahl's SDC with "ah" stammers and speech editing forming the major grouping. A third category, language editing, was added by Klein and Wolitsky (1970).

The results indicated that under WNM, compared to normal conditions, there were significant increases in unweighted and weighted drive, loosened self-boundaries, and morality references. In general the masking condition produced an amplification of associative content, particularly in relation to appetitive and drive ideation. The findings on formal speech characteristics showed that the amount of "ah" utterances and speech editing were negatively correlated with the amount of weighted-drive expression. Language editing, which is mainly a measure of the qualifications on content, was negatively correlated with drive expression. These results, coupled with the fact that under WNM subjects were able to perform successfully tasks normally susceptible to interference from arousal (e.g., correct color naming for stimuli discrepantly labeled, subtracting backwards from 100 by 3s), provide some support for the view that vocal masking leads to disinhibition of content in overt speech and, therefore, a suppression of a monitoring function.

In Holzman and Rousey's (1970) experiment, the main dependent variables were responses to Thematic Apperception Test (TAT) cards and Holzman Inkblot Test (HIT) responses under WNM and normal conditions. The TAT responses were scored by trained double-blind judges for impulsive and defensive expression. The HIT was scored for the use of color as a determinant. The results indicated that generally with both tests the effects of WNM were enhanced when WNM followed normal conditions rather than when it preceded them. In either order, however, subjects showed greater impulse-dominated themes under WNM than under normal conditions. Predictions concerning the HIT responses were verified only for women, who had more color responses under WNM than under normal conditions. Men showed no effects for WNM on color response production in one experiment and a decrease in productivity in a replication. Overall, the authors pointed out that there is no evidence that WNM interferes with thought organization or reality attainment. It does appear that WNM increases drive-related fantasies, and the authors viewed this as supporting their contentions concerning the monitoring function of speech.

As with the experiments on self-confrontation, in these instances there may be questions concerning the reliability and validity of the tests used as dependent measures. Indirect support for the findings presented above comes from an experiment that used more objective scoring techniques. Holmes and Holzman (1966) had subjects talk about an embarassing situation in nonsense language, under WNM and normal conditions, in a counterbalanced design. The dependent variables were length of speaking time, latency to first utterance, average number of syllables spoken per 15 sec and the number of English words spoken. The results indicated that under WNM, subjects spoke for a greater length of time, the average number of syllables was larger, and more English words intruded into their stories. Latency was not significantly different between the two conditions. Whereas the experiments reported above were principally concerned with the effects of WNM on disinhibiting the content of speech, this experiment indicated that WNM may influence other variables in a disinhibiting manner.

C. The Aversiveness of Self-Confrontation

The evidence reviewed so far indicates that feedback of the self leads to autonomic arousal, negative self-evaluations, defensive reactions, and constrictions on ideational content. The evidence from vocal masking experiments indicates that WNM is associated with greater drive-related fantasies and a general disinhibition of ideational content. Subjects' phenomenological reports of what they experience during self-confrontation generally describe negative affective states of increased anxiety. One might expect, therefore, that self-confrontation would be aversive and that subjects would avoid situations that would elicit self-directed attention.

In a study that examined this issue, Duval, Wicklund, and Fine (cited by Duval and Wicklund, 1972, pp. 16–21), by manipulating beliefs about the self and self-confrontation conditions, found that individuals avoid self-confrontation when given negative feedback about the self. Subjects reported to experimenters and were told that the experimenters required from them only some demographic background information and requested that they participate afterwards in a different experiment concerned with visual perception. The background information was necessary to complete a follow-up related to findings concerning creativity and intelligence tests given to subjects weeks earlier. After answering six questions, subjects were given false feedback on the results of those tests. Half the subjects were told they were in the upper 10th percentile of their college class and half were informed that they were in the lower 10th percentile. Following this, subjects were led to a cubicle for the perception experiment. The subjects were seated at a table, and half of them had a mirror facing them and a television camera directed at the backs of their heads. The other half had the back of the mirror facing them and the camera turned toward a corner of the room. All were informed that the mirror and the camera would be used in the experiment. The experimenter faked surprise that the individual running the perception experiment was not in the cubicle. The subjects were requested to wait about 5 minutes (a clock was on the table) for the individual running the perception experiment to arrive. After that time, subjects were instructed to look for the experimenter in another room in the building. The dependent measure was the latency of the subjects' departure from the cubicle. No subject was allowed to wait more than 10 minutes.

The results indicated that subjects who were in the self-confrontation condition (mirror and camera facing them) and who were also in the high cognitive-discrepancy condition (negative false feedback) left the room significantly earlier than subjects in any of the other three combinations. Avoidance was determined by the interaction of level of discrepancy and self-confrontation condition.

Gibbons and Wicklund (cited in Wicklund, 1975) found that when male subjects experienced social rejection by a female confederate, they spent less time in listening to tapes of their own voices than subjects who had received highly positive feedback. Avoidance of self-confrontation was interpreted as particularly likely when subjects are characterized by internal negative discrepancies.

A difficulty that has characterized much of the research on self-confrontation is that the direction of the subjects' attention has been inferred only on the basis of experimental manipulations. It has been assumed that when subjects are positioned in front of a mirror or listen to tape playbacks of their own voices, attention is focused inward. Two experiments reported by Davis and Brock (1975) provide some evidence that this assumption is valid and that self-confrontation can be aversive.

Davis and Brock (1975) had subjects attempt to determine the English translations of pronouns in foreign languages. Self-confrontation manipulations involved in one experiment the presence of absence of a camera directly facing the subjects and in the second experiment the positioning of subjects so that they faced either the front or the back of a mirror. In both experiments, subjects were given either positive or negative false feedback concerning their perform- ance on a bogus test of creativity prior to the experiment. The results indicated that under positive feedback conditions, the self-confronted subjects emitted more first-person pronouns than the other groups. There were no differences between positive and negative false feed- back groups in the no-camera and no-mirror conditions. Self-con- fronted subjects given negative false feedback emitted fewer first- person pronouns that self-confronted subjects given positive false feedback.

The Duval, Wicklund, and Fine (as cited in Duval and Wicklund, 1972), Gibbons and Wicklund (1976), and Davis and Brock (1975) studies suggest that self-confrontation can be aversive and can lead to avoidance responses. Although Duval and Wicklund (1972) have argued that negative affect is invariably produced when individuals are self-confronted, it appears that experimental manipulations of congitions concerning the self are effective in determining whether or not self-confrontation will be avoided.

D. Social Psychological Effects of Self-Confrontation

Interest in the self-confrontation experience would be minimal if the influence of the experience was both transitory and restricted to a few physiological and psychological changes. Holzman and Rousey (1966) noted that reactions to "my voice" on semantic differentials given five minutes after the subjects heard brief playbacks of their own voices returned to prestimulus levels. The authors viewed the affective changes due to self-confrontation as short-lived, with reac- commodation occurring quickly. However, there is a good deal of evidence indicating that for a range of social behaviors, self-confronta- tion has dramatic effects. It may be the case that evaluations of one's voice return quickly to prestimulus levels, but there is also reason to assert that other consequences of self-confrontation are quite broad and continue for some period of time.

Duval and Wicklund (1972), in their book *A Theory of Objective Self Awareness*, have presented the most comprehensive theory of the social psychological effects of self-confrontation. They have argued that stimuli in the environment will focus an individual's attention either outward, toward objects in the environment, or inward, on the self. Attention directed outward is labeled *subjective self-awareness*. When attention is directed inward and the self is perceived as an object, the state is labeled *objective self-awareness*. Duval and Wicklund have claimed that the direction of attention cannot be simultaneously focused on the environment and the self. In this, they differ from Holzman, (e.g., Holzman and Rousey, 1966), who argued that individuals are continually self-monitoring. In addition, Duval and Wicklund have asserted that when an individual is in a state of objective self-awareness, the individual will evaluate perceptions of the self and behavior in terms of the individual's standards of correctness. This examination will generally produce discrepancies between perceptions and standards of correctness and result in negative affect. Similar to cognitive dissonance theory (Festinger, 1957), Duval and Wicklund's theory assumes that discrepancies or dissonance lead to their own reduction. In Duval and Wicklund's framework, the individual either avoids objective self-awareness by distracting attention (and thereby become subjectively self-aware) or attempts to behave in a way that is consistent with the standards of correctness.

Duval and Wicklund have drawn on several of their own experiments, which use self-confrontation techniques, and many experiments by other investigators, which may be interpreted as manipulating these dimensions, to demonstrate how their theory can account for distinct types of social behavior. Several studies have recently been published that further test the adequacy of this theory (e.g., Insko, Worchel, Songer, and Arnold, 1973; Liebling and Shaver, 1973; Storms, 1973).

These experimental investigations have indicated that the phenomena of communication sets and deindividuation, as well as conformity, attribution processes, cognitive dissonance, and social facilitation, may be mediated by direction of attention. We do not attempt here to evaluate these studies or the theories they have generated. The interested reader is directed instead to reviews of this literature by Duval and Wicklund (1972) and by Wicklund (1975). However, it is quite clear that social psychological effects of self-confrontation indicate that the direction of attention of conscious awareness may have broad implications for behavior. As many psychological experiments employ manipulations, such as the presence of an audience, which may alter direction of attention and promote self-confrontation, the investigation and control for such effects would seem requisite.

E. *Self-Confrontation and States of Awareness*

The issue concerning whether the correlates and consequences of self-confrontation differ as a function of the state of awareness of confronted individuals has not received much empirical investigation. One would think, however, that states of awareness do exert powerful influences on reactions to self-confrontation. In dreams, it is often reported that the central character is the self, yet it does not appear that the affective and cognitive reactions found when individuals are forced to attend selectively to the self in waking states characterize what occurs during dreaming.

Castaldo and Holzman (1967, 1969) have provided some evidence for this view. In two experiments, they presented voice tapes of self and others to sleeping subjects. The tapes consisted of four neutral words, played on a tape loop. EEG activity and gross body movement were measures of stage of sleep. The dependent variables were the dream reports of subjects, free associations after dreaming, and dream mentations measured on control nights, nights when the voice of another was presented, and nights when the voice of the self was presented. In the original experiment and its replication, Castaldo and Holzman found that double-blind ratings of the dreams of subjects after hearing their own voices were heavily weighted on assertive, active, and independent dimensions. The dreams following the voices of others were weighted on passive and dependent dimensions.

The total number of subjects in both studies was small ($N = 20$), making for only relative confidence in these results. Nevertheless, the uniformity of the differential reactions of subjects to experimental conditions was striking. Although the dependent measures used in these studies do not correspond to those that have been investigated in awake subjects, the flavor of these results suggests that affective and cognitive reactions to self-confrontation during sleeping states are different from, if not opposite to, the reactions to self-confrontation during waking states.

F. Individual Differences in Reactions to Self-Confrontation

Duval and Wicklund's (1972) theory of objective self-awareness places little emphasis on the role of individual differences in predicting reactions to self-confrontation. Although they have acknowledged that individual differences may exist, they view these differences as extending only to the frequency and duration of the individual's self-confrontation experiences. Even these factors, it is maintained, are of limited theoretical interest:

> This is not to deny that such differences exist, in that some people surely spend a greater proportion of time focusing on themselves than others. But theoretically these differences have as their source the person's immediate situation and anticipation of situations that arouse the state;

thus, in the last analysis, it is the environment we should inspect if we
want to know something about the frequency and duration of someone's
objective self-awareness. (p. 222)

Experiments that have manipulated the aversiveness of self-
confrontation and the effects of self-confrontation on task performance
suggest, however, that individual differences in personality variables
may be significant in predicting the direction and the intensity of the
effects of self-confrontation. Studies by Duval, Wicklund, and Fine
(cited in Duval and Wicklund, 1972, pp. 16–21) and Davis and Brock
(1975) found that attention to the self is avoided when subjects are
given false feedback about personal attributes and are self-confronted.
Liebling and Shaver (1973) found that self-directed attention has a
detrimental effect on task performance when subjects are under high
evaluatory conditions. If individuals differ in the degree to which they
hold discrepant cognitions about the self or in the way they assess the
evaluatory nature of situations, one would expect that they would also
differ in their reactions to self-confrontation.

An experiment by Sackeim (1974) was designed to test the notion
that individual differences in cognitive discrepancy are related to the
intensity of reactions to self-confrontation. *Cognitive discrepancy* was
defined as any conflict within an individual concerning an aspect of
self. The individual may perceive a conflict between the self-ideal and
the self-image, the self-image and the objective self, the objective self
and moral values, etc. In this perspective, anything that an individual
worries about, dislikes, or is dissatisfied with concerning the self
would count as an instance of cognitive discrepancy.

Previous to the experimental session, subjects had filled out the
Eysenck Personality Inventory (EPI) (Eysenck and Eysenck, 1963) and
the assimilation scale (McReynolds and Acker, 1966), a test of trait
anxiety. Ten items from the neuroticism scale of the EPI had been
judged to load on the dimension of cognitive discrepancy. During the
experiment, subjects viewed videotapes of innocuous interviews of
themselves and a stranger, in counterbalanced order. As expected,
individuals showed significantly greater GSR reactivity in the self
condition, as opposed to the other condition. Neither the complete
neuroticism score, the extraversion score, nor the anxiety score
predicted levels of reactivity to the self. However, subjects who scored
above the mean on the cognitive discrepancy measure showed significantly greater reactivity than subjects below the mean. Furthermore,
double-blind ratings of subjects' postexperimental responses to a
questionnaire concerned with reactions to the video stimuli indicated
that those subjects with negative reactions to the self evidenced
greater reactivity to stimuli of the self. These subjects also loaded

significantly higher on cognitive discrepancy than subjects with positive or neutral reactions to the self. There is then some evidence to support the notion that discrepancies between individuals' perceptions of the self and their expectations lead to the psychophysiological changes characteristic of self-confrontation and that their loading on a variable, purporting to measure cognitive discrepancy, predicts the intensity of such reactivity.

Recently, it has been proposed that the frequency and duration of states of self-awareness may reflect individual differences in dispositional variables. Fenigstein, Scheier, and Buss (1975) have developed a scale of self-consciousness, which contains reliable subscales measuring tendencies to attend to inner thoughts and feelings (private self-consciousness), tendencies to have an awareness of self as a social object (public self-consciousness), and tendencies to experience discomfort in the presence of others (social anxiety). Experimental investigations of the validity of these measures and their usefulness in predicting outcomes of self-confrontation have only just begun. The issues examined by Fenigstein *et al.* (1975) are distinct from those examined in the Sackeim (1974) study. Whereas the former investigators have been concerned with individual differences in the susceptibility to experiencing self-confrontation as a function of types of stimuli, the latter investigation was concerned with individual differences in variables that predict the intensity of reactions to self-confrontation, once attention is directed to the self.

G. A Theoretical Integration of Studies of Self-Confrontation

There have been numerous investigations of the correlates and consequences of self-confrontation. To date, the results of studies that have examined psychophysiological and psychological effects of self-directed attention have not been integrated with the results of studies that have centered on the social behavioral effects of self-confrontation. A theoretical integration of the diverse findings in these areas will hopefully contribute to an understanding of the processes underlying self-confrontation and have significant implications for the study of the nature of consciousness.

Holzman (e.g., Holzman and Rousey, 1966) and Duval and Wicklund (1972) have viewed self-confrontation manipulations as heightening self-monitoring. This position is supported by evidence from a number of studies. For instance, Davis and Brock (1975) found that subjects use more first-person pronouns when guessing the nature of pronouns in a foreign language if they are given positive false feedback about the self and are self-confronted. Pryor, Gibbons, and Wicklund (cited in Wicklund, 1975) obtained low correlations between subjects' reports of their sociability and behavioral measurements. However, when subjects made ratings while facing a mirror, the correlations were much higher. The changes in self-esteem found after self-confrontation manipulations (e.g., Boyd and Sisney, 1967; Ickes, Wicklund, and Ferris, 1973; Wicklund, 1975) further suggest that individuals attend to salient aspects of the self when self-confronted.

A question that comes to the fore concerns the fact that in normal conversation individuals can be said to be continually self-monitoring. The self-regulatory role of speech has been emphasized by theorists in several areas of psychology. Freud (1895/1966) argued that ideas are engendered with reality by their coding in overt speech. Vygotsky (1962) maintained that speech serves a central mediating function in connecting thoughts to actions. Indeed, Luria (1961) has written, "speech enters integrally into the structure of mental processes and . . . it is a powerful means of regulation of human behavior" (p. 50). One wonders why the cognitive, affective, and behavioral consequences of self-confrontation do not seem to take place during the normal circumstances of self-monitoring. Duval and Wicklund (1972) assumed that attention is discontinuously distributed either to features of the environment or to the self. Self-confrontation manipulations direct attention to the self, and self-awareness, in their formulation, is an all-or-none phenomenon, differing between individuals only in duration and frequency. In this respect, Duval and Wicklund's theory is incompatible with the notion that, at least on some level, individuals may be continually self-monitoring. Holzman (e.g., Holzman and Rousey, 1966), on the other hand, argued that self-confrontation heightens ongoing self-monitoring processes. An analogy related to this position is that of an individual who is writing a paper and the same individual proofreading the paper. In the first case, the individual is principally concerned with the work of expression but is also aware of what is being written, although mistakes will be made. The proofreader, who is freer to deploy attention to the material, is likely to find errors that escaped the writer. The Holzman position is more amenable to the view that in everyday conversation we are engaged in a self-monitoring process.

The aspects of the self that are being monitored during self-confrontation have not been directly investigated. However, an examination of the cognitive, affective, and behavioral correlates and consequences of self-confrontation and the types of manipulations that affect their expression may provide some indication of the content of the monitoring process. We know that self-confrontation is associated with increased physiological arousal, negative self-evaluations, and constrictions of ideational themes. Furthermore, self-confrontation is frequently aversive, and the extent to which self-confrontation is avoided or interferes with task performance can be manipulated if the subjects are given negative false feedback about the self or if they are placed in highly evaluative situations. Taken as a whole, the evidence suggests that individuals when self-confronted perceive aspects of themselves that they do not like. It is further suggested that the perception of such discrepancies is aversive and is reflected in heightened anxiety. This position is congruent with the findings of Sackeim (1974), which indicated that individual differences in cognitive discrepancy, a measure of the degree of internal conflict, predicted individual differences in the magnitude of psychophysiological reactivity to self-confrontation and the type of self-evaluations subjects made after such confrontation.

The claim that the self-confronted individual perceives internal discrepancies is in harmony with the theories advanced by Holzman and by Duval and Wicklund. Holzman went further to claim that the perceived discrepancies are of a specific nature. He argued that the self-confronted individual perceives aspects of the self that are censored incompletely and are not expressed intentionally. However, Holzman did not provide any direct evidence for this view, and the finding that WNM is associated with a disinhibition of drive expression only marginally supports it. The effects of self-confrontation manipulations and WNM cannot be directly compared because of the asymmetry in these procedures. While self-confrontation manipulations presumably direct attention to the self, WNM not only interferes with such attention but establishes a new stimulus context.

Duval and Wicklund also presented a more specific view as to the nature of the discrepancies perceived during self-confrontation. They argued that individuals when self-confronted examine the differences between actual and ideal or aspired-for levels of performance. They also did not provide any direct evidence to support this interpretation, but the fact that self-confrontation manipulations can enhance task performance, cognitive dissonance reduction, and transmitter effects furnishes some indirect support for their view. However, in the self-confrontation manipulations employed in the series of studies by Holzman and co-workers, by Sackeim (1974), and by Gur and Sackeim (1976), subjects were not required to engage in any tasks during or after self-confrontation, and yet pronounced effects were demonstrated. It may be that the types of discrepancies proposed by Duval and Wicklund come into play when self-confronted individuals are required to engage in specific tasks during or immediately after self-confrontation. Indeed, if self-confrontation is viewed as heightening self-monitoring processes, then any behavior that can be evaluated by the self-confronted individual is likely to be influenced by the self-confrontation manipulations. We suggest that in the Duval and Wicklund experiments, the discrepancies that were perceived were partly a function of the contexts in which self-confronted subjects were placed.

As those psychologists who have written about self-confrontation have agreed that the self-confronted individual perceives discrepancies of a cognitive nature, it is not surprising that increased anxiety is an outcome of the confrontation. Brown (1965) has noted that all balance theories claim that dissonance is arousing. The view that anxiety is a consequence of failure to integrate information into an adequate self-concept or a predictive model is central to the ideas of Goldstein (1939), Robers (1951), May (1950), and Mandler and Watson (1966). Since it is well documented that anxiety exerts a curvilinear effect on performance, it is questionable whether one needs to postulate that the facilitating effects of self-confrontation on task performance are a direct function of individuals perceiving discrepancies between actual and desired levels of performance and that decrements are a function of individuals directing too much attention to these discrepancies. A more parsimonious account may be to view the levels of anxiety engendered by attention to internal discrepancies as influencing levels of performance.

While it may be true that levels of anxiety mediate task performance, there is little reason to believe that increased anxiety directly enhances conformity, transmitter, and cognitive dissonance effects. In accounting for these effects, Duval and Wicklund may have overlooked some relevant findings from their own studies. Duval and Wicklund (1972, 1973) found that self-confrontation increases attribution of personal responsibility for behaviors with positive and negative outcomes. This conceptual readiness for self-confronted individuals to assume responsibility for behavior may be a function of the general principle that individuals attribute greater causal efficacy to stimuli that are focal in attention (Arkin and Duval, 1975; Storms, 1973), or it may be due to the fact that when self-confronted, individuals perceive aspects of themselves that they find surprising. When confidence in self-knowledge is shaken, individuals may be more willing to view the self as responsible for a diverse range of behaviors. Furthermore, it is known that situations that are highly evaluative accentuate the effects of self-confrontation (Liebling and Shaver, 1973). The studies of conformity, communication sets, and cognitive dissonance that have employed self-confrontation manipulations may be interpreted as also placing subjects in evaluative positions. In situations in which individuals can assume responsibility for behavior and are evaluated, it is likely that any manipulations that increase self-monitoring and attributions of responsibility will exert strong effects on behavior. For instance, Costanzo and Shaw (1966) and Costanzo (1970) found that the tendency to assume personal responsibility for behavior is highly related to tendencies to engage in conformity behavior.

This account of self-confrontation and its effects would be incomplete if the issue of individual differences were not considered. It has been argued that self-confronted individuals perceive discrepancies in their cognitions about the self. Certainly, individuals may be said to differ in the degree to which they are cognitively discrepant. Sackeim (1974) found that individual differences on such a measure predicted differences in the magnitude of psychophysiological reactivity to self-confrontation and negative self-evaluations after self-confrontation. Furthermore, it is likely that individuals differ in the direction of their cognitive discrepancies. That is, some people may overestimate their abilities, skills, attributes, etc., while others may underestimate themselves on these dimensions. It would be predicted that for both groups, self-confrontation is aversive, provided that it is the perception of discrepancy, and not its direction, that leads to the aversive properties of self-confrontation. However, it may be the case that the direction of discrepancies mediates changes in self-esteem following self-confrontation. For instance, Ickes and Wicklund (cited in Duval and Wicklund, 1972, pp. 24–27), employing female undergraduates as subjects, and Alkire and Brunse (1974), using patients in marital therapy as subjects, found decreases in self-esteem following self-confrontation. Boyd and Sisney (1967), however, when self-confronting male inpatients on a psychiatric ward, found increased levels of self-esteem.

In summary, the position we wish to advance is that individuals differ in the degree to which they hold discrepant cognitions about the self. When self-confronted, individuals exhibit heightened self-monitoring and perceive these internal discrepancies. These reactions result in increased physiological arousal, negative affect, and a constriction of ideational content. The anxiety engendered by self-confrontation at first facilitates task performance and at high levels produces decrements. When self-confronted, individuals also assume greater personal responsibility for behavior. When placed in situations that are of an evaluative nature, the self-confronted individual, because of increased self-monitoring and willingness to assume personal responsibility, attempts to reduce discrepancies between the self and the environment. In this respect, the self-confronted individual shows enhanced conformity, communication set, and dissonance reduction effects. Finally, self-confrontation produces significant changes in self-esteem, the direction and intensity of which may be a function of individual differences in the direction and degree of cognitive discrepancy.

We have argued above that it is inappropriate to equate states of awareness with the contents of awareness. As James pointed out, it is a common fallacy to extrapolate from what individuals are conscious of to what is the nature of consciousness. Experimental investigations of self-confrontation have centered on manipulations of the contents of consciousness. Attention is directed either inward to the self or outward to the environment. However, it has been asserted (e.g., Duval and Wicklund, 1972) that such manipulations not only alter the contents of awareness but also are successful in producing changes in states of consciousness. The fact that confrontation with stimuli of the self has psychophysiological, cognitive, affective, and behavioral consequences that differ markedly from those associated with confrontation with stimuli of others provides some support for such a view. Differential reactions to stimuli of self and others are found in both waking and sleeping subjects, suggesting that the state of self-monitoring produced by self-confrontation is not restricted to or dependent on conscious awareness. Intuitively, there are further grounds for arguing that the changes in awareness resulting from self-confrontation reflect changes in states of consciousness and not only changes in the contents of awareness. Individuals may attend exclusively to a task or they may attend to themselves participating in the task. It is hypothesized that self-directed attention is expected to introduce a metacognitive state that results in changes not only in the response systems discussed above but also in other areas, such as the perception of time. The ability to engage in metacognitive acts is dependent on a conceptual differentiation between the self and the environment. It is noteworthy that in order for chimpanzees to identify visual images in mirrors with their own bodies, long exposure or training is required (e.g., Gallup, 1970). However, it is clear that chimpanzees and other lower animals are capable of becoming aware of objects in the environment. The development of a self-concept may be a necessary precondition for metacognition of self-consciousness.

The claim that self-confrontation results in changes in states of consciousness requires further investigation. Experiments on self-confrontation have contrasted the reactions of individuals when they are exposed either to the self or to neutral others. In order to determine whether self-confrontation produces a distinct metacognitive state that is specific to awareness of the self, it is necessary that future investigations employ methodologies in which reactions to the self are compared to reactions to nonneutral others and, in particular, to reactions to aversive, significant others.

If it is shown that self-confrontation is reflected in a distinct metacognitive state, issues concerning the function of such a state of consciousness become central. Psychologists for the most part have not examined naturally occurring instances of self-consciousness or self-directed attention but have artificially produced these states in subjects by the use of audio- and videotape playbacks and evaluative audiences. It has been noted that when individuals are self-confronted in the laboratory, they are likely to attend to those aspects of themselves about which they are cognitively discrepant. We suggest that in naturally occurring situations, individuals become self-conscious or self-confronted when they become aware of discrepancies between the needs and/or wants of the self and environmental situations. The test-anxious individual who observes the self writing an examination instead of focusing directly on the test may do so because of fears or worries concerning failure (Wine, 1971). In this respect, it may be the case not only that self-confrontation results in heightened awareness of discrepancies about the self but also that such cognitive discrepancies may initiate self-confrontation. This position is in line with Freud's (1923/1961) claim that the concept of the self develops as a reaction to discrepancies between internal needs and external reality. The metacognitive state of self-consciousness may serve a self-regulatory role. Individuals, when self-confronted, are more likely to perceive both internal conflicts and discrepancies between the self and the environment. Furthermore, as Holzman argued, self-monitoring may serve not only to alert the individual to internal and external conflict but also as a means of safeguarding against the emission of undesirable behavior.

Evidence has been presented above that indicates that the hypothesized metacognitive state engendered by self-confrontation is frequently aversive. Heightened self-monitoring of psychological conflicts is found to be an unpleasant experience. That animals avoid what is aversive is a basic assumption of almost all psychological theories (e.g., Freud, 1930/1961; Hull, 1943; Irwin, 1971). Logically, an individual may avoid awareness of aversive stimulation either by leaving the field or by selective awareness of aspects of the internal or external environment. We have argued that the concept of self-deception is the superordinate category of instances of motivated selective transparency in consciousness. If self-deception exists, it might be demonstrated in examples of avoidance of the metacognitive state of the self-consciousness produced by self-confrontation.

IV. THE EXPERIMENTAL INVESTIGATION OF SELF-DECEPTION

> "The discovery of a deceiving principle, a lying activity within us, can furnish an absolutely new view of all conscious life." (Jacques Rivére, cited in Fingarette, 1969)

A. Studies of Nonrecognition of the Self

Presenting necessary and sufficient criteria for the ascription of self-deception and providing a unitary account of the nature of self-confrontation establish a foundation for the experimental investigation of self-deceptive behavior in the avoidance of the self-monitoring engendered by self-confrontation. An issue we have posed for investigation concerns whether instances of nonrecognition of the self should be viewed as instances of self-deception.

To examine this hypothesis we conducted an experiment (Gur and Sackeim, 1976) that involved a simple identification task. Sixty subjects were presented with audiotapes of self and others. The tapes were structured into five blocks of trials, with each block containing six voices. The voice of the self appeared once within each block and the temporal durations of voice stimuli increased with each block (2, 4, 6, 12, and 24 sec). Subjects were asked to identify each stimulus as soon as possible after onset by pressing one of six buttons in front of them. Three buttons referred to the choice of the self at varying levels of certainty and three buttons referred to the choice of the other, at varying levels of certainty. The reaction times of responses and GSR were continually monitored.

Few previous studies have investigated instances of nonrecognition of the self. Wolff (1943) presented subjects with sets of stimuli consisting of voice tapes, film clips, and photographs of self and others. Subjects were asked to write personality sketches based on the composite sets of stimuli. Despite the fact that an extraordinarily high proportion of subjects did not recognize the stimuli of the self, these subjects nevertheless wrote their most extreme sketches, either positive or negative, in reaction to stimuli of the self. These results were replicated by Huntley (1940). High rates of nonrecognition of the self have characterized almost all studies involving audiotape feedback (e.g., Holzman and Rousey, 1966; Holzman *et al.*, 1966; Huntely, 1940; Wolff, 1943). The lowest rate of nonrecognition reported to date was in the Olivos (1967) study, where false negative responses—that is, incorrect identifications of stimuli of the self as stimuli of others— constituted 45% of the responses to stimuli of the self. The previously reported high rates of nonrecognition of the self may have been due to the fact that the quality of the audio presentations often was not optimized and the instructions to subjects concerning the identification of stimuli sometimes were not explicit. Since our interest in nonrecognition of the self centers on the issue of self-deception, we attempted to minimize all errors in identification that would be due to factors other than self-deception.

B. The Demonstration of the Existence of Self-Deception

Supporting the general finding that confrontation with the self is psychophysiologically arousing, we found that subjects evidenced greater changes in skin conductance after onset of the voices of the self than after voices of others (see Figure 1). In addition, subjects were also slower in their identifications of stimuli of the self as opposed to stimuli of others (see Figure 2).

The first criterion for ascribing self-deception requires evidence that the individual holds two contradictory beliefs (p and not-p). Our identification experiment provided evidence relating to the beliefs of the subject. If one affirms that a given stimulus is the voice of another individual, a statement has been made concerning a particular belief. Demonstrating that a contradictory belief is also held is more difficult. However, inferences concerning beliefs need not be based only on self-reports. The behavioral correlates of beliefs can be measured, and when reliable indices are found, beliefs may be attributed on the basis of these indices (Armstrong, 1968; Quinton, 1973). This methodology, as employed in the detection of lying by the use of psychophysiological measurements, has been discussed by Lykken (1959, 1974) and Orne, Thackray, and Paskewitz (1972), among others. Similar procedures have been used in subception experiments (Dixon, 1971; Eriksen, 1956, 1958; Lazarus and McCleary, 1951). In the present investigation, a psychophysiological index (GSR) was used.

In relation to nonrecognition phenomena, the self-report of the subject is used to determine that one particular belief is held. The behavioral indices, measured while the self-report is made, are used to indicate whether a contradictory belief is also held. The evidence that the contradictory belief is truly contradictory must come from a

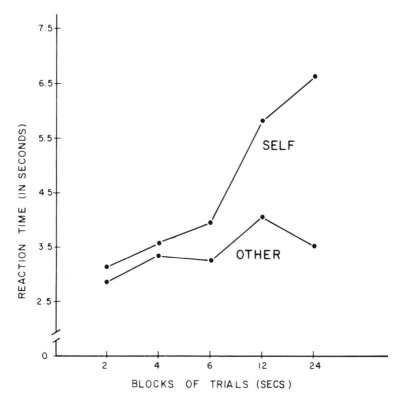

FIGURE 2.   Reaction times (in seconds) to audio stimuli of self and other, as a function of block of trials.

comparison of the topographies of the behavioral correlates of this belief with those of subjects who have recognized their own voices. That is, if the behavioral correlates of a subject who affirms that not-p (e.g., nonrecognition) are identical to those who affirm that p (e.g., recognition), the conclusion is that the subject who affirms that not-p also believes that p.

This type of argument has been used in other contexts. In eye-blink conditioning experiments, the "same" reponses may be either voluntary or involuntary. One means that has been used to discriminate between these types of behavior has been to examine the different physical features of the responses. Kimble (1964) argued that the voluntary blink, for example, differs in form and latency from the involuntary, conditioned blink. In the present context, uniformity of topography was used to infer identical beliefs, while differences in topography led to the opposite conclusion.

Further evidence for the assertion that a subject who affirms belief p can also be attributed belief not-p would come from discovering that the variables that predict the behavioral correlates of not-p in subjects who outwardly affirm that not-p and those variables that predict the behavioral correlates of not-p in subjects who outwardly affirm that p are identical. In this regard as well, the methodology does not differ from that of the conditioned eye-blink situation. Peak (1933) and Grant (1968) attempted to distinguish voluntary from involuntary, conditioned blinks by showing differential reactions to experimental manipulations.

The proposal, then, for establishing the first criterion was to demonstrate that the topographies of the behavioral correlates of incorrectly claiming that a stimulus is another (false negative) are identical to those when the stimulus is correctly identified as the self (true positive). Likewise the topographies of the behavioral correlates of incorrectly identifying a stimulus as the self (false positive) should be demonstrated to be identical to those when the stimulus is correctly identified as another (true negative). Furthermore, if it were shown that the variables that predicted the behavioral correlates did so with regard to stimulus condition and not with regard to self-reports, the conclusion that the subject holds two contradictory beliefs would be strengthened.

The results bearing on these predictions are presented in Figure 3. Levels of reactivity for both true positive and false negative responses differed significantly from those for both true negative and false positive responses. Furthermore, true positive responses did not differ significantly from false negative responses, nor did true negative and false positive responses differ significantly from each other on this measure.

The methodology employed to show that some subjects held contradictory beliefs was similar to that used in earlier studies of subception (Lazarus and McCleary, 1951) and subliminal perception (Dixon, 1971). A major criticism of this research was offered by Eriksen (1956, 1958), when he argued that differences found between the verbal reports and psychophysiological responses of subjects are often an artifact of the substantial but imperfect correlation between the two response systems. He pointed out that the lack of a perfect correlation would naturally lead to some instances where psychophysiological responses would be associated with correct identifications while verbal reports would be in error. In addition, Eriksen presented some of his own results that showed that in identification tasks, verbal reports are far more accurate overall in identifications of stimuli than are psychophysiological responses.

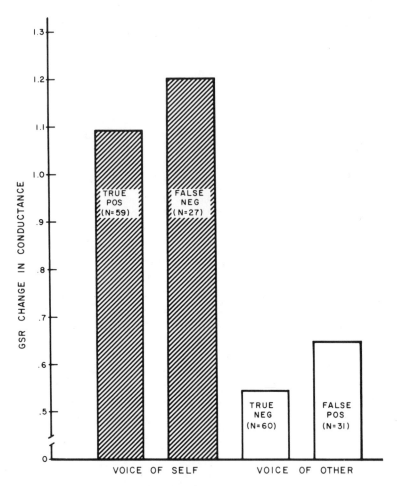

FIGURE 3. Subjects' mean levels of psychophysiological reactivity (in micromhos) for true positive, false negative, true negative, and false positive responses.

Studies of subception and subliminal perception have tradition-ally used either weak supraliminal or subliminal stimuli. As our experiment employed strong supraliminal stimuli that were affectively charged (i.e., the voices of self), it was felt that Eriksen's criticisms would not apply to the findings of this study. Indeed, a point-biserial correlation of identifications of self and other with psychophysiologi-cal reactivity on trials of the self indicated that there was no relation-ship between the verbal reports and reactivity for these trials. A similar analysis for trials of other also showed that there was no relationship between the two response systems on trials of other

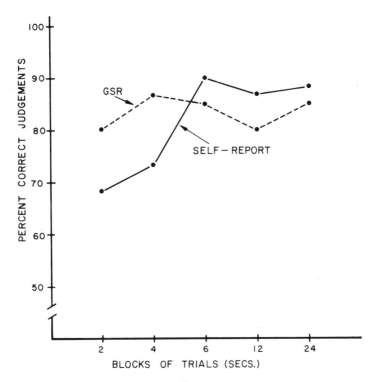

FIGURE 4. Accuracy of identifications of audio stimuli of the self for GSR and self-report responses, as a function of block of trials.

voices. In addition, accuracy rates for the two response systems were computed and are presented in Figure 4.[1] Overall, psychophysiological responses provided correct identifications on 83% of the trials, while the self-reports of subjects were correct on 81% of the trials. These results indicate that the verbal report and psychophysiological response systems were independent.

In summary, the first criterion was fulfilled by a demonstration that on trials of errors in identification, psychophysiological reactivity paralleled the reactivity of trials of correct identification. Furthermore, we found that psychophysiological and self-report responses were independent. The second criterion, that the contradictory beliefs be

[1] Mean change in conductance scores were computed for trials of other within each of the five blocks and subtracted from change in conductance scores for the trial of the self in each block. As no practice trials were given to subjects prior to experimental trials, reactivity scores for the first two trials of other voices (in the first block) were dropped from the analysis.

held simultaneously, was fulfilled by our taking self-report and psychophysiological measures contemporaneously.

In the present context, demonstration of the third criterion required that subjects be shown to be unaware that they had committed errors. In studies of learning without awareness, as well as in other areas of investigation, fulfillment of a similar criterion of nonawareness has proved to be particularly difficult. This is the case primarily because experimenters have relied on obtrusive postexperimental reports of subjects for indices of awareness. Martin *et al.* (1974) wrote, "The most pressing methodological problem with the present studies is the one that plagues all studies of learning without awareness. There seems to be no entirely defensible method of assessing subject awareness after the experiment" (p. 604). To fulfill the third criterion, and to avoid this difficulty in our study, we took one obtrusive and developed two unobtrusive measures of awareness. It was expected that if subjects were unaware of making misidentifications of stimuli of the self, then on a postexperimental questionnaire, subjects who had given false negative responses would report that the self was present on the tape for fewer trials than subjects who did not make these errors. The results supported this prediction. However, the reciprocal situation, in which subjects who made false positive responses reported more trials of the self than subjects who did not commit these errors, was predicted not to hold because it was expected that not all false positive responses would qualify as instances of self-deception. The fact that subjects have greater prior experience with the voice of the self, whether recorded or otherwise, suggested that some false positive responses would reflect artifactual influences, such as degree of experience with tape playbacks. As expected, subjects who made false positive responses did not differ from subjects who did not commit such errors in recalling the number of trials in which the self was a stimulus for identification. Subjects who made false positive responses did differ from subjects who did not make such errors in that they did have less prior experience with audio playbacks. This was not true of the subjects who made false negative responses.

The first unobtrusive measure of nonawareness was concerned with reaction time on the trial of other following presentation of the self. It was predicted that if subjects were aware that the previous stimulus was the self, they would show savings by responding faster on these trials. It was found that reaction times on trials following true positive responses were faster than on the remaining trials of stimuli of others. If subjects were unaware that the self had been the stimulus for identification when they gave false negative responses, it was predicted that they would show no savings on trials of other following false negative responses. Indeed, the results indicated that reaction time on trials following false negative responses were not different from the remaining trials of other.

The second unobtrusive measure of nonawareness related to reaction time and levels of certainty when subjects "broke through" the hypothesized self-deception. It was predicted that if subjects were truly unaware that the self was the stimulus for identification when false negative responses were made, they should also show longer reaction times and less certainty on trials where they gave true positive responses than subjects who had not committed such errors. Again, the results supported these predictions, and at least in terms of false negative responses, the third criterion of nonawareness was fulfilled.

We had regarded the fourth criterion as the most difficult to establish, and this study took only initial steps toward this goal. The false negative response may be viewed as an avoidance of the negative consequences provoked by self-confrontation. In this respect, it might have been predicted that subjects who made false negative responses loaded highly on the dimension of cognitive discrepancy. However, our position is that self-deception is not a stimulus-bound response but may be viewed as a generalized response set. It was predicted that the tendency to be self-deceived would depress measures of psychopathology and that therefore subjects who made false negative responses would score, at best, at the mean on such measures. However, the motivational determinants of the false positive response were considered as opposite in direction to those of the false negative response. Subjects who gave false positive responses could, if anything, be said to seek self-confrontation and were predicted to have low scores on the dimension of cognitive discrepancy. Prior to the experimental session, subjects had filled out a number of personality forms. It was found that for the two measures of cognitive discrepancy (the items from the EPI employed by Sackeim, 1974, and the worry scale of the Pre-Examination Questionnaire of Liebert and Morris, 1967), subjects who made false positives had lower scores than subjects who did not commit such errors.

In order to test whether the tendency to engage in self-deception could be measured by a paper-and-pencil inventory and to strengthen the motivational account, the self-deception questionnaire (Gur and Sackeim, 1975) was constructed. Questions on this inventory were specifically worded so that they centered on statements judged to be universally true and also psychologically threatening to subjects. It was found that subjects who committed false positive or false negative errors scored higher on this measure of self-deception than subjects who did not make these errors. It was particularly important to find that subjects who had high rates of denying general and threatening psychological statements also made errors in the identification of audio stimuli, not only because it supported the motivational account for such errors but also because it supported the view that individual differences in the tendency to be self-deceived exist and are measurable.

C. The Ascription of Self-Deception

The new data that have been presented support the claim that there is a phenomenon that fits the concept of self-deception. Positive evidence was found for fulfilling the four criteria for ascription. The psychophysiological correlates of responses of nonrecognition do not differ from those correlates of responses of correct identification. In this regard, the evidence supports the attribution of contradictory beliefs. The fact that the psychophysiological correlates were measured at the same time that the subjects delivered their identifications fulfills the criterion of simultaneity. Obtrusive and unobtrusive measures indicated that, at least for false negative responses, subjects are not aware of holding contradictory beliefs. In support of the requirement that the act of nonawareness be motivated, it was found that individuals who gave false positive responses scored lower on measures predicting the aversiveness of self-confrontation than individuals who did not make false positive responses. Finally, evidence was obtained in support of the view that self-deception is a generalized response set and that the tendency to reject threatening statements about the self is related to the tendency to commit errors in the identification of voices.

It might be possible that our results are a function of artifacts in our procedures or are susceptible to alternative interpretation. For instance, one might argue that the self-reports or identifications of stimuli by subjects were unreliable measures of their beliefs. It could be contended that the subjects, at times, were aware of the correct identifications but consciously lied in producing false negative or false positive responses. In our view, this position is untenable. Our subjects were given no reason to lie to the experimenters, and they appeared cooperative and interested in performing to the best of their abilities. Most subjects expressed dismay and chagrin when they were informed in the debriefing after the experimental session that they had committed errors. Most importantly, two of our measures of the awareness of misidentifications were unobtrusive. No subject could be expected to deceive the experimenters not only in communicating identifications but also in consciously manipulating a complex set of measures that are dependent on differences in reaction times over a series of trials.

We have examined our results in relation to other possible artifacts or alternative explanations (Gur and Sackeim, 1976). Frequency of previous exposure to playbacks was not associated with the number of false negative responses, although it did predict the number of false positive responses. At least some false positive responses should be considered as "errors" or false alarms and not as instances of self-deception. The results bearing on levels of certainty of responses showed that no coherent account of the role of certainty could be made as a mediating variable, producing the observed relationships. Indeed, we found that the level of certainty for false negative responses did not differ significantly from the level of certainty for true positive responses. Subjects who gave false negative responses were no more nor less likely to make false positive responses than subjects who did not give any false negative responses. Similarly, subjects who made false positive responses were no more nor less likely to make false negative responses than subjects who did not make any false positive responses. In the present study, 18.7% of the trials of self involved false negative responses, the lowest rate yet to be reported in the literature. Rates of false positive responding have not been reported. The rate of false positive responding in the present investigation was 3.8%. The failure to find support for an alternative explanation and the evidence that the methodology employed in the present investigation was successful in minimizing the frequency of instances of nonrecognition lends further credence to the claim that the existence of self-deception as an experimentally real phenomenon has been demonstrated.

Self-deception has been a popular topic in philosophical and literary writings (e.g., Camus, 1956; Fingarette, 1969; Gide, 1955; Sartre, 1958). As we have pointed out, psychologists have frequently employed the concept in providing explanations for a diverse range of behaviors. Given this interest in self-deception, it is somewhat surprising that there have been no previous experimental investigations of the ontological status of the concept. Now that there is some evidence that self-deception can be demonstrated, several questions concerning the nature of self-deception and the implications of the findings concerning self-deception for theories of consciousness come to the fore.

V. SELF-DECEPTION, FUNCTIONAL BRAIN ASYMMETRY, AND CONSCIOUSNESS

On the basis of our logicolinguistic analysis of the criteria necessary and sufficient for the ascription of self-deception, we have
contended that the self-deceived individual simultaneously holds two
contradictory beliefs and is unaware of holding one of these beliefs.
Further, in order for the individual to be characterized as self-
deceived, the lack of awareness of one of the beliefs must be
motivated. If one accepts the criteria we have offered for the ascription
of self-deception and if one accepts the results we have presented as
demonstrating the existence of self-deception, then the conclusion
must be reached that consciousness should be attributed the properties of motivated selective transparency. In holding such a view of
consciousness, we maintain that the processing of information and the
products of such processing, at times, may not be subject to awareness. A major factor determining which cognitions will be subject to
awareness is the motivational context of the individual. We will
presently discuss the role of motives in producing self-deceptive
behaviors and individual differences in the tendency to be self-
deceived, and we will present some new findings that bear on these
issues. On the basis of studies of functional brain asymmetry and
hemisphericity, we suggest that there are grounds for the hypothesis
that functional differences between the two hemispheres may be
implicated in the mechanisms underlying self-deception. We conclude
with an overview of the work we have presented here and with a
discussion of the implications of our modes of investigation for the
study of consciousness.

A. Motives and Individual Differences in Self-Deception

Wisdom (1967), in writing about the essential contribution of
Freud's idea of the unconscious, stated that what characterizes this
idea "is that in it the unconscious is dynamic and rooted in the
emotions and that this gives rise to all the richness of conscious life.
For such an idea there are scarcely any precursors" (pp. 190–191).
Similarly, the concept of self-deception requires a dynamic view of
consciousness. Not only is consciousness seen as selectively transparent, but also the very transparency and lack of it are motivated.

The fact that studies of subliminal perception and subception (cf.
Dixon, 1971) have often found only weak and transient effects may be
the result of a failure to account for the dynamic and motivational

facets of awareness. These studies traditionally have attempted to demonstrate processing of information that is out of awareness. The manipulations that have been used in such demonstrations have centered on the intensity of incoming perceptual stimuli. It is suggested here that an alternate and perhaps more promising approach for demonstrations of selective awareness of processing is to tie the contents of the processing to the motivational concerns of the individual. In this respect, awareness and nonawareness of stimulation and processing are not viewed as a static property of consciousness, solely determined by the intensity of stimulation, but as a dynamic and variable behavior, subject like most of behavior to motivational considerations.

The investigation of the motivational determinants of self-deception in the Gur and Sackeim (1976) experiment was incomplete. To bolster our account of the reasons why individuals are self-deceived in their errors of self-recognition, it should be shown further that the frequency of self-deceptive behavior varies with changes in motivational context. Freud (1915/1957) argued that repression acts in a highly individual manner and that whether or not an idea will be repressed is a function of the degree of distortion of that idea. He also argued that "The same result as follows from an increase or a decrease in the degree of distortion may also be achieved at the other end of the apparatus, so to speak, by a modification in the condition for the production of pleasure and unpleasure" (pp. 150–151). Similarly, we view self-deception as mobile, and the frequency and nature of self-deceptive acts should be determined, in part, in our experimental situation by the aversiveness or lack of aversiveness of beliefs about the self. In addition, it should also be demonstrated that differential outcomes result when individuals identify themselves correctly and when they make errors. The consequences of engaging in self-deception should differ from the consequences of veridically representing internal reality in conscious awareness.

We have recently completed an experiment that addresses the first issue of the mobility of self-deceptive acts dependent on motivational contexts. The aversiveness of the self was manipulated by pretreatments with experiences of success or failure. Half the subjects were asked to solve the easiest verbal synonym problems from a standard test of verbal comprehension. Half the subjects were asked to solve the most difficult problems from the same test. All subjects then participated in a self-confrontation experiment similar to the one discussed above. Our results indicate that the subjects who received pretreatments of success made more false positive errors than the subjects who received pretreatments of failure. The latter group committed more false negative responses than the former group, and the differences between the two groups are significant. There is evidence, then, for the claim that variations in the aversiveness of the self result in differences in the frequency and direction of self-deceptive acts regarding recognition of the self.

The findings of Wolff (1943) and Huntley (1940) are relevant to the suggestion that there are differential outcomes as a consequence of recognition or nonrecognition of the self. They found that subjects who failed to identify themselves when self-confronted wrote more extreme (positive or negative) character sketches than they wrote when confronted with stimuli of strangers. We are currently investigating changes in self-concepts following instances of recognition and nonrecognition of the self. It may be the case that types of affects and ideations found after failures in identification are markedly different from those found when there is an awareness of self-confrontation.

Considerations of the motivational components of self-deception are intimately tied to the issue of individual differences in the tendency to be self-deceived. As Pynchon (1963) has written, sometimes "the motive is part of the quarry" (p. 362). In our first study, it was hypothesized that the individuals who would find self-confrontation most aversive would commit false negative responses. However, the premeasure of the aversiveness of the confrontation was a self-report inventory of psychopathology, and it was also hypothesized that individuals who were high in the tendency to be self-deceived would have depressed scores on a psychopathology measure. The assumption behind this view was that self-deception is not a stimulus-bound phenomenon but a generalized response set, or characteristic defense, the frequency of its use varying among people. In support of this view, it was found that the tendency to deny psychologically threatening statements was associated with the frequency of false negative and false positive responses. Furthermore, we have found that high scores on the SDQ are negatively correlated with a number of tests of psychopathology (see Table 1).

These findings are in line with the contention of Meehl and Hathaway (1946), who argued that the effects of self-deception are of greater importance in influencing personality inventory scores than the effects of conscious lying. As a generalized response set, self-deception may influence behavior in contexts other than personality testing. For instance, Mischel (1974) argued that the "neurotic paradox" reflects a motivated attempt by individuals to keep specific ideas out of awareness and that all neurotic behavior is self-deceptive. The phenomena found in cognitive dissonance experiments may be likewise accounted for in terms of self-deceptive acts. Since it may be

TABLE 1

Intercorrelations among Measures of Psychopathology, Self-Deception, and Other-Deception[a]

	MSQ[b]	EPI—N	EPI—L	BECK	SDQ	ODQ
MSQ	×	0.65[c]	−0.16[d]	0.72[c]	−0.48[c]	−0.22[c]
EPI—N		×	−0.12	0.55[c]	−0.34[c]	−0.18[e]
EPS—L			×	−0.06	0.24[e]	0.57[c]
BECK				×	−0.34[c]	−0.10
SDQ					×	0.28[c]
ODQ						×

[a] N = 250 undergraduates at the University of Pennsylvania.
[b] MSQ: Total score on the Manifest Symptom Questionnaire.
EPI—N: Eysenck Personality Inventory—Neuroticism scale.
EPI—L: Eysenck Personality Inventory—Lie Scale.
BECK: Beck Depression Inventory.
SDQ: Self-deception Questionnaire.
ODQ: Other-deception Questionnaire.
[c] $p < 0.001$.
[d] $p < 0.05$.
[e] $p < 0.01$.

possible (as evidenced by the SDQ) to measure relative tendencies to employ self-deception, we now have an opportunity to examine not only individual differences in self-deception but also the influence of self-deception on broad ranges of behavior.

B. Mechanisms Underlying Self-Deception: The Hemisphericity Hypothesis

Once it is accepted that self-deception exists, the question may be asked as to what are the mechanisms and structures that make self-deception possible. The findings with patients who have undergone cerebral commissurotomy suggest that functional differences between the two hemispheres may be implicated in self-deception (Fingarette, 1969). Sperry (1968) has presented evidence that these patients have two separate streams of consciousness. Indeed, these patients may be shown to hold contradictory beliefs and nonawareness of one of these beliefs. In a dramatic demonstration, Sperry presented a female commissurotomy patient with a picture of a nude, tachistoscopically projected to the right hemisphere. The patient reacted by giggling and blushing but could give no explanation for her reaction. When pressed, she said, "Dr. Sperry, you've got some funny machine!" Even though such observations were made with people whose inter-hemispheric neuronal connections had been severed, the inhibitory functions of the corpus callosum suggest that in normal people, the transfer of information between the two hemispheres is sometimes blocked.

More evidence linking self-deception with hemispheric functioning is found in studies of functional brain asymmetry in neurologically intact populations. Such studies, using a diversity of techniques, have converged in their results with studies of split-brain and unilaterally brain-damaged patients. A number of dichotomies have been offered as describing the essence of the differences found between the two hemispheres. The early verbal (left) versus spatial (right) dichotomy was refined in terms of dichotomies such as analytic–synthetic (Levy, 1969), propositional–appositional (Bogen, 1969), logical and rational versus holistic and intuitive (Ornstein, 1972), and serial–parallel (Cohen, 1973; Gur and Hilgard, 1975). These characterizations of dichotomies are in no way mutually exclusive and do not reflect basic disagreements over fact or theory. Rather, they seem to convey differences in emphasis and perspective. Most investigators in the field would probably agree to the following statement regarding the functional differences between the hemispheres:

The left hemisphere seems to serve functions primarily associated with propositional and logical ideation; it approaches problems analytically and processes information serially. These features probably account for its superior proficiency in verbal comprehension. The right hemisphere, by contrast, serves functions primarily associated with appositional and intuitive ideation, seems to approach problems in a synthetic fashion, and processes information in a parallel mode. These features are likely to account for its superiority in the comprehension of spatial relations and pictorial stimuli.

Along with the discovery of functional differences between the two hemispheres within a person, evidence has started to accumulate suggesting individual differences in the tendency to use right versus left hemispheric modes of information processing and problem solving. Thus, Bogen (1969) observed individual differences in what he called hemisphericity. Ornstein (1972) talked about individual differences in logical versus intuitive cognitive styles, and Bakan (1969) offered the typology of "right hemisphere" and "left hemisphere" people. Since *hemisphericity* seems to be the shortest and most concise word to characterize this dimension of individual differences, we will use it from now on as a descriptive term to denote the possible tendency of an individual characteristically to use one hemisphere more than another (Gur and Gur, 1976; Gur, Levy, and Gur, 1977).

Cerebral asymmetries affect not only the perceptual world but the motoric one as well. A series of experiments, conducted during the past two decades, has investigated the variety of conditions under which conjugate lateral eye movements occur in human subjects. Characteristic direction of eye movement has been offered as a metric of individual differences in hemisphericity. Teitelbaum (1954) was the first to report that when a subject is faced by a questioner, he usually breaks eye contact following the presentation of a question and moves his eyes either to the right or to the left. This phenomenon was later investigated more thoroughly by Day (1964; 1967a,b; 1968), who found that the direction in which the eyes move is fairly consistent for a given individual. His investigations have also revealed various differences between "left-movers" and "right-movers," primarily in the experience of anxiety, in verbal and cognitive styles, and in a number of personality measures. Bakan and his colleagues (Bakan, 1969; Bakan and Shotland, 1969; Bakan and Svorad, 1969) substantiated these findings and established a number of additional indications that these groups of subjects differed in cognitive and conative organization. The pattern of these differences led Bakan (1971) to conclude that eye-movement directionality reflected hemisphericity.

In 1972, Kinsbourne and, independently, Kocel, Galin, Ornstein, and Merrin reported findings that appeared to contradict this position. They recorded eye movements of subjects as they responded to verbal, spatial, and numerical questions and found that subjects showed a significant tendency to move their eyes to the right for verbal problems, to the left for spatial problems, and in no consistent direction for numerical problems. Schwartz, Davidson, and Maer (1975) found further that eye movements to the left were associated with responses to emotional problems, whether of a verbal or of a spatial nature. This latter study supports the view that the right hemisphere is primary in the processing of emotional material. The claim that individuals characteristically display undirectional eye movements that reflect individual differences in hemisphericity appeared inconsistent with the findings that direction of eye movements is a function of the type of problem presented to subjects.

The apparent inconsistency in results was resolved in a study by Gur, Gur, and Harris (1975) that demonstrated that the direction of eye movements during problem solving can be influenced by the amount of stress imposed on the subject. When stress is minimal, as when the experimenter is seated behind the subject and cannot be viewed, eye movements are related to problem type. When stress is increased, as when subjects directly face an attractive experimenter of the opposite sex, the same subjects tend to move their eyes consistently in one direction, either left of right, regardless of problem type. In stressful situations, the frequency of inappropriate eye movements relative to problem type increases. Gur *et al.* (1975) found that in these instances quality of performance deteriorated. The investigators reasoned that problem saliency decreased under stress and subjects resorted to stereotypic response modes, which reflected their individual differences in hemisphericity.

In a number of subsequent studies by R. E. Gur, R. C. Gur, and their colleagues, it has been found that hemisphericity is a good predictor for a wide range of personality traits, including hypnotic susceptibility (Gur and Gur, 1974; Gur and Reyher, 1973), type of defense mechanisms employed (Gur and Gur, 1975), and self-reports of psychopathological symptoms (Gur and Gur, 1975; Gur, Sackeim, and Gur, 1976). The nature of personality correlates associated with differences in hemisphericity is consistent with our knowledge of right and left hemisphere functioning. Thus, for example, left hemisphericity subjects (right movers) tend to intellectualize and use defense mechanisms such as projection, while right hemisphericity subjects (left movers) are more emotional and tend to use holistic defense mechanisms such as repression.

There is also some suggestive evidence that hemisphericity and functional brain asymmetry may be implicated in subliminal perception. Although it is likely that the left hemisphere, for most people, is more susceptible to subliminal perception of verbal stimuli and the right hemisphere is more likely to process spatial stimuli out of awareness (Henley and Dixon, 1974), individual differences in overall susceptibility to subliminal perception have also been observed. Allison (1963) found that when pictorial stimuli were used, subliminal effects were found only when subjects were encouraged to use cognitive sets that were intuitive and holistic in emphasis. When subjects were encouraged to employ cognitive sets that were logical and analytic in emphasis, subliminal effects could not be found. Gordon (1967), in a *post hoc* analysis of results from an experiment using verbal stimuli, discovered that art students, but not science and engineering students, showed subliminal effects. It is hypothesized that subliminal perception of either verbal or pictorial stimuli is characteristic of left-movers (right hemisphericity people).

These lines of research bear on the issue of self-deception. Split-brain patients may be shown to hold contradictory beliefs and not be aware of one of the beliefs. Conjugate lateral eye movements have been associated with individual differences in emotionality, defensive style, and psychopathology. Susceptibility to subliminal stimulation also may be related to hemispheric activation and to individual differences in hemisphericity. It would seem likely, then, that functional differences between the two hemispheres provide possible mechanisms for the occurrence of self-deception. Indeed, both Orn-stein (1972) and Galin (1974) have suggested that the blockage of information from entering the left hemisphere provides the neurologi-cal underpinnings of repression.

C. Overview

It is widely agreed among psychologists that investigations of concepts of defensive behavior, such as repression, generally have been unsuccessful in demonstrating the construct validity of such concepts (e.g., Eysenck and Wilson, 1973; Hilgard, 1973; Holmes, 1974). We have argued that such investigations have been plagued by significant conceptual and methodological difficulties. Rarely have investigators explicitly outlined requirements for demonstrating the existence of a construct. Furthermore, in attempting to come to an understanding of the nature of consciousness, researchers have fre-quently committed what James termed the "psychologist's fallacy" of equating the contents of consciousness with the nature or structure of consciousness. Studies of defensive behavior and processing of infor-mation out of awareness may be criticized for often failing to attune methodologies to the motivational and idiosyncratic properties of the phenomena under investigation. Obtrusive measures, clearly suscepti-ble to the demand characteristics of experimental situations, have often been employed to determine the awareness or lack of awareness of cognitions or beliefs.

We have offered the concept of self-deception as a superordinate category, of which repression and other defense mechanisms (cf. Hilgard, 1949) are special instances. We began our investigation of self-deception with a logicolinguistic analysis of the concept. Our concern, at that point, was not to demonstrate the existence of self-deception but rather to determine what is meant by the concept. We argued that the concept of self-deception did not entail a paradox if it were assumed, at the very least, that consciousness is not transparent. On the basis of the logicolinguistic analysis, four criteria were pre-sented as necessary and sufficient for the ascription of self-deception.

Having established these criteria, we searched for a methodology that would allow for their operationalization in scientifically objective measures and that at the same time would be sensitive to the idiosyncratic nature of defensive behavior. We reviewed studies of the effects of self-confrontation. It was concluded that confrontation with the self resulted in psychophysiological, cognitive, conative, and behavioral consequences that differed markedly from confrontation with others. We argued that self-confrontation engenders a metacognitive state that is inherently different from the normal consciousness of the environment and that since this metacognitive state is often found to be aversive, individuals are motivated in their nonrecognition of the self.

On the basis of our review of studies of self-confrontation, we operationalized the four criteria for the ascription of self-deception in an experimental situation in which subjects were required to identify audio stimuli of self and others. Self-reports and psychophysiological measures were used as indices of the beliefs of subjects. Obtrusive and unobtrusive measures were employed to investigate the criterion of the nonawareness of beliefs. We examined loadings on measures of psychopathology, in particular the dimension of cognitive discrepancy, in providing a motivational account of errors in the identification of audio stimuli. As it was found that the four criteria for the ascription of self-deception were fulfilled in this study, it was concluded that self-deception is an experimentally real phenomenon.

We felt that the weakest point in our demonstration of the existence of self-deception resided in the correlational nature of the measures of the motivational context of self-deceptive behaviors. To bolster our account, we conducted a second experiment in which the motivation of subjects was manipulated by pretreatments of success and failure. It was discovered that such pretreatments resulted in differential directions for errors in the identification of audio stimuli of self and others. The demonstration of the existence of self-deception raises many issues, particularly concerning the possible mechanisms that underlie self-deceptive behavior. We reviewed studies of functional brain asymmetry and hemisphericity and suggested that functional differences between the two hemispheres may provide possible mechanisms for the occurrence of self-deception. Most importantly, however, the demonstration of the existence of self-deception calls for the acceptance of the view that consciousness is nontransparent and that at times the very selectivity in transparency is motivated.

The methodology employed in this work was somewhat unusual. Our investigation began with a purely logicolinguistic analysis of the meaning of a concept. Then, an attempt was made to discover experimentally whether a phenomenon existed that could fit the criteria for ascribing this concept. At the outset, this attempt was viewed as a high-risk type of operation—a long shot. However, the probability of success for such an approach may have been initially underrated. Skinner (1938), the *prima facie* operationalist, wrote:

> The relation of an organism to environment must be supposed to include the special case of the relation of scientist to subject matter. If we

contemplate an eventual successful extension of our methods, we must suppose ourselves to be describing an activity of which describing is itself one manifestation. It is necessary to raise this epistemological point in order to explain why it is that popular terms so often refer to what are later found to be "experimentally real entities." The reason is that such terms are in themselves responses of a generic sort: they are the responses of the population of which the experimenter is a member. Consequently, when the organism under investigation fairly closely resembles man (for example, when it is a dog), the popular term may be very close to the experimentally real entity. (p. 43)

Perhaps this statement is particularly true when the behavior under consideration is particularly human.

ACKNOWLEDGMENT

Many people have contributed to various phases of our investigations and have commented on our work. In particular we thank Henry Gleitmen, Ernest R. Hilgard, Leonard Horowitz, Gary E. Schwartz, and Donna M. Zucchi for their comments and suggestions.

REFERENCES

ALKIRE, A. A., AND BRUNSE, A. J. Impact and possible casualty from video-tape feedback in marital therapy. *Journal of Consulting and Clinical Psychology*, 1974, *42*, 203–210.

ALLISON, J. Cognitive structure and receptivity to low intensity stimulation. *Journal of Abnormal and Social Psychology*, 1963, *67*, 132–138.

ANASTASI, A. *Psychological testing*, New York: Macmillan, 1961.

ARKIN, R. M., AND DUVAL, S. Focus of attention and causal attributions of actors and observers. *Journal of Experimental Social Psychology*, 1975, *11*, 427–438.

ARMSTRONG, D. M. *A materialist theory of the mind*. London: Routledge & Kegan Paul, 1968.

BAILEY, G. G., AND SOWDER, W. T. Audiotape and videotape self-confrontation in psychotherapy. *Psychological Bulletin*, 1970, *74*, 127–137.

BAKAN, P. Hypnotizability, laterality of eye movement and functional brain asymmetry. *Perceptual and Motor Skills*, 1969, *28*, 927–932.

BAKAN, P. The eyes have it. *Psychology Today*, 1971, *4*, 64–69.

BAKAN, P., AND SVORAD, D. Resting EEG alpha and asymmetry of reflective lateral eye movements. *Nature*, 1969, *223*, 975–976.

BAKAN, P., AND SHOTLAND, J. Lateral eye movement, reading speed, and visual attention. *Psychonomic Science*, 1969, *16*, 93–94.

BEKESY, G. V. The structure of the middle ear and the hearing of one's own voice by bone conduction. *Journal of the Acoustical Society of America*, 1949, *21*, 217–232.

BOGEN, J. E. The other side of the brain, II: An appositional mind. *Bulletin of the Los Angeles Neurological Societies*, 1969, *34*, 135–162.

BOYD, H. S., AND SISNEY, V. V. Immediate self-image confrontation and changes in self-concept. *Journal of Consulting Psychology*, 1967, *31*, 291–294.

BREHM, J. W. *A theory of psychological reactance.* New York: Academic Press, 1966.

BROWN, R. *Social psychology.* New York: The Free Press, 1965.

BRUNER, J. S., AND POSTMAN, L. Perception, cognition, and behavior. *Journal of Personality,* 1949, *18,* 14–31.

CAMUS, A. *The fall.* New York: Vintage Books, 1956.

CANFIELD, J. V., AND GUSTAFSON, D. F. Self-deception. *Analysis,* 1962, *23,* 32–36.

CARVER, C. S. Facilitation of physical aggression through objective self-awareness. *Journal of Experimental Social Psychology,* 1974, *10,* 365–370.

CASTALDO, V., AND HOLZMAN, P. S. The effects of hearing one's own voice on sleep mentations. *Journal of Nervous and Mental Disease,* 1967, *144,* 2–13.

CASTALDO, V., AND HOLZMAN, P. S. The effects of hearing one's own voice on dream content: A replication. *Journal of Nervous and Mental Disease,* 1969, *148,* 74–82.

CHERRY, C. *On human communication.* Cambridge, Mass.: MIT Press, 1957.

COHEN, G. Hemispheric differences in serial versus parallel processing. *Journal of Experimental Psychology,* 1973, *97,* 349–356.

COSTANZO, P. R. Conformity development as a function of self-blame. *Journal of Personality and Social Psychology,* 1970, *14,* 366–374.

COSTANZO, R. R., AND SHAW, M. E. Conformity as a function of age level. *Child Development,* 1966, *37,* 967–975.

COYNE, L., AND HOLZMAN, P. S. Three equivalent forms of a semantic differential inventory. *Educational and Psychological Measurement,* 1966, *26,* 665–674.

DANET, B. N. Self-confrontation in psychotherapy reviewed. *American Journal of Psychotherapy,* 1968, *22,* 245–258.

DAVIS, D., AND BROCK, T. C. Use of first person pronouns as a function of increased objective self-awareness and performance feedback. *Journal of Experimental Social Psychology,* 1975, *11,* 381–388.

DAY, M. E. An eye-movement phenomenon relating to attention, thought and anxiety. *Perceptual and Motor Skills.* 1964, *19,* 443–446.

DAY, M. E. An eye-movement indicator of individual differences in the physiological organization of attentional processes and anxiety. *The Journal of Psychology,* 1967a, *66,* 51–62.

DAY, M. E. An eye-movement indicator of type and level of anxiety. Some clinical observations. *Journal of Clinical Psychology,* 1967b, *23,* 433–441.

DAY, M. E. Attention, anxiety and psychotherapy. *Psychotherapy: Theory, Research and Practice,* 1968, *5,* 146–149.

DEMOS, R. Lying to oneself. *Journal of Philosophy,* 1960, *57,* 588–595.

DESCARTES, R. [Meditations on first philosophy.] In E. S. Haldane and G. R. T. Ross (Ed. & Trans.), *The philosophical works of Descartes.* Cambridge: Cambridge University Press, 1967. (originally published in 1641.)

DIBNER, A. S. Ambiguity and anxiety. *Journal of Abnormal and Social Psychology,* 1958, *56,* 165–174.

DICKINSON, W. H., AND RAY, T. S. Immediate effects of body image confrontation with chronic schizophrenic women. Paper read at Oklahoma State Psychological Association, Oklahoma City, October, 1965.

DIXON, N. F. *Subliminal perception: The nature of a controversy.* London: McGraw-Hill, 1971.

DUVAL, S., AND WICKLUND, R. A. *A theory of objective self awareness.* New York: Academic Press, 1972.

DUVAL, S., AND WICKLUND, R. A. Effects of objective self-awareness on attribution of causality. *Journal of Experimental Social Psychology,* 1973, *9,* 17–31.

ERDELYI, M. H. A new look at the new look: Perceptual defense and vigilance. *Psychological Review*, 1974, *81*, 1–25.

ERICKSEN, C. W. Subception: fact or artifact? *Psychological Review*, 1956, *63*, 74–80.

ERIKSEN, C. W. Unconscious processes. In M. R. Jones (Ed.), *Nebraska Symposium on Motivation*, Vol. 6. Lincoln: University of Nebraska Press, 1958.

EYSENCK, H. J., AND EYSENCK, S. B. G. *Eysenck Personality Inventory*. London: University of London Press, 1963.

EYSENCK, H. J., AND WILSON, G. D. *The experimental study of Freudian theories*. New York: Barnes & Noble, 1973.

FENIGSTEIN, A., SCHEIER, M. F., AND BUSS, A. H. Public and private self-consciousness: Assessment and theory. *Journal of Consulting and Clinical Psychology*, 1975, *43*, 522–527.

FESTINGER, L. *A theory of cognitive dissonance*. Evanston, Ill.: Row, Peterson, 1957.

FINGARETTE, H. *Self-deception*. London: Routledge & Kegan Paul, 1969.

FREUD, S. [Project for a scientific psychology.] In J. Strachey (Ed. and Trans.), *The complete psychological works of Sigmund Freud*, Vol. 1. London: Hogarth, 1966. (Originally written in 1895.)

FREUD, S. [On the history of the psychoanalytic movement.] In J. Strachey (Ed. and Trans.), *The complete psychological works of Sigmund Freud*, Vol. 14. London: Hogarth, 1957. (Originally published in 1914.)

FREUD, S. [Repression.] In J. Strachey (Ed. and Trans.), *The complete psychological works of Sigmund Freud*, Vol. 14. London: Hogarth, 1957. (Originally published in 1915.)

FREUD, S. [The ego and the id.] In J. Strachey (Ed. and Trans.), *The complete psychological works of Sigmund Freud*, Vol. 19. London: Hogarth, 1961. (Originally published in 1923).

FREUD, S. [Civilization and its discontents.] In J. Strachey (Ed. and Trans.), *The complete psychological works of Sigmund Freud*, Vol. 21. London: Hogarth, 1961. (Originally published in 1930.)

FRYREAR, J. L., NUELL, L. R., AND RIDLEY, S. D. Photographic self-concept enhancement of male juvenile delinquents. *Journal of Consulting and Clinical Psychology*, 1974, *42*, 915.

GALIN, D. Implications for psychiatry of left and right cerebral specialization. *Archives of General Psychiatry*, 1974, *31*, 572–583.

GALLUP, G. G. Chimpanzees: Self-recognition. *Science*, 1970, *161*, 86–87.

GARDINER, P. L. Error, faith and self-deception. *Proceedings of the Aristotelian Society*, 1970, *50*, 221–243.

GIBBONS, F. X., AND WICKLUND, R. A. Selective exposure to self. *Journal of Research in Personality*, 1976, *10*, 98–106.

GIDE, A. *The counterfeiters*. New York: Modern Library, 1955.

GOLDSTEIN, K. *The organism, a holistic approach to biology*. New York: American Book Company, 1939.

GORDON, G. Semantic determination by subliminal verbal stimuli: A quantitative approach. Unpublished doctoral dissertation, University of London, 1967.

GRANT, D. A. Adding communication to the signaling property of the CS in classical conditioning. *Journal of General Psychology*, 1968, *79*, 147–175.

GUR, R. C., AND GUR, R. E. Handedness, sex and eyedness as moderating variables in the relation between hypnotic susceptibility and functional brain asymmetry. *Journal of Abnormal Psychology*, 1974, *83*, 635–643.

GUR, R. C., AND HILGARD, E. R. Visual imagery and the discrimination of differences between altered pictures simultaneously and successively presented. *British Journal of Psychology*, 1975, *66*, 341–345.

GUR, R. C., AND SACKEIM, H. A. The Manifest Symptom Questionnaire, with scales to measure self- and other-deception. Unpublished manuscript, University of Pennsylvania, 1975.

GUR, R. C., AND SACKEIM, H. A. Self-deception: A concept in search of a phenomenon. Manuscript submitted for publication, 1976.

GUR, R. C., SACKEIM, H. A., AND GUR, R. E. Classroom seating and psychopathology: Some initial data. *Journal of Abnormal Psychology*, 1976, *85*, 122–124.

GUR, R. E., AND GUR, R. C. Defense mechanisms, psychosomatic symptomatology, and conjugate lateral eye movements. *Journal of Consulting and Clinical Psychology*, 1975, *43*, 416–420.

GUR, R. E., AND GUR, R. C. Correlates of conjugate lateral eye movements in man. In S. Harnad (Ed.), *Lateralization in the nervous system*. New York: Academic Press, 1976.

GUR, R. E., GUR, R. C., AND HARRIS, L. J. Cerebral activation, as measured by the subjects' conjugate lateral eye movements, is influenced by experimenter location. *Neuropsychologia*, 1975, *13*, 35–44.

GUR, R. E., LEVY, J., AND GUR, R. C. Clinical studies of brain organization and behavior. In A. Winokur and A. Frazer (Eds.), *Biological bases of psychiatric disorders*. New York: Spectrum, 1977.

GUR, R. E., AND REYHER, J. The relationship between style of hypnotic induction and direction of lateral eye movement. *Journal of Abnormal Psychology*, 1973, *82*, 499–505.

HENLEY, S. H. A., AND DIXON, N. F. Laterality differences in the effect of incidental stimuli upon evoked imagery. *British Journal of Psychology*, 1974, *65*, 529–536.

HILGARD, E. R. Human motives and the concept of the self. *American Psychologist*, 1949, *4*, 374–382.

HILGARD, E. R. A neodissociation interpretation of pain reduction in hypnosis. *Psychological Review*, 1973, *80*, 396–411.

HOLMES, C., AND HOLZMAN, P. S. Effect of white noise on disinhibition of verbal expression. *Perceptual and Motor Skills*, 1966, *23*, 1039–1042.

HOLMES, D. S. Repression of interference: A further investigation. *Journal of Personality and Social Psychology*, 1972, *22*, 163–170.

HOLMES, D. S. Investigations of repression: Differential recall of material experimentally or naturally associated with ego threat. *Psychological Bulletin*, 1974, *81*, 632–653.

HOLT, R. R., AND HAVEL, J. A method for assessing primary and secondary process in the Rorschach. In M. A. Rickers-Ovsiankina (Ed.), *Rorschach psychology*. New York: Wiley, 1960.

HOLZMAN, P. S., BERGER, C., AND ROUSEY, C. Voice confrontation: A bilingual study. *Journal of Personality and Social Psychology*, 1967, *7*, 423–428.

HOLZMAN, P. S., AND ROUSEY, C. The voice as a percept. *Journal of Personality and Social Psychology*, 1966, *4*, 79–86.

HOLZMAN, P. S., AND ROUSEY, C. Monitoring, activation, and disinhibition: Effects of white noise masking on spoken thought. *Journal of Abnormal Psychology*, 1970, *75*, 227–241.

HOLZMAN, P. S., ROUSEY, C., AND SNYDER, C. On listening to one's own voice: Effects on psychophysiological responses and free associations. *Journal of Personality and Social Psychology*, 1966, *4*, 432–441.

HOWIE, D. Perceptual defense. *Psychological Review*, 1952, *59*, 308–315.

HULL, C. L. *Principles of behavior*. New York: Appleton-Century, 1943.

HUNTLEY, C. W. Judgments of self based upon records of expressive behavior. *Journal of Abnormal and Social Psychology*, 1940, *35*, 398–427.

ICKES, W. J., WICKLUND, R. A., AND FERRIS, C. B. Objective self awareness and self esteem. *Journal of Experimental Social Psychology*, 1973, *9*, 202–219.

Innes, J. M., and Young, R. E. The effect of presence of an audience, evaluation apprehension, and objective self-awareness on learning. *Journal of Experimental Social Psychology*, 1975, *11*, 35–42.

Insko, C. A., Worshel, S., Songer, E., and Arnold, S. E. Effort, objective self-awareness, choice, and dissonance. *Journal of Personality and Social Psychology*, 1973, *28*, 262–269.

Irwin, F. W. *Intentional behavior and motivation: A cognitive theory*. Philadelphia: Lippincott, 1971.

James, W. *The varieties of religious experience*. New York: Longmans, Green, 1902.

James, W. *The principles of psychology*. New York: Dover, 1950. (Originally published in 1890).

Kimble, G. A. Categories of learning and the problem of definition. In A. W. Milton (Ed.), *Categories of human learning*. New York: Academic Press, 1964.

Kinsbourne, M. Eye and head turning indicates cerebral lateralization. *Science*, 1972, *176*, 539–541.

Klein, G. S. On hearing one's own voice: An aspect of cognitive control of spoken thought. In N. D. Greenfield and W. C. Lewis (Eds.), *Psychoanalysis and current biological thought*. Madison: University of Wisconsin Press, 1965. Pp. 245–273.

Klein, G. S., and Wolitzky, D. L. Vocal isolation: Effects of occulding auditory feedback from one's own voice. *Journal of Abnormal Psychology*, 1970, *75*, 50–56.

Kocel, K., Galin, D., Ornstein, R., and Merrin, E. Lateral eye movement and cognitive mode. *Psychonomic Science*, 1972, *27*, 223–224.

Lader, M., and Marks, I., *Clinical anxiety*. London: William Heinemann, 1971.

Lazarus, R. S., and McCleary, R. A. Autonomic discrimination without awareness: A study of subception. *Psychological Review*, 1951, *58*, 113–122.

Levy, J. Possible basis for the evolution of lateral specialization of the human brain. *Nature*, 1969, *224*, 614–615.

Liebert, R. M., and Morris, L. W. Cognitive and emotional components of test anxiety: A distinction and some initial data. *Psychological Reports*, 1967, *20*, 975–978.

Liebling, R. A., and Shaver, P. Evaluation, self-awareness, and task performance. *Journal of Experimental Social Psychology*, 1973, *9*, 297–306.

Luchins, A. S. On an approach to social perception. *Journal of Personality*, 1950, *19*, 64–84.

Luria, A. R. *The role of speech in the regulation of normal and abnormal behavior*. New York: Liveright, 1961.

Lykken, D. T. The GSR in the detection of guilt. *Journal of Applied Psychology*, 1959, *43*, 385–388.

Lykken, D. T. Psychology and the lie detector industry. *American Psychologist*, 1974, *29*, 725–738.

Mahl, G. F. Measuring the patient's anxiety during interviews from "expressive" aspects of his speech. *Transactions of the New York Academy of Sciences*, 1959, *58*(ser. 2), 402–405.

Mandler, G., and Watson, D. L. Anxiety and the interpretation of behavior. In C. D. Spielberger (Ed.), *Anxiety and behavior*. New York: Academic Press, 1966. Pp. 263–288.

Martens, R. Palmar sweating and the presence of an audience. *Journal of Experimental Social Psychology*, 1969, *5*, 371–374.

Martin, D. G., Hawryluk, G. A., and Guse, L. L. Experimental study of unconscious influences: Ultrasound as a stimulus. *Journal of Abnormal Psychology*, 1974, *83*, 589–608.

May, R. *The meaning of anxiety*. New York: Ronald, 1950.

McREYNOLDS, P., AND ACKER, M. On the assessment of anxiety, II: By a self-report inventory. *Psychological Reports*, 1966, *19*, 231–237.

MEEHL, P. E., AND HATHAWAY, S. R. The K factor as a suppressor variable in the Minnesota Multiphasic Personality Inventory. *Journal of Applied Psychology*, 1946, *30*, 525–564.

MILLER, B. Actor and observer perceptions of the learning of a task. *Journal of Experimental Social Psychology*, 1975, *11*, 95–111.

MISCHEL, T. Understanding neurotic behavior: From "mechanism" to "intentionality." In T. Mischel (Ed.), *Understanding other persons*. Totowa, N.J.: Rowman & Littlefield, 1974.

MORAY, N. *Listening and attention*. London: Penguin Books, 1972.

MURPHY, G. Experiments in overcoming self-deception. *Psychophysiology*, 1970, *6*, 790–799.

MURRAY, H. A. Studies of stressful interpersonal disputations. *American Psychologist*, 1963, *18*, 28–36.

OLIVOS, G. Response delay, psychophysiologic activation and recognition of one's own voice. *Psychosomatic Medicine*, 1967, *29*, 433–440.

ORNE, M. T., THACKRAY, R. I., AND PASKEWITZ, D. A. On the detection of deception: A model for the study of the physiological effects of psychological stimuli. In N. S. Greenfield and R. A. Sternbach (Eds.), *Handbook of psychophysiology*. New York: Holt, Rinehart & Winston, 1972.

ORNSTEIN, R. E. *The psychology of consciousness*. San Francisco: W. H. Freeman & Co., 1972.

OSGOOD, C. E., SUCI, G. J., AND TANNENBAUM, P. H. *The measurement of meaning*. Urbana: University of Illinois Press, 1957.

PADEN, R. C., HIMELSTEIN, H. C., AND PAUL, G. L. Videotape versus verbal feedback in the modification of meal behavior of chronic mental patients. *Journal of Consulting and Clinical Psychology*, 1974, *42*, 623.

PEAK, H. An evaluation of the concepts of reflex and voluntary action. *Psychological Review*, 1933, *40*, 71–89.

PENELHUM, T. Pleasure and falsity. In S. Hampshire (Ed.), *Philosophy of mind*. New York: Harper & Row, 1966.

PLATO [*Cratylus*]. In R. Jowett (Ed. and Trans.), *The dialogues of Plato*, Vol. 3. Oxford: Clarendon Press, 1953. (Originally published circa 386 B.C.)

PLATO [*The Republic*]. In R. Jowett (Ed. and Trans.), *The dialogues of Plato*, Vol. 4. Oxford: Clarendon Press, 1953. (Originally published circa 359 B.C.)

PYNCHON, T. *V*. New York: Bantam Books, 1963.

QUINTON, A. *The nature of things*. London: Routledge & Kegan Paul, 1973.

ROGERS, C. R. *Client-centered therapy*. Boston: Houghton Mifflin, 1951.

ROUSEY, C., AND HOLZMAN, P. S. Recognition of one's own voice. *Journal of Personality and Social Psychology*, 1967, *6*, 464–466.

ROUSEY, C., AND HOLZMAN, P. S. Some effects of listening to one's voice systemically distorted. *Perceptual and Motor Skills*, 1968, *27*, 1303–1313.

SACKEIM, H. A. A theory of the self-confrontation experience. Unpublished manuscript, Oxford University, 1974.

SACKEIM, H. A., AND GUR, R. C. Necessary and sufficient criteria for ascribing self-deception. Manuscript submitted for publication, 1976.

SARTRE, J. P. *Being and nothingness: An essay on phenomenological ontology*. Trans. by H. Barnes. London: Methuen & Col, 1958.

SCHWARTZ, G. E., DAVIDSON, R. J., AND MAER, F. Right Hemisphere lateralization for emotion in the human brain: Interactions with cognition. *Science*, 1975, *190*, 286–288.

SCHWARTZ, G. E., FAIR, P. L., SALT, P., MANDEL, M. R., AND KLERMAN, G. L. Facial muscle patterning to affective imagery in depressed and nondepressed subjects. *Science*, 1976, *192*, 489–491.

SIEGLER, F. A. Demos on lying to oneself. *Journal of Philosophy*, 1962, *59*, 469–475.

SKINNER, B. F. *The behavior of organisms*. New York: Appleton-Century, 1938.

SPERRY, R. W. Hemispheric deconnection and unity in conscious awareness. *American Psychologist*, 1968, *23*, 723–733.

STORMS, M. D. Videotape and the attribution process: Reversing actors' and observers' points of view. *Journal of Personality and Social Psychology*, 1973, *27*, 165–175.

TEITELBAUM, H. A. Spontaneous rhythmic ocular movement: Their possible relationship to mental activity. *Neurology*, 1954, *4*, 350–354.

VERWOERDT, A., NOWLIN, J. B., AND AGNELLO, S. A. A technique for studying effects of self-confrontation in cardiac patients. *Health Sciences TV Bulletin*, 1965, *2*, 1–6.

VYGOTSKY, L. S. *Thought and language*. Cambridge, Mass.: MIT Press, 1962.

WASON, P. C., AND JOHNSON-LAIRD, P. N. *Psychology of reasoning: Structure and context*. Cambridge, Mass.: Harvard University Press, 1972.

WICKLUND, R. A. Objective self-awareness. In L. Berkowitz (Ed.), *Advances in experimental social psychology*, Vol. 8. New York: Academic Press, 1975.

WICKLUND, R. A., AND DUVAL, S. Opinion change and performance facilitation as a result of objective self awareness. *Journal of Experimental Social Psychology*, 1971, *7*, 319–342.

WICKLUND, R. A., AND ICKES, W. J. The effect of objective self awareness on predecisional exposure to information. *Journal of Experimental Social Psychology*, 1972, *8*, 378–387.

WINE, J. Test anxiety and direction of attention. *Psychological Bulletin*, 1971, *76*, 92–104.

WISDOM, J. O. Psychoanalytic theories of the unconscious. In P. Edwards (Ed.), *The encyclopedia of phislosphy*, Vol. 8. New York: Macmillan, 1967.

WOLFF, W. *The expression of personality*. New York: Harper, 1943.

WUNDT, W. *An introduction to psychology*. New York: Arno Press, 1973. (Originally published in 1912).

5   *Visceroception, Awareness, and Behavior*

GYÖRGY ÁDÁM

I. VISCEROCEPTION AND PSYCHOPHYSICS

Taking into consideration the Sherringtonian classification of receptors, one notes that the power law of psychophysics is absolutely inapplicable to only one class of sensory organs, the *visceral receptors;* that is, their impulse flow to the brain does not generally evoke any sensation. The title of the present section should be somewhat thought-provoking because it challenges the classical concepts of neurophysiology. Some 15 or 20 years ago, even handbooks and textbooks of sensory physiology refused to recognize visceral sensation as an independent psychophysiological phenomenon.

Does visceral perception exist at all? The answer to this question seems not so simple. If we analyze in detail the main characteristics of visceral input to the brain, the existence of inborn sensations starting from our internal organs seems to be problematic. The main role of visceroceptive information sent to the brain must be the *homeostatic* function, but we are presently in possession of a body of evidence that demonstrates the *extrahomeostatic* activity of this afferent system. Visceral sensory impulses reach the brain and may have a marked influence on behavior (Ádám, 1967). The common feature of both homeostatic and nonhomeostatic influences is well known to physicians and surgeons: Visceroception is not perceived except in some emergency situations (painful stimuli, hunger, thirst, etc.).

The crucial problem of visceral input is thus that of consciousness. The stimulation of several visceral receptors in the range of physiological intensities does not evoke any subjective sensations. Our previous investigations have demonstrated that, for example, nonpainful duodenal stimulation can deeply modify the electrical activity of the brain

GYÖRGY ÁDÁM · Department of Comparative Physiology, Eötvös Loránd University, Budapest, Hungary.

without causing any feeling of pressure or discomfort (Ádám, Preis-ich, Kukorelli, and Kelemen, 1965).

The classical law of psychophysics is consequently inapplicable to visceroception. If, however, we look at the Fechner–Stevens law, $\psi = k.\phi^n$, using a roundabout approach—for example, instead of subjective verbal account (ψ) applying the observation of behavior and/or electrical activity of the brain—some basic psychophysical approximations can be made. At present, we are far from applying the power law concerning central events, but because of the fundamental congruity between neural activity and perceptual intensity (Stevens, 1971), this bypass may be fruitful in the future.

For the moment, we are in possession of two sets of data using this byway: one concerning the *threshold* problem and the other regarding the *discrimination* of visceral input. Both groups of results may be starting points to future detailed investigation of the psychophysical law concerning visceroception (Ádám, 1974).

II. THE VISCEROCEPTIVE THRESHOLD

As far as the threshold problem is concerned, we have collected data proving that visceral afferent impulses exert a *dual influence* on the brain activity, depending on the intensity and duration of the stimuli. Kukorelli and Juhász (1976) in our laboratory have shown that intestinal or splanchnic stimuli *above* the splanchnoabdominal threshold level trigger arousal and desynchronization, whereas visceral stimuli *below* that level induce hypersynchronization. Even more, a

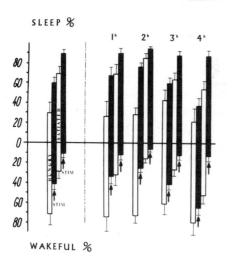

FIGURE 1. Shift of sleep–wakefulness cycle in a group of five cats with chronically implanted cortical electrodes and isolated intestinal loop before and after repetitive visceroceptive stimulation. The control percentage values of the starving and fed animals are represented by white columns. The black columns represent the range of the sleep–wakefulness cycle due to electrical stimulation of the mucosa of the isolated loop. *Left to right:* average values of the four-hour recording and separate values of each hour successively. The arrows indicate the intestinal stimulus (Kukorelli and Juhász, unpublished data).

TABLE 1
The Dual Role of Visceral Input to the
Brain

Visceral Input
Below   Viscerosomatic threshold
↓
EEG synchronization
Sleep induction
Above   Viscerosomatic threshold
↓
EEG desynchronization
Arousal

habituated suprathreshold stimulus elicits the same response as a subthreshold one.

In another series of experiments on chronic cats, Kukorelli and Juhász have demonstrated that weak repetitive stimulation of the intestinal wall produces a shift of the wakefulness–sleep balance toward the direction of sleep in both starving and satiated animals (Figure 1). As far as the different stages of sleep are concerned, this shift enhances primarily the slow-wave period (on account of the paradoxical sleep).

Consequently, it can be stated, that the effect of the visceral influence on the brain electrical activity is entirely dependent on the parameters of the stimuli. Under physiological conditions, a weak train of impulses (below the viscerosomatic threshold) elicits synchronization and sleep, and a more intense train evokes arousal (Table 1). We presume that these latter impulses are suitable for psychophysical measurements, since the former, weak input is unable to maintain the minimum level of wakefulness necessary for behavioral responses.

III. VISCERAL DISCRIMINATION

The recording of behavioral reactions proved to be an adequate although rough approach to the study of visceral discrimination, which by itself can initiate further and more delicate psychophysical studies.

In series of experiments on dogs with chronic ureteral fistulae published a number of years ago (Ádám and Mészáros, 1957), it was proved that the animal can discriminate between the stimulation of

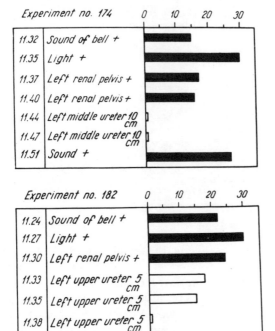

Figure 2. Irradiation of the renal pelvic conditional reflex upon stimulation of the proximal portion of the ureter and its absence upon stimulation of the middle portion of the ureter in dog Vihar with ureteral fistulae. The conditional salivary response is represented in units of the Hanicke–Kupalov scale. Black horizontal columns, positive (reinforced) conditional response; white horizontal columns, negative (discriminative) conditional response. First vertical row, time of stimulation; second vertical row, type of stimulus (Ádám and Mészáros, 1957).

the renal pelvis and a segment of the ureter situated 10 cm below and cannot distinguish at the same time another site situated only 5 cm from the pelvis (Figure 2). By the application of the same alimentary classical conditioning method, it has been shown that the dog can discriminate between stimuli arriving from the left and right kidneys (Ádám, Mészáros, and Zubor, 1957).

Subsequently, we extended the investigations to discrimination by applying the operant conditioning technique. In the first series of experiments (Slucki, Ádám, and Porter, 1965), we have obtained evidence that rhesus monkeys with a surgically prepared isolated intestinal loop discriminated between the presence and absence of the intestinal stimulus. Recently, these studies have been repeated with my collaborator György Bárdos on rats with chronically operated isolated intestinal loop, with weak electrical stimulation of the intestinal mucosa used as SΔ (Figure 3). Thus, the weak electrical stimulation of the gut has been used as a discriminative stimulus for lever pressing. The results have proved that rats, similarly to monkeys, succeed in discriminating between the presence and absence of the visceral stimulus (Bárdos and Ádám, 1978).

A third approach used to demonstrate visceral discrimination possibilities in both dogs and humans has been the so-called habituation discrimination test. When the intestinal stimulus (inflation of a balloon, which causes EEG arousal) was repeated several times, the arousal diminished step by step, and habituation occurred. In this stage of habituation, a second balloon was inflated, which was situated 15 cm from the first one. The realization of one of two alternatives was tested. Desynchronization would mean, we postulated, that the brain could discriminate between the impulses coming from the two intestinal segments situated 15 cm apart (Figure 4). The persistence of habituation, on the other hand, would indicate a lack of discrimination. The topical discrimination property of the brain has been successfully proved in 8 patients of the 14 tested (Preisich and Ádám, 1964). As for our dog experiments, in a group of 9 animals, every dog with a chronically isolated intestinal loop showed discrimination when the two balloons were situated *more than 5 cm* apart (Ádám, Heffler, Kovács, Nagy, and Szigeti, 1965; Moisseeva and Ádám, 1966).

To summarize our results, we have demonstrated visceral discrimination using *three different methods* (Table 2). Classical conditioning in dogs enabled us to demonstrate both topographic and intensity differentiation; the operant technique made it possible to prove the presence or absence of the visceral stimulus; and finally the EEG habituation test gave further evidence of topical discrimination. All

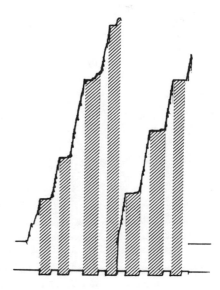

Figure 3. Cumulative curve of operant behavior of rat "Cicero" with chronically operated isolated intestinal loop following discriminative training of nonpainful stimulation of the isolated gut. The zigzag line and the dark columns indicate the intestinal stimulus.

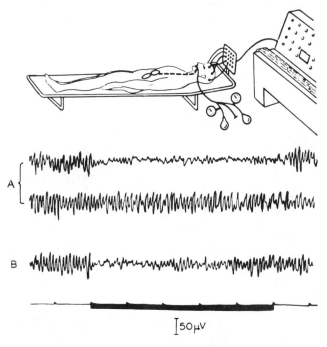

FIGURE 4. Duodenal discrimination test in humans. Distension of balloon A caused desynchronization, which was soon habituated. Inflation of balloon B under such circumstances led to blocking of the alpha rhythm. Top: schematic representation of the experimental procedure. Bottom: time curve and duration of visceral stimulation, thick block (Preisich and Ádám, 1964).

TABLE 2
Different Methodical Approaches of
Visceroceptive Topographic and
Intensity Discrimination

Visceroceptive Discriminative Tests

1. Classical Conditioning
   Topical discrimination +
   Intensity discrimination +

2. Operant Conditioning
   Intensity discrimination +

3. EEG Habituation
   Topical discrimination +

three techniques may serve in the future as starting points for more detailed and sophisticated indirect psychophysical investigations.

IV. VISCERAL PERCEPTION

What about *direct* examination of the relation of the magnitude of visceral stimulations and the central sensations elicited by them? In other words, is it possible to teach the subjects to perceive more and more visceral events? After such a learning procedure would it be possible to investigate the power law of psychophysics?

Considering that human infants become aware of rectal and vesical stimuli most probably by means of a learning process necessary for their adaptation to human society, a series of experiments has been undertaken with volunteers to determine whether unconscious visceral stimuli could be rendered conscious by conditioning. Some years ago, by means of verbal feedback we succeeded in teaching a group of subjects to perceive duodenal stimuli that prior to conditioning had been unconscious (Ádám, 1967). Recently, we continued these studies with a second series of experiments on 16 women subjected to bipolar stimulation of the cervix uteri, a treatment reported to be effective in cases of infertility (Kukorelli, Ádám, Gimes, and Tóth, 1972).

Electrical stimulation of the cervix uteri elicited electrographic arousal in all of the 16 experimental subjects with well-developed alpha activity. Some of the subjects reported feeling stimulation of more than 15 cps frequency. Therefore we always applied lower frequencies. During repeated stimulations with identical parameters, the desynchronizing effect rapidly decreased, especially during repetitive stimulations at frequencies below 10 cps. The stimuli, habituated after several repetitions, were presented in trains of 1–5 min duration. In this case, an enhancement of synchronization consisted of an increase in the amplitude of alpha waves; further, in some cases a decrease of the EEG frequency was observed.

The analogy is evident with our results on cats, mentioned before, on the *double nature* of visceral input to the brain: arousing and hypnogenic.

In a second stage of these experiments, conditioning procedure was undertaken in 6 patients to determine whether they could be taught to perceive unconscious uterine impulses by means of verbal feedback (Table 3). Starting from the level of the subjective sensation of discomfort, the voltage of the successive trains of uterine impulses

TABLE 3
Effect of Selective Attention and Verbal Feedback on the Perception of Visceroceptive Impulses Elicited by Electrical
Stimulation of the Cervix Uteri (Kukorelli et al., 1972)

Number of subject	Sensation threshold before association, volt	Verbal association												Alpha desynchronizing threshold, volt	Sensation threshold after association, volt
		V	No.	V	No.	V	No.	V	No.	V	No.	V	No.		
1	8.0	7.5	9 / 9	7.0	12 / 21	6.5	19 / 40	6.0	30 / 70					5.0	6.5 — 1.5 / 1.5
2	8.5	8.0	10 / 10	7.5	21 / 31	7.0	25 / 56	6.5	30 / 86					6.5	7.0 — 1.5 / 0.5
3	9.5	9.0	8 / 8	8.5	13 / 21	8.0	18 / 39	7.5	21 / 60	7.0	23 / 83	6.5	30 / 113	6.0	7.0 — 2.5 / 1.0
4	7.5	7.0	6 / 6	6.5	5 / 11	6.0	19 / 30	5.5	15 / 55	5.0	30 / 85			4.1	5.5 — 2.0 / 1.4
5	8.0	7.5	30 / 30											6.0	8.0 — — / —
6	6.5	6.0	30 / 30											4.5	6.5 — — / —
Mean	8.3	7.8	8 / 8	7.3	12 / 21	6.8	20 / 41	6.3	18 / 57					5.4	6.5 — 1.8 / 1.1

was lowered step by step, the frequency of 3 cps being preserved. Each visceral stimulation was accompanied by verbal feedback ("The uterine stimulus is now applied" or "You now feel vibration in your abdomen," etc.). After 10–50 of such associative trials, the subjects became aware of the stimulus at a voltage much lower than the initial subjective threshold (of course, without verbal reinforcement at this point). In some cases, the threshold of perception was found to be very close to the level at which EEG desynchronization—the so-called objective threshold—originally occurred. In these cases, a considerably higher number of associations was needed (Figure 5). In other words, by using verbal feedback, we found it possible to teach the women to notice—to bring into consciousness—afferent uterine stimuli that prior to conditioning had been unconscious.

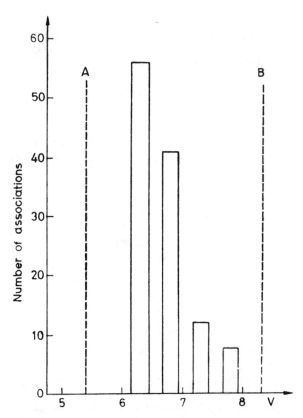

FIGURE 5. Relation between the sensation threshold (B) and the number of verbal associations (ordinate). Abscissa: voltage of uterine stimulation; A: alpha desynchronizing threshold. Each column represents the average of data on six subjects (Kukorelli *et al.*, 1972).

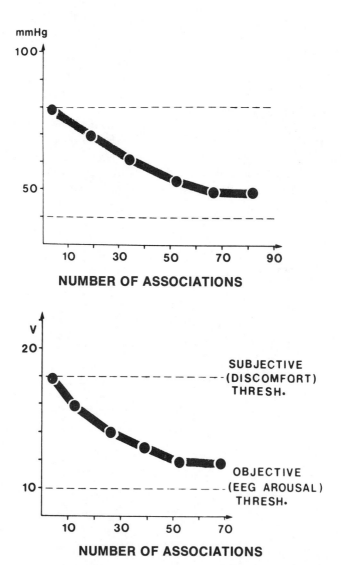

FIGURE 6. Visceral perception curves. The upper (duodenal) and the lower (uterine) diagrams represent the process of converting unconscious stimuli into conscious awareness by verbal feedback. Unconscious visceral stimuli, when reinforced by verbal feedback, are brought to consciousness by learning; the subjective pain-threshold approaches the objective one. Abscissa: number of associations; ordinate: intensity of visceral stimuli.

In conclusion, from our two series of experiments applying duodenal or uterine stimulation combined with verbal feedback, some important statements seem to be evident:

1. By using verbal feedback, it is possible to teach human subjects to notice and perceive visceral stimuli that prior to conditioning were unconscious (Figure 6).

2. The success of the training is dependent on the parameters of the visceral stimulus applied, among other factors. Weak stimuli have hypnogenic rather than arousing effect; thus, these cannot figure as the basis of feedback training.

3. Visceral perception is reached always at a somewhat higher stimulus-intensity level than the objective threshold, causing manifest arousal before the training is started.

It is difficult at the present time to explain the mechanism of the results of our feedback experiments. It is, however, obvious that the verbal control has been the essential factor in bringing the subsensory visceral impulses into consciousness. But how this perceptive mechanism works and what structures are involved, we do not know at present.

V. Conclusions: The Possible Roles of Visceroception

Let us return to the problem of psychophysics. At the beginning of this paper, it was emphasized that the classical law of psychophysics is inapplicable to visceroception *directly*. It is applicable only if some sort of bypass is used. But after presenting the evidence on learning to perceive visceral events, we may reconsider this statement. Namely, the possibility cannot be excluded that such learned sensations may serve as appropriate background for the detailed analysis of the dependence of the sensation on the parameters of the stimuli applied.

We must draw attention to the observation that the intensity of the visceral input is an essential factor in this respect. Stimuli weaker than the viscerosomatic threshold are not effective; they cannot be rendered conscious by training; and they will have, in all probability, a hypnogenic effect. On the other hand, stimuli more intense than the pain threshold evoke the feeling of discomfort (nociceptive stimuli, of course, do not fall within the range of psychophysical examination) (Figure 7).

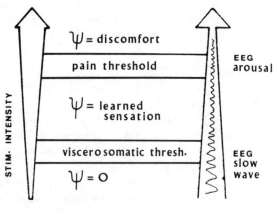

FECHNER - STEVENS LAW:

$$\Psi = k \cdot \Phi^n$$

Ψ = behavioral and/or
electrical responses

FIGURE 7. Intensity arrow (left) representing the intensity continuum of visceral stimulation from the point of view of the power law of psychophysics. The low intensities do not cause any sensations ($\psi = 0$), they merely take part in homeostatic regulatory functions and sleep induction. Higher intensities—that is, between viscerosomatic and pain thresholds—may serve as the background of visceroceptive conditioning and cause desynchronization of the EEG (right arrow).

To conclude, the different functions of visceral input are summarized on Table 4 in the light of our own data.

Most of these mechanisms take place unconsciously. First of all, the main inborn function of visceral afferents is related to homeostatic regulation of the same visceral functions from which these sensory pathways arise. Without any doubt, it can be stated that all the other roles of visceroception—that is, the extrahomeostatic functions—may be regarded as accessory, supplementary ones.

In earlier years, it was demonstrated by Bykov, Airapetyants, and our own group that visceral impulses can control animal and human behavior. Moreover, they can figure as starting points for an unconscious learning process. Interoceptive conditional reflexes may play an essential role in the life of the organism, in both visceral and somatic functions.

The conscious visceroceptive mechanisms include the initiation of emergency functions. This perceived input develops in early childhood by way of conditioning.

Finally, one of the most fascinating roles of visceroception may be related to visceral perception. Some evidence has been presented in this paper concerning the possibility of perception through learning by means of verbal feedback. Does this technique have any theoretical or practical importance, or is it merely an attractive laboratory artifact? Let us be rather optimistic in this respect and anticipate the gradually growing significance of visceral perceptive learning experiments.

But as far as the application of visceral perceptive learning in everyday psychological and medical practice is concerned, we must be extremely careful and cautious (Figure 8). Depending on the typology (personality) of the subjects, visceral perception might prove to be beneficial to one group of humans and damaging to another group. All depends on the personality, the type, and the psychological features (e.g., suggestibility) of the organism. Thus, the application in therapy of any visceral learning procedure must be preceded not only by intensive research in this field but also by careful investigation of

TABLE 4

The Possible Roles of Visceroception in Homeostatic and Extrahomeostatic Regulatory Functions of the Organism

1.	Unconscious	
	1.1.	Homeostatic regulation
		(control of visceral functions)
		(inborn)
	1.2.	Control of behavior
		1.2.1.—Control of states of awareness
		1.2.2.—Initiation of visceral learning
		1.2.3.—Control of operant behavior
		1.2.4.—Control of somatic learning
		(learned)
2.	Conscious	
	2.1.	Control of emergency states
		2.1.1.—Control of hunger
		2.1.2.—Control of thirst
		2.1.3.—Initiation of defecation
		(learned)
	2.2.	Visceral perception
		2.2.1.—(Laboratory artifact?)
		2.2.2.—Initiation of self-control
		benefaction for one human type
		damage for another human type
		(learned)

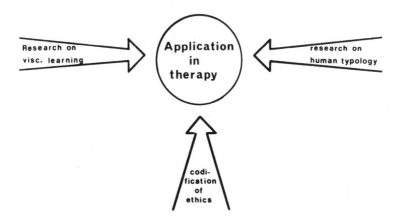

Figure 8.   In addition to intensive research in the field (left arrow), the application in practice of human visceral learning must be preceded, by research on human typology (right arrow) as well as by codification of the ethics (center arrow).

human typology (personality). Last but not least, juridical measures should be taken in order to prevent the misuse of this exceptional technique and to facilitate its real application for the benefit of human physical and mental health.

References

Ádám, G. *Interoception and behaviour: An experimental study.* Budapest: Akadémiai Kiadó, 1967.

Ádám, G. Interoceptive stimuli and learning. In *Proceedings of the International Union of Physiological Sciences,* Vol. 10. New Delhi, Association of Physiologists and Pharmacologists of India, 1974.

Ádám, G., Heffler, J., Kovács, Á., Nagy, A., and Szigeti, Á. Electrographic test for the discrimination of intestinal stimuli. *Acta Physiologica Academiae Scientiarum Hungaricae,* 1965, 27, 145–147.

Ádám, G., and Mészáros, I. Contributions to the higher nervous connections of the renal pelvis and the ureter. *Acta Physiologica Academiae Scientiarum Hungaricae,* 1957, 12, 327–334.

Ádám, G., Mészáros, I., and Zubor, L. On the joint function of the cerebral hemispheres in connection with renal pelvic and ureteral symmetric afferent impulses. *Acta Physiologica Academiae Scientiarum Hungaricae,* 1957, 12, 335–339.

Ádám, G., Preisich, P., Kukorelli, T., and Kelemen, V. Changes in human cerebral electrical activity in response to mechanical stimulation of the duodenum. *Electroencephalography and Clinical Neurophysiology,* 1965, 18, 409–411.

Airapetyants, E. S. [*Higher nervous activity and the receptors of inner organs*] Leningrad: Soviet Academic Publishing House, 1952. (In Russian.)

BÁRDOS, G., AND ÁDÁM, G. Visceroceptive control of operant behavior in rats. *Physiology and Behavior*, 1978. In press.

BYKOV, K. M. *The cerebral cortex and the internal organs.* New York: Chemical Publishing, 1957.

KUKORELLI, T., ÁDÁM, G., GIMES, R., AND TÓTH, F. Uteral stimulation and vigilance level in humans. *Acta Physiologica Academiae Scientiarum Hungaricae*, 1972, *42*, 403–410.

KUKORELLI, T., AND JUHÁSZ, G. Electroencephalographic synchronization induced by stimulation of small intestine and splanchnic nerve in cats. *Electroencephalography and Clinical Neurophysiology*, 1976, *41*, 491–500.

MOISSEEVA, N. A., AND ÁDÁM, G. [Electroencephalographic investigation of interoceptive impulses in kittens.] *Doklady Akademii Nauk SSSR*, 1966, *167*, 482–485. (In Russian.)

PREISICH, P., AND ÁDÁM, G. La discrimination nonconsciente des stimuli duodénaux: le test de différentiation d'habituation électroencéphalographique. *Acta Gastro-Enterologica Belgica*, 1964, *27*, 625–629.

SLUCKI, H., ÁDÁM, G., AND PORTER, R. W. Operant discrimination of an interoceptive stimulus in rhesus monkeys. *Journal of Experimental Analysis of Behavior*, 1965, *8*, 405–414.

STEVENS, S. S. Sensory power functions and neural events. In W. R. Loewenstein (Ed.), *Principles of receptor physiology: Handbook of sensory physiology*, Volume 1. Berlin-Heidelberg-New York: Springer Verlag, 1971. Pp. 226–242.

6   *Stimulus-Bound Behavior and Biological Self-Regulation: Feeding, Obesity, and External Control*

JUDITH RODIN

One challenge of contributing to this series is that it provides the incentive to try to reconceptualize work on the eating behavior of humans in terms of consciousness and self-regulation. In animals, eating is one behavioral component of long-term weight regulation and energy balance and, as such, is part of an exquisitely precise biological feedback system. However, in humans, eating often occurs for reasons other than the regulation and maintenance of body weight, and thus the biologically determined system can be overcome or at least disturbed. For example, people often overeat when food is plentiful; they take dessert when there is no longer a physiologic need; they eat at certain times of the day whether or not there is actual depletion. If biological regulation is disturbed by the impact of these external stimuli upon feeding, how do people actually regulate their body weight? The answer is that many do not, and some become overweight.

For numerous overweight and normal weight individuals too, the regulation of feeding is consciously initiated and restrained. Information from internal physiological states representing depletion and satiation—especially metabolic and neural signals—undoubtedly influences this process to some extent. However, there is no clear evidence as yet that the conscious experience of hunger is well correlated with identifiable physiological indicators of depletion on the one hand or with amount eaten on the other. Moreover, regardless of which internal events might stimulate the subjective state of

JUDITH RODIN · Department of Psychology, Yale University, New Haven, Connecticut.

215

hunger, other cognitive factors such as time of day, setting, and amount of food available are at least as likely as hunger to influence the initiation and cessation of eating.

It is important to notice a major distinction between the type of external or cognitive information described above and the external information often thought about when one is dealing with issues of consciousness and self-regulation, for example, in biofeedback conditioning procedures. In the latter case, the subject is given visible or audible external feedback cues based on some change in internal physiological processes. Awareness of and attention to the external signal allows the person to control and/or alter the internal state to which it is linked. By contrast, in the naturally occurring process that has evolved with regard to eating, many of the external conscious signals are not derived at all from conditions of the physical state of the organism. Thus, the biobehavioral process regulating eating has a third variable—the external environment—that may sometimes create havoc in an ecology of abundance. One can, however, conceive of the ecological value of responsiveness to environmental cues under conditions of scarcity. In this instance, regulation needs to be based on the availability of food in the environment rather than on internal need states. The metabolic systems would have to adapt to environmentally influenced feeding in order for the organism to survive. This example is provided to suggest that externally controlled eating may sometimes have positive as well as negative consequences for the organism. In both cases, however, the degree of one's reliance on external cues to eat makes inroads on the impact of more biological stimuli for feeding. Let us first consider what we mean by cues for eating in humans.

I. CUES FOR EATING

In purely biological terms, hunger is assumed to be the expression of a current or incipient deficiency in energy supply to working tissues, and satiety or loss of appetite is the anticipation of the correction of that deficiency. Thus the sensations that an individual habitually experiences when he has an appetite or satisfies it are, at least in part, presumed to be the identifiable subjective correlates of a potentially high or low energy supply. This view assumes that the motivation to eat food results from the effect of energy-relevant states of the stomach, the liver, the intestines, and body tissue on cerebral activity (Booth and Mather, 1977; Friedman and Stricker, 1976). However, surprisingly, there is as yet no clear evidence that the conscious experience of hunger is well correlated with these physiological indicators of depletion. In part, this is true because conscious sensations labeled as hunger or appetite also derive from purely cognitive or social cues. Thus, deciding when to eat can be strongly influenced by the presence of food, meal times, assessments of appropriate intake, expectation of further food availability, social facilitation, palatability of food, thoughts about food, beliefs about prior intake, and the range of available alternative behaviors. The cessation of feeding is also influenced by cognitive and social cues such as prescriptions about meal size, the palatability of the food, decisions to employ voluntary control, the size of servings, and the place where the food is eaten.

As an example of how cognitive cues can influence eating, let us consider time of day. To assess the impact of mealtime upon eating, Schachter and Gross (1968) tested subjects in two different experimental situations. In the first, a large wall clock was speeded up, leading subjects to believe that an hour had passed and that it was close to dinnertime. In the other condition, the clock was slowed down, so that subjects believed that dinnertime was still over an hour away. In both conditions, the actual amount of time that had passed was identical. Subjects were college undergraduates, who normally took their meals in dormitories, where mealtimes were standardized. Schachter and Gross (1968) found that subjects did use cues from the passage of time to regulate consciously their eating and that this use of cues differed for overweight and normal weight subjects. The overweight group ate, on the average, almost twice as much when they believed that it was dinnertime as they did when they thought that it was not yet close to the dinner hour. For normal weight subjects, the reverse was more true. They ate somewhat less near dinnertime than earlier, and many reported curtailing their intake because it was close to mealtime and they did not wish to spoil their appetite. In a subsequent study, Rodin (1975a) demonstrated that the perception of the passage of time itself is subject to external and cognitive influences, such as how boring or interesting ongoing events are. These time-relevant judgments influence both the initiation of eating and the amount consumed, especially but not exclusively for overweight individuals.

To assess the effects on consumption of seeing and thinking about food, Ross (1974) seated participants in his study before a table on which chessmen, candlesticks, marbles, a toy car, and cashew nuts were placed. During the experimental session, the table was either brightly illuminated with a 40-watt unshaded white bulb or dimly lit with a 7.5-watt shaded red bulb. The difference in illumination provided the manipulation of cue salience, that is, the visual salience of the cashew nuts on the table. Ross varied cognitive salience—the degree to which the subjects thought about the nuts—in three ways, by instructing them to consider cashews, marbles, or anything they chose. Subjects were encouraged to do whatever they liked with the several items on the table: play with the marbles, touch the candlesticks, eat the nuts. Unknown to them, the experimenter simply weighed the nuts at the end of each session.

Participants in Ross's study ate significantly more when the lights were brightly focused on the nuts than they did when the cashews were less visible under dim illumination. Those instructed to think about cashews also ate many more nuts than did subjects who were permitted to think about anything. In both cases, the effects were particularly strong for overweight subjects.

In a second phase of the study, all subjects played an absorbing guessing game. The cashews were left, fully visible, on the table, and the amount eaten was once again determined. As before, overweight subjects ate significantly greater amounts than normals, but they were subsequently unable to report accurately how much they had eaten. This degree of inaccuracy was in fascinating contrast to the first phase, in which they correctly recalled how much they had eaten. These data suggest that when food is freely available, overweight people who are distracted by interesting activities may overeat without conscious awareness. Indeed, many diet programs aimed at modifying the eating behavior of overweight people recommend not eating during other activities such as watching television or reading, precisely because they are trying to bring eating under more conscious control. As the Ross data indicate, short-term regulation can break down when the externally responsive individual does not consciously attend to the social and cognitive cues that influence his eating. Nonetheless, it is clear from the first part of Ross's study that regulation based on attention to external nonphysiologic cues may also lead to overeating and must necessarily be less precise than regulation based on internal, biologically initiated signals.

II. INDIVIDUAL DIFFERENCES IN ATTENTION AND RESPONSIVENESS TO EXTERNAL CUES

If, in some people, eating is more compelled by prominent external cues than eating in others, even without their conscious awareness, how might these individuals be different? Is their physiology faulty, or should we think of this fact in motivational, perceptual, or information-processing terms? To answer this question, our strategy at one stage of our investigations was simply to gather as many possibly relevant facts as we could in the hope that the sheer accumulation of information would eventually force a more conceptually precise picture of the phenomenon.

In a series of small studies, we first compared the performance of obese and normal weight subjects on tasks that, in the literature of experimental psychology, have been assumed to indicate something about the likelihood that a stimulus will trigger a response. We reasoned that if the obese are generally more responsive to salient stimuli than are normals, they should react more quickly to external cues, take in more environmental stimuli, remember them better, and so forth. To test these possibilities, we measured the reaction time latencies of obese and normal subjects, their immediate recall for items presented briefly on a slide, and their threshold for the recognition of tachistoscopically presented stimulus material. We found that, on the average, overweight subjects had a quicker mean latency to respond to complex external stimuli; lower (i.e., more sensitive) tachistoscopic recognition thresholds; and better immediate recall for food- and non-food-relevant cues than normals (Rodin, Herman, and Schachter, 1974; Rodin, Slochower, and Fleming, 1977). In addition, overweight subjects were generally more distracted than normals by prominent irrelevant stimuli (Rodin, 1973; Rodin and Slochower, 1974), which appears to be owing to an inability to divide their attention between two or more compelling sources of stimulus input (Rodin and Goodman, 1976, note 1).

These first indications that the abberant eating behavior of the obese may be a special case of a much broader phenomenon were particularly intriguing, for if they were correct, there were major implications for our conception of the nature and origin of obesity. It seemed important, then, to investigate the general externality notion on as wide a variety of non-food-related behaviors as possible. Other experiments were then conducted that further tested the generalizability of the external sensitivity ideas in a variety of experimental contexts having nothing to do with consumatory behavior. Experiments demonstrated that time perception (Pliner, 1974; Rodin, 1975a), emotionality (Pliner, 1974; Rodin, Elman, and Schachter, 1974), and current thoughts (Rodin, 1973) were all more directly influenced by prominent external stimuli in overweight people, on the average, than in normals. Finally, overweight individuals generally required idea-generating external stimuli to produce original images, and when such cues were absent, they reported relatively few internally produced images (Pliner, 1974; Rodin and Rubin, 1976, note 2).

What form might such a difference in information processing

take, if it does exist? General measures of personality or cognitive style such as introversion–extraversion, internal–external locus of control, and field dependence–independence have not reliably proved to differentiate weight groups (Karpowitz and Zeis, 1975; Schachter, 1971). However, one should not confuse constructs that are descriptively linked to external responsiveness with those that are conceptually related. For example, behavioral responsiveness to prominent environmental cues does not mean that one necessarily anticipates reinforcements from luck or circumstance rather than from one's own efforts or capacities. This misunderstanding is a problem with some attempts to study the generalized construct of external responsiveness (cf. Nisbett and Temoshok, 1976).

Rather than a reliance on generalized questionnaires or on tests that seem descriptively linked, the process of external responsiveness might be more clearly explicated by the testing of subjects in situations where there are complex and potentially competing external and internal processing demands. For example, the self-generated private events, memories, fantasies, and related facets of the stream of consciousness may represent a competing stimulus field with information derived from the external environment (Singer, 1966, 1975). Indeed, to prevent overloading of the visual system, people may often move their eyes from rich external stimuli when they wish to clear channel space for internal processing, such as imagery or extended searches through long-term memory.

Rodin and Singer (1976) examined patterns of lateral eye-shift when subjects were responding to questions requiring reflection and self-generated imaginal processes. We studied eye movement for two reasons. First, differential engagement of the hemispheres of the brain is presumably manifested during thought by lateral eye-shift in the direction contralateral to the hemisphere primarily involved in the cognitive task. Second, as noted above, eye shift away from rich external stimuli occurs during complex internal processing. The eye-shift data demonstrated that overweight subjects were more likely to process reflective material in the verbal mode than through imagery. In addition, the obese appeared to have a greater need to avoid the rich environmental stimuli of the human face in order to process internal imagery material or verbal sequences stored in long-term memory.

Some broader cognitive implications of this study may be cited here briefly. Perhaps the key issue is that the very processes of storage and retrieval are active ones that almost continuously compete for attention with the processing of new, externally derived information. Recent experimental evidence suggests that the same sensory mechanisms and neural pathways may be involved in producing private images or fantasies as in processing externally derived content (Atwood, 1971; Antrobus, Singer, Goldstein, and Fortgang, 1970; Segal and Fusella, 1970). Fortunately most physical environments we confront are relatively redundant and so we can rely on well-established "plans" (Miller, Galanter, and Pribram, 1960) for steering ourselves through them and still attend also to private events—anticipations, memories, fantasies. The face of another person, however, conveying as it does so much information, presents an additional environmental complexity that must be "gated out" (usually by a shift of regard toward a more neutral stimulus field) if one is attempting concurrently to review elaborate private material.

Some people who have developed skill in attending to private processes may find it less necessary actually to move their eyes. They may have found other means of gating out the face before them or some other complex stimulus field (Singer, Greenberg, and Antrobus, 1971). However, this does not seem to be true for many overweight individuals. Not only did they appear less practiced in using visual imagery as they themselves indicated in their questionnaire responses, but they also found it more necessary to look away from the face toward a "blank" stimulus field in order to process complex material. Some overweight subjects may be a part of a class of individuals who, whether constitutionally or through early learning, have failed to develop fully their capacities for imagery and their ability to carry on extended searches of their long-term memory system while confronted by complex external environments. They may appear more sensitive to external cues but may also suffer from too limited an ability to use their own private anticipations or visual memories as an additional resource in cognitive control of their overt behavior.

III. GENERALIZABILITY OF THE OBESITY-EXTERNALITY FINDINGS

It is clear that the studies described thus far were correlational. Nonetheless, they provided crucial descriptive data that allowed us subsequently to move to questions of causal relationships. For example, while conducting these studies, we considered questions of generalizability regarding the populations from which subjects had been drawn. For the most part, all of the early work on obesity and external responsiveness tested moderately overweight (+15–40% overweight), college-age, white students. Thus, there were several issues, outlined below, about the generality of these effects.

A. Degree of Overweight

Both we (Rodin, Herman, and Schachter, 1974) and Nisbett (1972) had obtained data from a few greatly obese subjects indicating that they were no more responsive to food and nonfood external stimuli than normal weight individuals. During the course of our subsequent studies we tested the external responsiveness of several hundred participants who varied in degree of overweight. In each study, there were individuals in every weight category who were extremely responsive and those who were not. Across all weight groups, degree of overweight was almost totally unrelated to degree of external responsiveness. Using externality scores standardized on the entire sample in each study, we did find, however, that when group averages were compared, moderately overweight subjects were more external than either the normals or the extremely obese. This finding was consistent from study to study and was true for palatability ratings of increasingly sweet-tasting glucose solutions (Rodin, Moskowitz, and Bray, 1976) and milk shakes (Rodin, 1975b); responsiveness to preloads of varying caloric density (Rodin, Moskowitz, and Bray, 1976), and eating and noneating responses to manipulations of external cue salience (Rodin, Slochower, and Fleming, 1977). Moderately overweight subjects also appeared most willing to work to obtain a highly preferred milk shake when permitted to sample it first. However, the actual ease or difficulty of ingesting the milk shake (manipulated by straw width) once they had obtained it had a greater impact on their preference ratings and level of consumption than it did for either normals or the extremely obese (Rodin, 1975b).

Since the experiments that have studied the relationship between obesity and externality have varied greatly in how overweight the subjects were, some of the conflicting results reported in the literature may be more understandable. Moreover, since we have demonstrated in our recent studies that there are some externally responsive individuals in every weight category, it may be insufficient to group subjects only on the basis of weight.

B. Age and Socioeconomic Status

The use of summer camps for normal weight and overweight girls extended the range of subjects tested to as young as 9 years old. The use of an outpatient hospital clinic (Rodin, Bray, et al., 1977; Bray et al., 1976) and a self-help weight control group (Rodin, Slochower, and Fleming, 1977) extended the range to people as old as 60. The latter two samples also included blacks, people of Latin and Oriental origin, and those with as little as ninth-grade education. In all cases, the generality of the externality–overweight relationship was maintained. On the average, moderately overweight subjects appeared more external than those who were either extremely obese or normal.

C. Age of Onset

Generally the camp and college samples have represented individuals with juvenile onset obesity. In the adult samples from the weight reduction clinics and self-help groups, it was possible to divide participants into adult (over 21) and juvenile (before 10 years old) onset obesity. We found (Rodin, Slochower, and Fleming, 1977) that mildly overweight women whose obesity began in childhood were more responsive to external stimuli than their obese counterparts. By contrast, there was a tendency for mildly overweight women with adult onset obesity to be less external than the greatly obese, adult onset group. It is clear that obesity is not a single syndrome but that there are a number of subtypes. The appropriate dimensions along which to define groups are still being formulated, but current evidence suggests that there may be important differences as a function of (1) age of development of obesity; (2) differences in eating patterns; (3) degree of overweight; (4) degree of externality; (5) genetic predisposition; and (6) cultural background and social class. These categories are not mutually exclusive, however.

IV. REGULATION AND EXTERNAL RESPONSIVENESS

Once we had isolated the variables that demonstrate a correlation between overweight and external responsiveness, the next question that we examined was whether there was a possible causal relationship. The first hypothetical causal association that we studied was that obesity *per se* or some correlate of adiposity makes a person responsive to external cues. If this were true, we should expect that the fatter people are, the more responsive they will be to external cues. As discussed above, this does not seem to be the case. Nonetheless, since these studies were correlational, we conducted a series of experiments examining the effects of weight loss upon external responsiveness.

Three outcomes were theoretically possible. First, if obesity itself is the cause of externality, weight loss should decrease responsiveness to external cues. It is true that increased body weight produces a variety of metabolic and endocrine abnormalities that return to normal when weight is reduced (Sims *et al.*, 1968, 1973). Second, it may be that external responsiveness leads to overeating and poor self-regulation rather than following from it, in which case weight loss in overweight persons should have no effect on their external responsiveness. Finally, if a deprivation syndrome is the critical cause of externality, weight loss, during which subjects are in a state of energy deficit, should increase external responsiveness. The last prediction is derived from Nisbett's (1972) observation that there are animal studies showing instances of external responsiveness in deprived organisms. Based on these data, he suggested that many obese individuals, under social pressure to reduce their weight, could be literally starving and consequently behave like any deprived organism, that is, be highly externally responsive. The supportive data for this hypothesis however are also mainly correlational and, for humans, were primarily limited to changes in taste responsiveness as a function of deprivation.

We tested female campers at an eight-week summer camp for weight reduction and adult women attending outpatient diet clinics and self-help clubs at the beginning and again at the end of their diet programs. These samples included people differing widely in degree of overweight and age of onset of the obesity (Rodin, Slochower, and Fleming, 1977; Rodin, Moskowitz, and Bray, 1976; Rodin, Bray, *et al.*, 1977). All subjects were tested on those measures of heightened external responsiveness that had most clearly discriminated between overweight and normal weight people in previous experiments. These measures included eating in response to high visual salience or good-tasting food cues and time perception, emotionality, and slide recall.

Responsiveness to non-food-relevant external cues remained virtually unchanged for most subjects, regardless of the amount of weight lost (from 1 to 78 lb). Similarly, after weight loss, subjects' consumption was not significantly more influenced by the manipulation of visual food cue salience, although the overall amount that they consumed did increase. Neither degree of initial overweight nor amount of weight lost were systematically related to changes that did occur. Interestingly, we also found that in those programs where patients were not locked away from food cues (e.g., in outpatient clinics), degree of externality was negatively correlated with reported ease on the program and actual weight loss.

Taken together, these data suggest that losing weight—at least with the amounts lost in the present studies and by restriction of intake as the method of weight loss—is unrelated to changes in external cue responsiveness. In other words, externality neither increases nor decreases systematically with weight loss. We concluded from these data that responsiveness to external, nonphysiological cues in the environment is not simply a function of degree of obesity *per se* nor of degree of energy depletion. While it is quite possible that overweight people are physiologically hungry, this does not appear to be a sufficient explanation for their external responsiveness. Indeed, in a study measuring the effects of short-term, 24-hour deprivation, similar results were obtained (Fleming, 1975). After a 24-hour fast, hungry normal weight individuals were not significantly more responsive to external food- and non-food-relevant stimuli than they were prior to deprivation. Finally, the failure to find changes in external responsiveness following weight loss is important, since we know that the metabolic abnormalities frequently associated with obesity (e.g., hyperinsulinemia, increased steroid levels) do return to more normal levels following weight loss (Horton, 1975). Therefore, it does not appear that these dysfunctions are causing external responsiveness.

While external cue responsiveness appeared generally quite stable for the measures that we used, we next questioned whether responsiveness to *all* cues would remain constant in the face of great changes in body weight. Here we were concerned specifically with a comparison between external cues such as visual stimuli and responsiveness to taste and other oropharyngeal stimuli such as smell or texture. In the early studies of Schachter (1968, 1971), Nisbett (1968, 1972), and their associates, good taste was considered an external cue in much the same way as the sight of good food or the time of day. But as Pfaffmann (1960) has suggested, the capacity of taste and other oropharyngeal stimuli to motivate behavior and to arouse feelings places them in close psychological relationship to pain and to the contact sensations and implies that they have strong projections to the limbic and brain-stem structures serving motivation and the emotions. The receptor sites of stimulation by taste and smell are also quite different than those of visual cues. For example, Rolls (1976) has recently reported specific and different neurons firing to the sight and to the taste of food in deprived animals. In addition, taste can serve as an unconditioned stimulus for learning and appears to have more direct biological significance for the organism (Garcia and Hankins, 1974; Rozin and Kalat, 1971).

It has been argued by Cabanac and his associates (1968, 1970, 1971) that taste responsiveness is an index of set point, or the level at which body weight is biologically determined for a particular organism. Specifically, Cabanac suggested that people at or close to set point would find otherwise pleasant-tasting sweet solutions to be aversive when they sampled them a few minutes after a gastric load of glucose. This suggestion implies that individuals further from set point would show both exaggerated responsiveness to cues and unresponsiveness to short-term changes in nutritional state. Nisbett (1972) has argued that many moderately overweight dieters belong in this latter group because their set point for adipose tissue may actually be higher; that is, they may have been "programmed" to be fat. In fact, both Nisbett (1972) and we (Rodin, 1975b) found that moderately overweight people were highly taste responsive and that the obese, who, according to Nisbett, have allowed their eating to bring them close to set point weight, were less so.

Thus, it may be that taste responsiveness is more directly wired to long- and/or short-term changes in the energy state of the organism than responsiveness to visual cues—and indeed reflects this state. (Booth, 1976, has suggested eliminating the need for a concept like set point, however, by simply saying that palatability recalibrates and is recalibrated by the satiety mechanism.) Here, then, would be a clear instance of the influence of physiological factors on a conscious factor—palatability—that affects self-regulation of eating. Visual–cognitive externality, on the other hand, may be unrelated to this aspect of the person's physiology but instead may reflect his level of arousal or arousability. It is easy to conceive of the biological significance of a second mechanism of this sort—one that alerts and turns on an organism, thus preparing it to seek and notice food.

To consider these hypotheses, the next study (Rodin, Slochower, and Fleming, 1977) tested overweight women who were members of various local weight reduction clubs. On the basis of pretesting, those who were highest and lowest in responsiveness to external, non-food-relevant cues were selected as subjects. A control group of normal weight women also participated. Subjects were tested at noon after having eaten breakfast before 8 A.M. and no lunch. Every subject participated in the study on four occasions, each separated by one day, at the beginning of her weight loss program. The order of the four conditions manipulating visual salience and palatability was counterbalanced.

A. Manipulation of Visual Salience

In the high-salience condition, a large serving dish of artificially sweetened ice milk was directly in front of each subject, and a tape recording, to which she listened through headphones, reminded her to concentrate on the taste of the ice milk, to think about its flavor and its texture, etc. In the low-salience condition, the serving dish was equally close to the subject but was placed away from her direct line of vision. The tape that played during this condition asked subjects to think about the taste of winter snow, the smell after it rains, etc.—in other words, about non-food-relevant stimuli. In all conditions, subjects were encouraged to eat as much ice milk as they wished, and they were told that it was low calorie and artificially sweetened. The flavor selected was of moderate palatability for that subject—rated as 6 on a 9-point scale. Pretesting indicated that most subjects still found ice milk rated as 6 palatable even after eating it for several days.

B. Manipulation of Taste

In the high-palatability condition, the ice milk was a flavor that, for that subject, was rated 9 on a 9-point scale. In the low-palatability group, the flavor was one that she rated as 3. In both conditions, the large serving dish was in front of them, but subjects were asked to think about the neutral stimuli, thus providing a cue of moderate external salience.

C. After Weight Loss

The exact procedure was replicated for all subjects after weight loss. Instead of choosing an arbitrary time period to retest subjects after weight loss, we instead tested each subject after a certain percentage of her body weight was lost. On the average it took 22 weeks (± 7.4) for subjects to reach this criterion reduction index of 60 ($\sim$15–20% of body weight).

The experiment examined how, *for a particular subject,* weight loss influenced consumption in response to conditions of high versus low salience (holding palatability moderate) compared to the conditions of high versus low palatability (holding salience moderate). Those overweight subjects who were selected on the basis of high responsiveness to non-food-relevant external stimuli were also more responsive to manipulations of visual cues for feeding than either low external overweight or normal weight subjects. Weight loss did not reliably change degree of responsiveness to the visual and cognitive salience manipulations for any group. The pattern of findings for the palatability manipulations was different in several respects. First, high and low external overweight groups were more responsive to differences in taste than the normals prior to weight loss, and they were not different from one another. Second, they became even more taste responsive following weight reduction. Generally, increased responsiveness was reflected in exaggerated consumption of the highly palatable food rather than increased rejection of the poor-tasting food. This finding parallels Booth's (1972) demonstration that, in animals, pleasant flavors become more pleasant but unpleasant flavors less unpleasant in hunger relative to satiety.

The subjects who were the most responsive to manipulations of visual salience were not the most responsive to differences in palatability. Neither degree of initial overweight nor length of time taken to reach the fixed weight-loss criterion was significantly correlated with heightened taste responsiveness before or after weight reduction.

The issue remains complicated since further evidence has demonstrated that perceived palatability is not influenced directly by weight loss *per se* but by the way in which the weight is lost. While obese dieters continued to find sweet-tasting substances more palatable than normals after weight loss, obese patients who lost weight as the result of surgical reduction of their intestine began to show responsiveness to sweet taste that essentially resembled normal weight curves (Rodin, Moskowitz, and Bray, 1976). They also showed changes in consumption that appeared modified on the basis of differences in the caloric value of a preload (Bray *et al.*, 1976), although their regulation was highly disturbed prior to surgery. These data from intestinal bypass patients and current hypotheses about feeding control (Friedman and Stricker, 1976; Novin, 1976) suggest that glucoreceptors at the site of the intestine may be involved in the short-term regulation of feeding and influence hunger and satiety by the changing response to sweet taste. It is significant to point out that while the bypass patients were tested for taste responsiveness to sweet, sour, salty, and bitter, only responsiveness to sweet changed following surgery (Rodin, Moskowitz, and Bray, 1976).

Given that external responsiveness does not appear to derive from adiposity or deprivation, the final causal possibility that we explored was that externality might precede and contribute to overeating in certain individuals. This hypothesis suggests that externality could increase weight if subjects were placed in an environment that was filled with potent food cues. To test this hypothesis, we again selected an eight-week summer camp for girls because of the constant environment (Rodin and Slochower, 1976). This was not a diet camp, so food was abundant, attractively prepared, and served "family style." Candy and other treats sent by parents were plentiful in each cabin and could also be purchased at any time at the camp canteen. It was predicted that the more external a child was, the more her eating behavior would be influenced by the shift to abundant food cues that coming to camp provided. This increased influence, in turn, would affect her weight. In contrast, nonexternal children were expected to maintain a relatively constant body weight independent of alterations in the environment. The strong test of this hypothesis was provided by a study of normal weight people with no overweight history.

The same measures of external responsiveness used in the earlier studies were given to all campers during the first week. Standardized externality scores for each subject were then correlated with weight change from the first to the final week divided by starting weight. There was a significant positive correlation between externality and this weight change measure, suggesting that the children who were most external subsequently gained the most weight. Activity level and emotional adjustment were not related to weight change.

That there are normal weight externals who behave as do the moderately obese lends further support to the proposition that externality is not purely a function of overweight but instead reflects an underlying tendency toward hyperresponsiveness that in a food-abundant setting could lead to weight gain. We do not yet know whether this responsiveness is genetically determined or due to early experience, but a two-factor process, requiring both external responsiveness and an abundant food environment, seems necessary for some forms of overweight to occur.

If external responsiveness is not innate, in what type of feeding situation might it be learned? In an interesting study, Gross (1968) directly manipulated the early environmental conditions of weanling rats by exposing them to conditions of both constant and randomly varied deprivation intervals. Animals fed on a schedule of random deprivation were expected to be in a state in which relatively constant energy depletion would be complicated by continual uncertainty regarding the future availability of food. In order to maximize the effects of the scarcity and unpredictability experienced by the animals, it was decided to expose them to these conditions for a considerable length of time. Evidence by Bruch (1973) and Keys, Brozek, Henschel, Mickelson, and Taylor (1950) indicates that exposure to prolonged deprivation often results, with humans, in a persistent tendency to overeat.

Gross created three groups of experimental animals immediately after weaning. One group was fed *ad libitum*, a second group was placed on a 22-hour deprivation schedule in which they were fed every 22 hours, and the third group was placed on a random deprivation schedule in which they fed on the average every 22 hours, but the feedings actually ranged from 8 to 48 hours of deprivation. All animals were kept on these schedules for 100 days. It was found that rats maintained under conditions of regular or randomly varied deprivation exhibited an increased degree of external control over their eating behavior, as compared with animals having abundant food constantly available. For example, these animals were highly responsive to variations in the taste and caloric density of their diet.

After the 100 days, the randomly and regularly deprived animals were placed on *ad lib* feeding, and Gross found that after this prolonged exposure to scarcity and unpredictability, the animals continued to exhibit externally oriented responses to dietary variations, even under conditions of abundance. Most interesting, the rats that had been randomly deprived also demonstrated a pattern of external control reflected in a nonconsumatory measure of responsiveness to external food cues. This was tested by measurement of the amount of time that they remained in contact with food in an open field, although they were not allowed to eat the food. We are currently conducting further studies with human infants to investigate the etiology of external responsiveness and its role in the development of feeding patterns and body weight. Let us next turn to some further ways in which external responsiveness might influence regulation, and the consequences of such influence.

V. THE INTERNAL–EXTERNAL DISTINCTION

As reviewed above, the studies of Schachter and his co-workers (1971, 1974) suggested a dichotomy between internal and external control of feeding. They argued that while the feeding behavior of normals is responsive to internal stimuli, overweight individuals are unresponsive to internal physiological cues for feeding and instead rely heavily on external cues in the environment. This view is cited in some form in almost every introductory psychology textbook, yet it now appears that the injunction of extreme discontinuity between internal–physiological and external–environmental stimuli may have been premature, especially with regard to eating behavior. Instead, feeding should be viewed as in integrated system of motivated behaviors that is not the addition of internal and external influences but the integration of sensory, cognitive, social, and physiological elements in a control system to which they are essential, even in abnormal conditions.

There are now many indications that the internal versus external view is far too simple a description of, or explanation for, even obese–normal eating differences. First, the development of this dichotomy was greatly influenced by the studies of Stunkard and Koch (1964), which reported high correlations between hunger and gastric contractions for normals but not for many overweight individuals. Schachter (1968) thus argued that the feeding behavior of normals was more influenced by internal signals like gastric motility but that motility was not a hunger cue for the obese. However, in reviewing the role of the gastrointestinal tract in the regulation of food intake, Janowitz (1967) concluded that while deficits of nutrients give rise to a complex of sensations that includes the epigastric hunger pang, gastric hunger contractions appear to be a dispensable component since feeding proceeds normally in their absence. In fact, he claimed that "at present no published data exist about any species that indicate whether or not food intake or other hunger-motivated behavioral parameters are actually correlated with gastric hunger contractions" (p. 220). Thus, relying on gastric motility as an important internal signal that might predict differential feeding behavior in overweight and normal weight persons was relying on a cue that does not appear to play a crucial role in the initiation of feeding.

The second kind of evidence for a lack of internal responsiveness in the obese came from studies demonstrating their failure to respond to caloric preloading as accurately as did normals (Nisbett, 1968; Pliner, 1974; Schachter, Goldman, and Gordon, 1968). However, it may simply be that the level of caloric preload used in these and other comparable studies was insufficient to be detected by the overweight subjects. For example, Nisbett has suggested that many overweight individuals are physiologically deprived by dieting or at least by conscious restraint of their eating. If they are literally starving, they would overeat whether they had already received 200 or 600 calories of a liquid or a sandwich, since none of these would be sufficient to satisfy their current nutritional needs. Thus, their short-term regulatory controls might be highly responsive to their internal physiological state at the moment.

One does not have to accept the Nisbett hypothesis to predict that overweight and normal weight individuals should not be equally responsive to preloading manipulations. The corpulent individual demonstrates a number of metabolic and endocrine abnormalities, generally as a result of overeating and adiposity (Sims, Danforth, Horton, Bray, Glennon, and Salans, 1973). Because of these weight-related metabolic differences, overweight individuals may be responding to different levels or kinds of internal signals. This response in turn could make them responsive to a different amount or type of caloric preload than normals.

Third, there is now a great deal of evidence that normals also show far from perfect internal regulation. Despite evidence that experimental animals are able to adapt relatively promptly and accurately to caloric dilution, studies with normal weight humans have shown that only some subjects are able to compensate over several days for changes in the caloric density of liquid diets, and in nearly all cases, consumption is sluggish and incomplete (Campbell, Hashim, and Van Itallie, 1971; Jordan, 1969; Spiegel, 1973; O. Wooley, 1971). That is, under the specific conditions of such experiments, internal signals do not appropriately guide eating behavior toward stable caloric intakes. Studies examining the short-term effects of caloric loading have also shown that adjustment on the basis of caloric signals may not occur when the sensory and cognitive cues related to the nutritional value of the preloads are held constant (Spiegel, 1973; S. Wooley, 1972). These results strongly suggest that most people— overweight and normal weight—cannot ordinarily perceive variations in deprivation level within the moderate or physiological range.

Recently, we have begun to consider whether external responsiveness might actually influence internal physical state, rather than exerting its effects exclusively on eating itself. First, we are assessing whether overweight people show greater arousal in response to potent external stimuli, suggesting that they are physiologically turned on by such cues, and second, whether their actual metabolic responses are also overresponsive to prominent external cues. Each of these effects has the potential to influence overeating and weight gain.

Activation and arousal are strongly linked to feeding and motivated behavior in all organisms (Stricker and Zigmond, 1976; Wolgin, Cytawa, and Teitelbaum, 1976), and there is extensive recent neurological and physiological data that bear on this issue. Very briefly, Teitelbaum and his co-workers suggest that sensory stimuli (taste, smell, sight of food) provide the background activation that maintains feeding behavior. In other words, in addition to their directing and incentive value, these sensory and external stimuli have a general activating component that energizes the animal. The recovery of feeding in animals with lateral hypothalamic damage, which initially produces aphagia, relies, according to Teitelbaum's view, on the recovery of endogenous activation. If there is a lack of tonic arousal, the activating function of external stimuli becomes even more important. Thus, he argued that arousal plays a crucial role in the control of feeding, and the lack of activation may be a contributing factor to the lack of interest in food seen in LH-lesioned animals. Arousing the animal in other ways—such as by tail pinch, a painful stimulus, or amphetamine—also leads to voluntary approach to food and vigorous feeding. In the course of recovery from LH damage, external stimuli also begin to activate feeding, just as do pain and amphetamine. Consequently, hyperactivation in response to external stimuli could, we suggest, lead to overeating.

The view takes on special significance in light of the recent data of Marshall (1975, 1976), who tested animals with unilateral ventromedial hypothalamic lesions. Since the neural region on one side of the brain is responsive to the external environment on the contralateral side, Marshall varied the location of food-dispensing dishes for these animals. He first found that 13 of the 14 rats with unilateral damage showed an increase in responsiveness to contralateral sensory stimuli of all kinds; they showed increased orienting, exaggerated response to whisker touch, head turning, increased biting of noxious stimuli, and aggressive responses to attack. Most important, in eating, the unilateral animals began taking a significantly greater proportion of their daily food from the contralateral food dish. This reaction suggests that the lesion itself was enhancing cue responsiveness. In other words, medial damage might produce hyperresponsiveness, which influences the animal's reactivity to external stimuli, which in turn influences feeding. Gibson and Gazzaniga (1971) noted a comparable finding in split-brain monkeys with unilateral hypothalamic damage. Such monkeys overate only when using the eye that projected to the hemisphere with the ventromedial lesion, suggesting that external visual cues were what influenced overeating.

These physiological data are consistent with earlier work (Schachter and Rodin, 1974) in which we compared the behavior of overweight humans to animals with electrolytic lesions in the ventromedial region of the hypothalamus. In this monograph, we suggested that both the VMH-lesioned rat and the obese human might share a pattern of hyperresponsiveness to the external cues associated with both food and nonfood stimuli. In our research on humans, we went on to investigate whether heightened external responsiveness could actually lead to overeating and consequent obesity and demonstrated that externality was an important predictor of overeating and weight gain, as described above.

These converging lines of evidence may be summarized as follows. Activation and arousal by external stimuli are related to the return of normal feeding in LH-lesioned animals, and hyperarousal in response to external stimuli appears to be related to overfeeding in VMH-lesioned animals. The neurochemical pathways involved in these responses are involved in the general arousal of the organism and its specific arousal in response to external stimuli. As Stricker and Zigmond have suggested (1976), an external stimulus would thus be seen as having two effects: a specific one that activates neurons that are involved in eliciting some appropriate motivational state and a nonspecific one that removes a "gate" and thereby permits such responses actually to occur. Thus, an individual could literally be "turned on" by an external stimulus.

At present, we are certainly not arguing for the underlying anatomical or neurochemical basis of these responses in humans. We are simply suggesting how external cues might arouse people and lead to overeating. Others have proposed (notably Maddi, 1968; Thayer, 1967) that there are individual differences with regard to both rate of activation change and level of activation. This difference may be especially important with regard to feeding, since, as McFarland (personal communication) has observed, from an ethological point of view rapid and/or excessive intake during arousal may represent an adaptive tendency to deal efficiently with food needs in the face of impending disruption or danger. Clearly, however, both the explanation and the significance of this phenomenon have yet to be determined.

Our second set of studies is examining the role of external stimuli in triggering those autonomic and endocrine responses that are involved in the metabolism of food. The studies are based on the hypothesis that the internal, physiological consequences of heightened responsiveness to external and sensory stimuli could themselves promote overeating and weight gain. For example, exaggerated responsiveness to external cues could trigger exaggerated internal responses such as insulin release. Insulin is an important mechanism in the promotion of overeating and in fat storage (Frohman and Bernardis, 1968). Indeed, those individuals who are externally responsive by our measures appear to show an increase in plasma insulin levels when they simply view a highly palatable food—such as a grilling steak—that they anticipate eating. The more palatable the stimulus, the larger the insulin response. A similar finding has been reported for salivation (Wooley and Wooley, 1973).

If people are more responsive physiologically as a function of palatability and if this response is stronger for externally responsive people, then it is clear how appetite could be stimulated and overeating result as a consequence of increased responsiveness to potent, palatable stimuli. Food industries have been attempting to fabricate palatable low-calorie analogues of certain calorically rich foods. However, it is not certain whether this approach would actually help overweight people to diet and lose weight. If the original internal-external formulation were entirely correct, obese people who are highly external should be just as satisfied by the calorically dilute food analogues as by the calorically concentrated original, so long as they tasted about the same. Thus, the external responsiveness of the obese in the absence of internal cues should allow them to meet their hedonic needs at a lower caloric price. On the other hand, on the basis of the hypotheses outlined above, we would expect the low-calorie good-tasting cues to stimulate metabolic responses and subsequent overeating in the same way as their high-calorie counterparts. Indeed, Nicolaidis (1969) reported the same metabolic effect for tongue stimulation with a nutritive or a nonnutritive sweet. Thus, a piece of diet chewing gum or a piece of rich-tasting low-calorie cake may stimulate hunger and food seeking or lead to greater consumption if food is already available. In fact, the richer looking and tasting the food stimulus—despite its actual caloric value—the more it might stimulate the appetite.

At the present time, we might logically ask whether making people aware of their external responsiveness would help. Perhaps, if we encouraged them to consciously restrain these tendencies—in other words, to place regulation under fully conscious control—they would do much better. In an interesting series of studies, Peter Herman and his colleagues (Herman and Mack, 1975; Herman and Polivy, 1975) demonstrated that people of all weight categories could easily be classified into those who consciously restrain their eating and responsiveness to external cues and those who do not. A simple questionnaire allowed assessment of these differences. They then placed both restrained and unrestrained eaters in the following situation (Herman and Mack, 1975). The study was presumably a taste experiment in which subjects were first required to taste 0, 1, or 2 large milk shakes. In the next phase of the study, subjects were encouraged to "taste" as much as they wanted from a large dish of ice cream.

The results showed a fascinating turn of events. When normally restrained eaters were required, as part of the study, to finish two large milk shakes, they subsequently ate greater amounts of ice cream in the following period than if they had consumed no milk shake or one only. Apparently having drunk so much milk shake, and perceiving themselves as already having overeaten, these normally restrained people gave up their restraint on consumption. Herman and his co-workers argued that this disinhibition effect is cognitive, since perceived and not real calories ingested produced the disinhibition of restraint. Subjects who reported less conscious restraint of their eating behaved in exactly the opposite fashion. For them, the greater amounts of milk shake *suppressed* ice cream consumption.

In another study, these investigators found that restrained subjects tend to overeat when anxious, possibly because strong emotions interfere with the self-control of the normally restrained eater. We have some data indicating that they tend to overeat when they are very happy as well. They also eat more when distracted and when intoxicated. These and similar findings suggest that while conscious restraint and self-control *can* influence weight loss and maintenance, it is a fragile sort of control that can be easily disrupted. In fact, the events that break down conscious restraint seem so numerous that we cannot rely on this process alone to control food intake.

From the studies described in the present paper, it seems clear that heightened external responsiveness contributes to the etiology and maintenance of overeating because it plays a crucial role in short-term self-regulation. Why this tendency makes some people overeat and not others, however, is an intriguing problem and one that we continue to study. Conscious control does not help and indeed may hinder the regulatory process, although certain conscious processes such as perception of palatability do seem more directly wired to the nutritional needs of the organism. The relationship of conscious factors to long-term weight regulation remains to be described and understood.

REFERENCES

ANTROBUS, J. S., SINGER, J. L., GOLDSTEIN, S., AND FORTGANG, M. Mind-wandering and cognitive structure. *Transactions of the New York Academy of Science,* 1970, *32,* 242–252.

ATWOOD, G. An experimental study of visual imagination and memory. *Cognitive Psychology,* 1971, *2,* 290–299.

BOOTH, D. A. Conditioned satiety in the rat. *Journal of Comparative and Physiological Psychology,* 1972, *81,* 475–481.

BOOTH, D. A. Approaches to feeding control. In T. Silverstone (Ed.), *Appetite and food intake.* Braunschweig: Pergamon Press, 1976.

BOOTH, D. A., AND MATHER, P. Prototype model of human feeding, growth, and obesity. In D. A. Booth (Ed.), *Hunger models: Computable theory of feeding control.* London: Academic Press, 1977.

BRAY, G. A., BARRY, R. E., BENFIELD, J., CASTELNUOVO-TEDESCO, P., AND RODIN, J. Intestinal bypass surgery for obesity decreases food intake and taste preferences. *Journal of Clinical Nutrition,* 1976, *29,* 779–783.

BRUCH, H. *Eating disorders.* New York: Basic Books, 1973.

CABANAC, M. Physiological role of pleasure. *Science,* 1971, *173,* 1103–1107.

CABANAC, M., AND DUCLAUX, R. Obesity: Absence of satiety aversion to sucrose. *Science,* 1970, *168,* 469–497.

CABANAC, M., MINARE, Y., AND ADAIR, E. Influence of internal factors on the pleasantness of gustative sweet sensation. *Communications in Behavioral Biology,* Part A, 1968, *1,* 77–82.

CAMPBELL, R. G., HASHIN, S. A., AND VAN ITALLIE, T. B. Studies of food-intake regulation in man: Responses to variations in nutritive density in lean and obese subjects. *New England Journal of Medicine,* 1971, *285,* 1402–1407.

FLEMING, B. Effects of short-term deprivation of the external responsiveness of overweight and normal-weight subjects. Unpublished senior honors thesis, Yale University, 1975.

FRIEDMAN, M., AND STRICKER, E. The physiological psychology of hunger: A physiological perspective. *Psychological Review,* 1976, *83,* 409–431.

FROHMAN, L. A., AND BERNARDIS, L. L. Growth hormone and insulin levels in weanling rats with ventromedial hypothalamic lesions. *Endocrinology,* 1968, *82,* 1125–1132.

GARCIA, J., AND HANKINS, W. G. The evolution of bitter and the acquisition of toxiphobia. In D. Denton (Ed.), *Fifth International Symposium on Olfaction and Taste,* 1974. Pp. 1–12.

GIBSON, A. R., AND GAZZANIGA, M. S. Hemispheric differences in eating behavior in split-brain monkeys. *Physiologist,* 1971, *14,* 150.

GROSS, L. The effects of early feeding experience on external responsiveness. Unpublished doctoral dissertation, Columbia University, 1968.

HERMAN, C. P., AND MACK, D. Restrained and unrestrained eating. *Journal of Personality,* 1975, *43,* 647–660.

HERMAN, C. P., AND POLIVY, J. Anxiety, restraint, and eating behavior. *Journal of Abnormal Psychology,* 1975, *84,* 666–672.

HORTON, E. Endocrine and metabolic alterations in spontaneous and experimental obesity. In G. A. Bray (Ed.), *Obesity in perspective.* Washington: U.S. Government Printing Office, 1975.

HORTON, E. S., DANFORTH, E., JR., SIMS, E. A., AND SALANS, L. B. Correlation of forearm muscle and adipose tissue metabolism in obesity before and after weight loss. *Clinical Research,* 1972, *20,* 548.

JANOWITZ, H. D. Role of the gastrointestinal tract in the regulation of food intake. In C. F. Code (Ed.), *Handbook of physiology: Alimentary canal,* Vol. 1. Washington: American Physiological Society, 1967. Pp. 219–224.

JORDAN, H. A. Voluntary intragastric feeding: Oral and gastric contributions to food intake and hunger in man. *Journal of Comparative and Physiological Psychology,* 1969, *68,* 498–506.

KARPOWITZ, D. H., AND ZEIS, F. R. Personality and behavior differences among obese and non-obese adolescents. In A. Howard (Ed.), *Recent advances in obesity research,* Vol. 1. London: Newman Publishing, 1975.

KEYS, A., BROZEK, J., HENSCHEL, A., MICKELSON, D., AND TAYLOR, H. *The biology of human starvation* (2 vols.). Minneapolis: University of Minnesota Press, 1950.

MADDI, S. R. *Personality theories: A comparative analysis.* Homewood, Ill.: Dorsey, 1968.

MARSHALL, J. Increased orientation to sensory stimuli following medial hypothalamic damage in rats. *Brain Research,* 1975, *86,* 373–387.

MARSHALL, J. Neurochemistry of central monoamine systems as related to food intake. In T. Silverstone (Ed.), *Appetite and food intake.* Braunschweig: Pergamon Press, 1976.

MILLER, G. A., GALANTER, E., AND PRIBRAM, K. *Plans and the structure of behavior.* New York: McGraw-Hill, 1960.

NICOLAIDIS, S. Early systemic responses to orogastric stimulation in the regulation of food and water balance: Functional and electrophysiological data. *Annals of the New York Academy of Sciences,* 1969, *157,* 1176–1203.

NISBETT, R. E. Taste, deprivation, and weight determinants of eating behavior. *Journal of Personality and Social Psychology,* 1968, *10,* 107–116.

NISBETT, R. E. Hunger, obesity, and the ventromedial hypothalamus. *Psychological Review*, 1972, *79*, 433–453.

NISBETT, R. E., AND TEMOSHOK, L. Is there an external cognitive style? *Journal of Personality and Social Psychology*, 1976, *33*, 36–47.

NOVIN, D. Visceral mechanisms in the control of food intake. In D. Novin, W. Wyrwicka, and G. A. Bray (Eds.), *Hunger: Basic mechanisms and clinical implications*. New York: Raven, 1976.

PFAFFMANN, C. The pleasures of sensation. *Psychological Review*, 1960, *65*, 253–268.

PLINER, P. On the generalizability of the externality hypothesis. In S. Schachter and J. Rodin, *Obese humans and rats*. Washington: Erlbaum/Halsted, 1974.

RODIN, J. Effects of distraction on the performance of obese and normal subjects. *Journal of Comparative and Physiological Psychology*, 1973, *83*, 68–78.

RODIN, J. Causes and consequences of time perception differences in overweight and normal-weight people. *Journal of Personality and Social Psychology*, 1975a, *31*, 898–910.

RODIN, J. The effects of obesity and set point on taste responsiveness and intake in humans. *Journal of Comparative and Physiological Psychology*, 1975b, *89*, 1003–1009.

RODIN, J., BRAY, G. A., ATKINSON, R. L., DAHMS, W. T., GREENWAY, F. L., HAMILTON, K., AND MOLITCH, M. Predictors of successful weight loss in an out-patient obesity clinic. *International Journal of Obesity*, 1977, *1*, 79–87.

RODIN, J., ELMAN, D., AND SCHACHTER, S. Emotionality and obesity. In S. Schachter and J. Rodin, *Obese humans and rats*. Washington: Erlbaum/Halsted, 1974.

RODIN, J., AND GOODMAN, N. R. Selective attention in overweight and normal weight individuals. Unpublished manuscript, Yale University, 1976.

RODIN, J., HERMAN, C. P., AND SCHACHTER, S. Obesity and various tests of external sensitivity. In S. Schachter and J. Rodin, *Obese humans and rats*. Washington: Erlbaum/Halsted, 1974.

RODIN, J., MOSKOWITZ, H. R., AND BRAY, G. A. Relationship between obesity, weight loss, and taste responsiveness. *Physiology and Behavior*, 1976, *17*, 591–597.

RODIN, J., AND RUBIN, S. Creativity differences in overweight and normal-weight persons. Unpublished manuscript, Yale University, 1976.

RODIN, J., AND SINGER, J. Eye-shift, thought, and obesity. *Journal of Personality*, 1976, *4*, 594–610.

RODIN, J., AND SLOCHOWER, J. Fat chance for a favor: Obese–normal differences in compliance and incidental learning. *Journal of Personality and Social Psychology*, 1974, *29*, 557–565.

RODIN, J., AND SLOCHOWER, J. Externality in the nonobese: The effects of environmental responsiveness on weight. *Journal of Personality and Social Psychology*, 1976, *33*, 338–344.

RODIN, J., SLOCHOWER, J., AND FLEMING, B. The effects of degree of obesity, age of onset, and energy deficit on external responsiveness. *Journal of Comparative and Physiological Psychology*, 1977, *91*, 586–597.

ROLLS, E. T. Neurophysiology of feeding. In T. Silverstone (Ed.), *Appetite and food intake*. Braunschweig: Pergamon Press, 1976.

ROSS, L. Effects of manipulating the salience of food upon consumption by obese and normal eaters. In S. Schachter and J. Rodin, *Obese humans and rats*. Washington: Erlbaum/Halsted, 1974.

ROZIN, P., AND KALAT, J. W. Specific hungers and poison avoidance as adaptive specializations of learning. *Psychological Review*, 1971, *78*, 459–486.

SCHACHTER, S. Obesity and eating. *Science*, 1968, *161*, 751–756.

SCHACHTER, S. *Emotion, obesity, and crime*. New York: Academic Press, 1971.

SCHACHTER, S., GOLDMAN, R., AND GORDON, A. Effects of fear, food deprivation, and obesity on eating. *Journal of Personality and Social Psychology*, 1968, *10*, 91–97.

SCHACHTER, S., AND GROSS, L. Manipulated time and eating behavior. *Journal of Personality and Social Psychology*, 1968, *10*, 98–106.

SCHACHTER, S., AND RODIN, J. *Obese humans and rats.* Washington: Erlbaum/Wiley, 1974.

SEGAL, S. J., AND FUSELLA, V. Influence of imaged pictures and sounds on detection of visual and auditory signals. *Journal of Experimental Psychology*, 1970, *83*, 458–464.

SIMS, E. A. H., DANFORTH, E., JR., HORTON, E. S., BRAY, G. A., GLENNON J. A., AND SALANS, L. B. Endocrine and metabolic effects of experimental obesity in man. *Recent Progress in Hormonal Research*, 1973, *29*, 457–496.

SIMS, E. A. H., GOLDMAN, R. F., GLUCK, C. M., HORTON, E. S., KELLEHER, P. C., AND ROWE, D. W. Experimental obesity in man. *Transaction of the Association of American Physicians*, 1968, *81*, 153–170.

SINGER, J. L. *Daydreaming.* New York: Random House, 1966.

SINGER, J. L. Navigating the stream of consciousness: Research in daydreaming and related inner experience. *American Psychologist*, 1975, *30*, 727–738.

SINGER, J. L., GREENBERG, S., AND ANTROBUS, J. S. Looking with the mind's eye: Experimental studies of ocular motility during daydreaming and mental arithmetic. *Transactions of the New York Academy of Sciences*, 1971, *33*, 694–709.

SPIEGEL, T. Caloric regulation of food intake in man. *Journal of Comparative and Physiological Psychology*, 1973, *83*, 24–37.

STRICKER, E. M., AND ZIGMOND, M. J. Brain catecholamines and the lateral hypothalamic syndrome. In D. Novin (Ed.), *Hunger: Basic mechanisms and clinical implications.* New York: Raven Press, 1976.

STUNKARD, A. J., AND KOCH, C. The interpretation of gastric motility, I: Apparent bias in the reports of hunger by obese persons. *Archives of General Psychiatry*, 1964, *11*, 74–82.

THAYER, R. E. Measurement of activation through self report. *Psychological Reports*, 1967, *20*, 663–678.

WOLGIN, D. L., CYTAWA, J., AND TEITELBAUM, P. The role of activation in the regulation of food intake. In D. Novin, W. Wyrwicka, and G. A. Bray (Eds.), *Hunger: Basic mechanisms and clinical implications.* New York: Raven Press, 1976.

WOOLEY, O. Long-term food regulation in the obese and nonobese. *Psychosomatic Medicine*, 1971, *33*, 436.

WOOLEY, S. Physiologic versus cognitive factors in short-term food regulation in the obese and nonobese. *Psychosomatic Medicine*, 1972, *34*, 62.

WOOLEY, S., AND WOOLEY, O. Salivation to the sight and thought of food: A new measure of appetite. *Psychosomatic Medicine*, 1973, *35*, 136.

7   *Operant Conditioning of Autonomic Responses: One Perspective on the Curare Experiments*

LARRY E. ROBERTS

I. INTRODUCTION AND BACKGROUND

Occasional reports of successful operant conditioning of autonomic responses in curarized rats have continued to appear in recent years (Cabanac and Serres, 1976; Gliner, Horvath, and Wolfe, 1975; Middaugh, Eissenberg, and Brener, 1975; Thornton and Van-Toller, 1973a,b). These reports have done little, however, to dispel the doubt that persists concerning the replicability of earlier research in this preparation by Miller and DiCara (Obrist, Black, Brener, and DiCara, 1974). One goal of the present chapter is to review recent efforts to obtain operant conditioning of autonomic responses in the curarized rat and to consider the interpretation of the original studies that seems to be necessitated by repeated failures to obtain learning. A further goal is to discuss the implications of these developments for the study of operant autonomic conditioning and self-regulation. The focus of the chapter is on the operant conditioning of autonomic responses rather than of electromyographic activity or central nervous system responding. Major emphasis is given to heart rate, since most of the attempted replications of operant conditioning in curarized rats have dealt with this response.

The issue of whether autonomic responses are operantly conditionable is seen in the present chapter as an issue pertaining to

LARRY E. ROBERTS · Department of Psychology, McMaster University, Hamilton, Ontario, Canada. The research reported here was supported by grants from the Ontario Mental Health Foundation (#345) and the National Research Council of Canada (#AO132). The chapter was written in the fall of 1976.

whether the properties of these responses can be altered by the establishment and manipulation of explicit relationships between autonomic responses and reinforcing events. Operant conditioning is said here to have taken place when changes in the response can be shown to be attributable to the relationship between the response and a reinforcer, rather than to some other feature of the experimental situation. The issue of whether operant conditioning has occurred is distinguished from questions pertaining to the mechanisms that are involved in the performance of learned visceral change (after Black, 1971). A change in visceral responding that is found to depend upon the relationship between the response and a reinforcer is attributed to operant conditioning, irrespective of whether the change was observed in an animal that was trained while in the normal state or while immobilized by a curariform drug.

Although a judgment concerning the problem of replication is obviously central to any assessment of the curare literature, the perspective that is developed in the present chapter has not been shaped wholly by this important issue. A more basic problem is that much of the earlier work on operant autonomic conditioning in both human subjects and curarized rats appears to have been based upon a view of neural organization and of operant conditioning that has been inimical to progress in this area of research. This problem can perhaps best be appreciated through an examination of the implications that the curare experiments were widely believed to have concerning (1) the mechanism of operant autonomic conditioning and (2) conceptions of the plasticity of visceral function.

A. The Mechanism of Operant Conditioning

Most observers agree that the initial impact of the curare experiments on the study of operant conditioning derived from the information these experiments were thought to have provided about the role of somatomotor processes in visceral learning. Curariform drugs produce flaccid paralysis by preventing the transmission of neural impulses across motor end-plates of the somatic and respiratory musculature (Koelle, 1970). It is therefore apparent that a demonstration of operant conditioning in the deeply curarized and artificially ventilated rat rules out the possibility that heart-rate changes might have been elicited by the performance of somatomotor or respiratory maneuvers with which these changes are frequently correlated in the normal state. However, paralysis controls only for the effects of proprioceptive and other consequences (for example, mechanical or metabolic) of

skeletal-motor and respiratory action. Nevertheless, several researchers went on to interpret operant heart-rate conditioning under curare
as strong presumptive evidence for the view that operant conditioning
was achieved without concomitant effects on somatomotor control
mechanisms. Katkin and Murray (1968) concluded that the curare
literature provided "the only truly convincing evidence of instrumental conditioning of ANS responses independent of possible mediators"
(Katkin and Murray, 1968, p. 64). The alternative hypothesis that
somatomotor mechanisms situated at higher levels of the brain may
have participated in the performance of heart-rate change was acknowledged in the early curare studies but was judged by Miller and
DiCara to have been "barely conceivable" (Miller and DiCara, 1967, p.
17; Miller, 1969).

The weakness of the latter judgment is that it ignores a substantial
body of evidence that indicates that somatomotor and cardiovascular
processes are integrated primarily at central levels of the brain, rather
than by proprioceptive or other feedback loops (see Smith, 1974, for a
review). It is further apparent that control of motor systems can be
established by operantly conditioning neural concomitants of them in
partially curarized and deeply curarized subjects (Black, 1967; Black,
Young, and Batenchuk, 1970; also see Koslovskaya, Vertes, and Miller,
1973) and that activation of these systems by an appropriate experimental manipulation exerts a measurable influence on heart rate in
curarized dogs (Black, 1974a), rats (Goesling and Brener, 1972), and
man (Freyschuss, 1970). Integrated central control of cardiovascular
function by motor processes is also suggested by recent reports that
human quadriplegics paralyzed by complete cervical lesions are nevertheless able to produce substantial changes in both heart rate and
blood pressure when instructed to attempt discrete movements of the
extremities (Freyschuss, 1970; Pickering, Brucker, Frankel, Mathias,
Dworkin, and Miller, 1977). These observations provide a basis for
severe criticism of curarization as an adequate control for total somatomotor involvement and serve to make the further point that participation of central motor systems in visceral learning under curare is
actually quite plausible on both conceptual and empirical grounds
(Black, 1967; Brener, Eissenberg, and Middaugh, 1974; Obrist, Webb,
Sutterer, and Howard, 1970).

Despite some reluctance to concede the point, this limitation of
the curare approach was acknowledged in early experiments on the
curarized rat and served as the basis for development of two additional research strategies that were designed to provide useful information. The first of these examined the relationship of heart-rate
responses to somatomotor and respiratory activity, to determine

whether these activities were affected by the operant conditioning procedure. Since the act of paralysis precluded observation of somatomotor and respiratory behavior during operant conditioning, DiCara and Miller (1969b) examined response relationships during a transfer test that was given in the normal state following prior operant conditioning under curare. The results of this study showed that rats that were trained to increase heart rate while curarized evidenced higher levels of motor activity and faster rates of respiration during the initial stages of the transfer test than did rats that were trained to decrease heart rate. These findings are obviously consistent with the view that central somatic and respiratory mechanisms are indeed affected when operant heart-rate conditioning is carried out under curariform paralysis. However, DiCara and Miller (1969b) also reported that continuation of operant conditioning in the normal state augmented bidirectional differences in heart rate, while bidirectional differences in respiratory function and motor activity diminished to statistical insignificance. This result is not easily explained by an appeal to a principle of cardiosomatic integration and suggests instead that correlated respiratory and motor responses were not required for the performance of heart-rate change (also see DiCara and Miller, 1969a). Unfortunately, the weight that should be given to the cardiosomatic dissociation evident in this study is unclear in view of the problem of replication surrounding the curare experiments. More recent evidence to be reviewed later in the chapter indicates that operantly conditioned changes in heart rate are closely related to respiratory and somatomotor function and are not easily dissociated from them (Black, 1974a; Obrist, Galosy, Lawler, Gaebelein, Howard, and Shanks, 1975).

The second research strategy examined the relationship of operantly conditioned changes in heart rate to other autonomic responses (for example, intestinal contractions) and determined whether the topography of cardiovascular operants could be shaped in highly specific ways (for example, blushing in one ear but not the other). This approach appears to have been based upon the assumption that motor processes exert a diffuse and undifferentiated influence on the activities of the viscera. Consequently, it was argued that if cardiovascular operants could be shown to be topographically specific (DiCara and Miller, 1968b; Fields, 1970a,b) and to occur independently of activities in other visceral response systems (Miller and Banuazizi, 1968), mediation of operant conditioning by somatomotor control mechanisms could be ruled out. The difficulty with this approach, however, is that the assumption necessary for it can be questioned by reference to a growing body of evidence that indicates that autonomic response systems are complexly organized and that the topography of autonomic activation is rather highly differentiated with respect to somatomotor function. There is, in fact, little empirical basis upon which to assume that intestinal motility is influenced by somatomotor arousal in curarized rat; in the absence of such data, the bearing of intestinal-cardiac dissociation on the issue of whether motor processes are involved in heart-rate conditioning is moot. It should further be noted that even autonomic systems that receive demonstrable somatomotor inputs, such as the electrodermal and the cardiac (Roberts, 1974), can be shown to be excited by different neural systems under some circumstances (Roberts and Young, 1971). Thus, dissociation of cardiac changes from an autonomic correlate will have little bearing on the role of motor processes in heart-rate performance, unless it is shown that the correlated response was sensitive to somatomotor influences under the conditions in which dissociation was obtained. Also germane to the present argument is the observation that localized augmentation of both vasomotor and electrodermal activity has been shown to occur when subjects engage in unilaterally specific somatomotor responding (Adams, Baccelli, Mancia, and Zanchetti, 1971; Culp and Edelberg, 1966; Edelberg, 1973; Ellison and Zanchetti, 1971; Roberts, L. E., 1970, unpublished results). These observations indicate that the patterning of peripheral autonomic activation in relation to such activity is rather precise. Reports of similar precision in the topography of operantly conditioned vasomotor responses (DiCara and Miller, 1968b) are not surprising in view of this patterning and may have little bearing on the question of whether motor processes are affected when operant control is established over this visceral response system.

These considerations indicate that bearing of the curare experiments on the issue of somatomotor mediation is less decisive than was originally believed. They also raise the further and provocative question of why this issue was the focus of so much concern, when other aspects of the phenomena of learned visceral control might have been more profitably pursued. The answer to this question appears to be that dissociation of cardiovascular operants from somatomotor processes was seen as pivotal to the status of these responses as members of an operant class (Katkin and Murray, 1968; Kimble, 1961). According to this conception of operant conditioning, the requirements for membership in an operant class stipulate not only that changes in responding must be shown to be attributable to the relationship between the response and a reinforcer but also that the response must be shown to occur without correlated changes in motor activities that might subsequently be found necessary for the performance of visceral change. Brener (1974) recently called attention to the inadequacy of this conceptualization of operant conditioning when he noted that many skeletal-motor behaviors that are ordinarily accepted as members of an operant class are not easily dissociated from correlated muscle and other activities that may be necessary for performance of the response in question. A conception of operant behavior that places topographical restrictions upon the form of the response appears on logical grounds to be quite arbitrary and is not easily defended against the argument that this characterization further implies the curious and untenable concept of an unmediated response (Brener, 1974; also see Black, 1971).

The approach taken by the curare studies to the conceptualization of operant behavior also appears to have derived in part from the aforementioned and erroneous conception of autonomic organization that was adopted by this work. The activities of the autonomic nervous system are closely integrated with other bodily processes and serve a variety of adaptive functions. Thus, it is apparent that integration of cardiovascular and motor activity meets an important metabolic need insofar as cardiovascular adjustments are required to supply the tissues with nutrients and to remove waste products produced by muscular activity. There are, however, occasions on which cardiovascular activation appears to be excited by other processes in the face of an impending metabolic load (Obrist, 1976). In these instances, cardiovascular adjustments do not appear to be closely related to concurrent motor activity, but this does not mean that the changes that occur are without correlated changes in other behavioral capacities of the organism. Complexity of organization is also characteristic of electrodermal activation, which has typically been depicted as a passive product of somatomotor and respiratory action in the literature on autonomic conditioning (for example, Smith, 1967). Although it is clear that sudomotor efferents are indeed integrated within neural systems that regulate motor behavior (Roberts, 1974), sudomotor outflow also appears to be modulated by neural systems that perform defensive (Roberts and Young, 1971) as well as perceptual (Edelberg, 1961) functions. Excitation of any of these systems by an appropriate behavioral manipulation produces a pattern of sudomotor events at the periphery that appears specifically adapted for the performance that is required (Edelberg, 1973). In view of this complexity of organization, it is unclear why dissociation of an autonomic response from motor activity should be held as a criterion for membership in an operant class, while dissociation from other correlates that may occur in different behavioral contexts is not. It should further be noted that the dissociations that were demonstrated in the curare literature were interpreted to mean that the effect of reinforcement was specific to efferent pathways that directly and uniquely innervated the response. While this conception can perhaps be entertained on theoretical grounds, it cannot be established by a focus merely upon somatomotor dissociation, and furthermore the likelihood of demonstrating specificity with respect to all adaptive functions appears on practical grounds to be exceedingly remote.

These considerations are sufficient to indicate that the bearing of the curare literature on the issue of whether somatomotor processes are involved in visceral learning has been overstated and largely misconceived. A demonstration of learning in the deeply curarized rat establishes nothing more than that changes in visceral activity have not been produced by proprioceptive or other effects of somatomotor or respiratory action. The possibility that central mechanisms that normally integrate these activities in the intact animal are involved in learning is not precluded by this demonstration; furthermore, the evidence that these mechanisms do in fact participate in operant conditioning is substantial. The analysis of specificity with respect to changes in other autonomic systems or with respect to the topography of the response is not directly relevant to the issue of somatomotor mediation and appears further to have been based upon a model of autonomic organization that is not in accord with the known facts pertaining to differences in the organization of visceral response systems and to the precise manner in which these systems are integrated with somatomotor and other behavioral activities. On the other hand, the analysis of specificity with respect to somatomotor behavior is clearly relevant to the issue of somatomotor participation in learning. However, data derived from this approach have been compromised by the problem of replication and appear in the light of recent research to have overstated the extent to which cardiac and somatomotor activities are dissociable in the normal state. Finally, there appear to be adequate grounds for rejecting the view that dissociation of a visceral response from motor activity is necessary if that response is to be allocated to an operant class. Topographical specification of the response is inconsistent with the practice that has been followed with respect to skeletal-motor behavior and appears further to have been proposed without sufficient appreciation for the complexity and integrated nature of visceral function.

B. Plasticity of Visceral Responding

A second and, in the opinion of this writer, more important reason for the impact of the curare literature on research in biofeedback concerns the rather remarkable properties that were evidenced by visceral operants in the curarized rat. The generality of the phenomenon appeared to have been well established by demonstrations of learning of several responses, including heart rate, blood pressure, gastric activity, stomach and intestinal contractions, renal blood flow, and vasomotor activity in the ear lobes (Miller, 1969). Visceral operants further appeared to have manifested properties that were generally held to be characteristic of operantly conditioned somatomotor responses. Included among these properties were acquisition of learned changes following positive as well as negative reinforcement (Miller and DiCara, 1967; DiCara and Miller, 1968a); highly specific reinforcement effects, including dissociation of the PP and PR intervals of the rat's electrocardiogram (Fields, 1970a,b; Miller and Banuazizi, 1968); bidirectional stimulus control of heart-rate changes and intestinal contractions (Banuazizi, 1972; DiCara and Miller, 1968a); retention of learning over a period of three months (DiCara and Miller, 1968c); and extinction of learned changes in heart rate when reinforcement was removed (DiCara and Stone, 1970; Fields, 1970a,b; Hothersall and Brener, 1969). This literature was also noted for the magnitude of the learned changes that was reported and for its extensive use of bidirectional and other control procedures that are necessary for the demonstration of response-contingent effects (Black, 1971). The emphasis given to the curare experiments in several review papers (for example, Harris and Brady, 1974; Katkin and Murray, 1968) leaves little doubt that these studies convinced many skeptics and provided a major source of support for the conclusion that autonomic responses are operantly conditionable. Research on operant autonomic conditioning in human subjects and on clinical applications, both of which predated the curare experiments, also appears to have been received with greater enthusiasm as a result of the phenomena reported in the curare literature. It was widely recognized that

> with the pioneering work of Miller and his colleagues (summarized in Miller, 1969) showing conclusively that autonomic responses can be controlled through operant conditioning without peripheral mediation, the whole repertoire of autonomic responses became potentially open to central, and possibly voluntary, control. (Blanchard and Scott, 1974, p. 273)

It is important to stress that the enthusiasm provoked for biofeedback research by the curare studies derived from more than a recognition that autonomic responses could be shaped by response-contingent reinforcement. Rather, it appears also to have derived from a conception of the plasticity of visceral function that was asserted vigorously by this literature. Whereas visceral activity had previously been regarded as closely integrated with somatomotor, emotional, and regulatory behavior, the alternative view asserted the potential independence of visceral function from these behavioral processes. Deeply implicit in this conception of plasticity was the notion that large and physiologically significant changes in autonomic responding could be shaped by operant conditioning and that the progress of such conditioning was largely unconstrained by intrinsic control mechanisms. DiCara and Stone (1970) speculated that visceral learning could be "carried far enough to create major physiologic changes in the internal environment" and offered data suggesting the plausibility of this view (DiCara and Stone, 1970, p. 359). Miller, DiCara, and Wolf (1968) proposed that operant conditioning might be a general phenomenon that serves to maintain homeostasis when innate homeostatic mechanisms are insufficient for this purpose. The effectiveness of operant conditioning when applied to diverse response systems, together with the specificity of learning and its apparent insensitivity to constraints, influenced heavily the view of Katkin (1971), who, after reviewing the curare experiments in an introductory textbook, concluded that

> the theoretical work has largely been done. The groundwork has been laid for an exciting future in which our innermost functions may be subject to modification by appropriate applications of external reward. Between now and 1984 you may well discover that you can voluntarily reduce your blood pressure, set your heart to beat at any rate you desire, and tell your kidneys just how fast to produce urine for your maximum convenience. (Katkin, 1971, p. 23)

There is little question that early applications of biofeedback training to the treatment of visceral pathology derived considerable impetus from the conception of autonomic plasticity that was implicit in the promise of these achievements (Miller, DiCara, Solomon, Weiss, and Dworkin, 1970).

Several recent developments have, however, given reason to reconsider the limits to which operant autonomic conditioning might conceivably be carried out. One of these developments concerns the mixed success that has been achieved in attempts to apply operant conditioning to the treatment of visceral pathology (for reviews see Blanchard and Young, 1973, 1974; Legewie, 1977). Much of the current effort in this area of research has been directed to determining whether the therapeutic effects that have been reported are in fact the product of learned changes in autonomic responding as opposed to some other effect of the treatment procedure, and to determining whether alternative forms of therapy might be equally or perhaps more effective than operant conditioning in the treatment of visceral disorder. However, of concern to the issue of plasticity is the fact that the magnitude of visceral control that has been established in recent work has frequently been modest, particularly in cardiovascular applications (for example, see Blanchard, and Young, 1973; A. H. Roberts, Schuler, Bacon, Zimmerman, and Patterson, 1975; Surwit and Shapiro, 1977). Furthermore, it is not clear whether patients who have learned to control visceral responding are able to perform their skills in those circumstances in which they are most likely to profit from them (Surwit, Shapiro, and Feld, 1976; Zeiner and Pollak, 1976). While most critics agree that biofeedback therapies offer promise and merit further study in the case of neuromuscular and possibly epileptic disorders (Blanchard and Young, 1974; Legewie, 1977), these observations give reason to reserve judgment on the issue of whether operant conditioning can generally be expected to establish control that is sufficient to yield therapeutic benefits in visceral applications.

Two further reasons to reconsider the plasticity of visceral function that are of particular concern in this chapter are as follows. First, there is a growing body of evidence that indicates that the results of the original curare experiments are unreplicable and that the remarkable phenomena depicted in this literature are unlikely to have been attributable to learning as was originally believed. The basis for this judgment, which is developed later in the chapter, is sufficiently strong to indicate that conclusions pertaining to the properties of visceral operants can no longer be defended by an appeal to this body of work. The second development concerns the results of recent studies in which operant autonomic conditioning was carried out in intact human subjects and animal preparations. Although these studies leave little doubt that visceral responses are operantly conditionable, the specificity of the learned changes that has been evidenced in them has fallen considerably short of that reported in the curare literature (for example, Brener, Phillips, and Connally, 1977; Lacroix and Roberts, 1976). More sophisticated attempts to dissociate cardiovascular operants from their somatomotor and autonomic correlates by means of disjunctive conditioning procedures (Black, 1974a; Schwartz, 1974) or by imposition of somatomotor constraints (Obrist *et al.*, 1975) have encountered only modest success and offer little support for the view that the progress of operant conditioning is largely unconstrained by visceral control mechanisms. These developments call attention to the question of plasticity and serve to indicate how little is known about the variables that maximize learned control and the circumstances under which such learning may be expressed. It is possible and perhaps likely that the phenomena reported in the curare literature served to eclipse the study of these issues, which are basic to conceptions of the organization and plasticity of the autonomic nervous system as well as to clinical applications.

The present chapter reviews selected evidence pertaining to the latter two developments. The issue of replication is considered in the next section of the chapter, where several experiments on operant heart-rate conditioning in the curarized rat that were undertaken in my laboratory are described. The following section reviews efforts undertaken elsewhere and examines the case against a learning interpretation of the original findings. An explanation of how these findings might have been obtained, on the other hand, is suggested in Section IV. The fifth section of the chapter examines the implications of these developments for basic and applied research in biofeedback and self-regulation. Recent research on the mechanism of operant heart-rate conditioning is discussed here, particularly with reference to the issue of whether operant conditioning may be employed to uncouple cardiovascular responses from somatomotor influences. Finally, it should be noted that the effort to produce operant autonomic conditioning in the curarized rat is continuing (Dworkin and Miller, 1977). Some comments on the relevance of this effort to basic issues in visceral learning are offered in the concluding section.

II. Some Experiments on Learning in the Curarized Rat

The experiments reported in this section of the chapter were undertaken in my laboratory in the fall of 1972 and were concluded in the spring of 1974. Experiments on operant conditioning utilized a nondiscriminative punishment procedure similar to that used by Fields (1970a,b), who presented extensive data indicating that such methods could be utilized to control selectively the PP, PR, and RR intervals of the rat's electrocardiogram. This work was designed to follow up earlier efforts in my laboratory by Wright (1974) and was not intended to duplicate the methods used by Fields (1970a,b). Nevertheless, the preparations and shaping procedures employed in the two sets of experiments appear to have been similar enough to address the issue of replication.

The shaping procedures used in the present experiments and in earlier work by Fields (1970a,b) are examples of a more general class of procedures defined by Platt (1973) as *percentile reinforcement schedules*. The defining property of these schedules is that they reinforce only those responses that exceed a predetermined portion of the animal's currently emitted response values. The differential between emitted and reinforced response values is specified as a percentile of the former and has been shown to be a major determinant of performance in studies in which percentile reinforcement has been applied to a variety of skeletal-motor operants, including interresponse times and response runs in the pigeon's key-peck response (Alleman and Platt, 1973; Kuch and Platt, 1976; Webster, 1976) and several quantitative features of bar pressing by rats (Platt, personal communication, 1976). It should be noted that the percentile criterion adopted in the present work (nominally the upper and lower 10% of emitted cardiac intervals; approximately 14% by actual measure) fell well within the range of criteria reported by Fields (1970a) to have produced cardiac conditioning in the curarized rat. Similar criteria have also proved highly effective for shaping quantitative characteristics of skeletal-motor behavior (Platt, 1973; Webster, 1976).

The research on operant heart-rate conditioning described below was preceded by several apparently successful experiments by DiCara and his colleagues (DiCara, 1971), in addition to the aforementioned studies by Fields (1970a,b). These studies are summarized, together with several other experiments that reported results in the direction of learning, in Table 1. Only experiments employing aversive conditioning procedures are included in the table, since it was this method of training that was used in our research. Inspection of Table 1 shows that although certain features, such as stimulus control of heart-rate changes, appeared on some occasions (for example, DiCara and Miller, 1968a, 1969b) and not others (for example, Thornton and Van-Toller, 1973a,b), in each experiment statistically reliable differences in baseline heart rate were observed between rats that were rewarded for increases or decreases in this response. It is also apparent that bidirectional differences were obtained over a wide (if not remarkable) range of punishment densities and a variety of shaping procedures, suggesting that the effect was robust and well buffered. The outcome of the research presented below, however, pointed to a different conclusion.

A. Operant Conditioning in the Curarized State

The preparation used in this research was similar to that employed in the early DiCara and Miller studies and may be described as follows. At the first sign of respiratory distress (usually 10–30 sec following injection), rats were transferred to a restraining platform, where connection was made with a face mask fashioned from a rubber balloon. A tight seal was achieved about the snout by a careful positioning of the rat's head followed by attachment of a Shuster clamp to an electrode assembly that had been cemented to the skull

TABLE 1

Experiments Reporting Statistically Significant Bidirectional Differences in the Direction of Learning during Avoidance Conditioning of Heart Rate in the Curarized Rat

Experiment	Shaping procedure	Shock density	Curare dosage respiration sample size[a]	Initial heart rate and % change[b]	Comment
DiCara and Miller, 1968a	Discrimination training with 100 shock, 100 safe, and 100 blank trials	One shock trial programmed every 90 sec on average; 0 to about 20 shocks/trial	1.2/1.2 70/1:1/20 6/6	410 + 13.4% 404 − 15.4%	Stimulus control observed on shock and safe trials; low shock density (cf. DiCara and Miller, 1968c; Fields, 1970a).
DiCara and Miller, 1968c	Discrimination training with 270 shock, 30 blank trials	Trials programmed every 30 sec on average; shocks/trial not reported	3.0/1.0 70/1:1/20 6/6	405 + 13.8% 418 − 17.0%	Extinction observed during retention test under curare 3 months later.
DiCara and Miller, 1969a	Discrimination training with 270 shock, 30 blank trials	Trials programmed every 30 sec on average; shocks/trial not reported	3.0/1.0 70/1:1/20 7/7	429 + 8.9% 418 − 12.4%	Rats trained initially in normal state; groups diverged during retention test under curare (cf. DiCara and Miller, 1968c).
DiCara and Miller, 1969b	Discrimination training with 270 shock, 30 blank trials	Trials programmed every 30 sec on average; shocks/trial not reported	3.0/1.0 70/1:1/20 8/8	415 + 6.3% 426 − 18.6%	Stimulus control observed but did not transfer to normal state.
DiCara and Weiss, 1969	Discrimination training with 270 shock, 30 blank trials	Trials programmed every 30 sec on average; shocks/trial not reported	3.0/1.0 70/1:1/15 7/7	395 + 8.9% 400 − 7.8%	Stimulus control observed under curare; increase rats appeared to freeze when tested in normal state.

TABLE 1. (Continued)

Experiment	Shaping procedure	Shock density	Curare dosage respiration sample size[a]	Initial heart rate and % change[b]	Comment
DiCara, Braun, and Pappas, 1970	Discrimination training with 135 shock, 15 blank trials	Trials programmed every 40 sec on average; shocks/trial not reported	2.0/1.0 70/1:1/15 6/6	407 + 1.2% 413 − 6.8%	Increase performance not significant; no mention of stimulus control; intact neocortex was necessary for learning.
Fields, 1970a	Nondiscriminative punishment training; constant criterion schedule	5–25% of all heartbeats shocked at start of training (estimate 20–115 shocks/min)	3.6/0.0 70/1:1/20 12/12[c]	459[d] + 9.8%[c] 459[d] − 10.5%[c]	PR interval also conditioned in a separate group.
Fields, 1970b	Nondiscriminative punishment training; percentile reinforcement schedule	5–25% of all heartbeats shocked throughout training (estimate 20–115 shocks/min)	3.6/0.0 70/1:1/20 12/12[c]	459[d] + 15.5%[c] 459[d] − 15.4%[c]	Extinction observed; PR interval conditioned independently of PP, RR; performance was a function of delay of reinforcement and percentile criterion.
Thornton, 1971 Experiment 1	Discrimination training with 80 shock, 80 safe, and 80 blank trials	Trials programmed every 20 sec on average; 0 to about 20 shocks/trial	0.6/0.6 70/1:1/14 6/6	396 + 14.8% 414 − 0.1%	No evidence of stimulus control; group difference in pattern of shock observed.

Reference	Training	Shock schedule	Curare/respiration/sample[a]	Heart rate[b]	Comments
Thornton and Van-Toller, 1973a	Discrimination training with 80 shock, 160 blank trials	Trials programmed every 20 sec on average; 0 to about 10 shocks/trial	0.6/0.6 70/1:1/14 4/2	472 + 8.5% / 468 − 4.5%	No evidence of stimulus control; immunosympathectomized rats did not learn.
Thornton and Van-Toller, 1973b	Discrimination training with 80 shock, 160 blank trials	Trials programmed every 20 sec on average; 0 to about 10 shocks/trial	0.6/0.6 70/1:1/14 5/5	455[e] + 9.5% / 473 − 4.0%	No evidence of stimulus control; group difference in pattern of shock observed; KCl on cortex prevented learning.
Wright, 1974, Experiment 4	Nondiscriminative punishment training approximating percentile reinforcement	Mean shock density 29 shocks/min; range 25–43 shocks/min	4.0/4.0[f] 70/1:1/12[g] 8/8	414 + 8.5% / 413 + 1.2%	Extinction observed 15 min after training; increase rats received more shock.
Gliner, Horvath, and Wolfe, 1975	Discrimination training for 90 min; estimate maximum of about 50 shock trials	Trials programmed every 90 sec on average; maximum of 5 shocks/ trial, at 15-sec intervals	3.0/1.0 60/1:1/19 8/8	437 + 4.0% / 436 − 9.0%	No evidence of stimulus control; increase rats received more shock; cardiac output measured.

[a] First entry is curare dosage [initial injection (mg/kg)/infusion (mg/kg/hr)]; second entry is respiration [rate (cpm)/inspiration-expiration ratio/peak inspiratory pressure (cm H_2O)]; third entry is sample size [number increase/number decrease].
[b] First entry is increase performance [heart rate in beats/min and percentage of change]; second entry is decrease performance.
[c] RR interval and PP interval groups combined.
[d] Initial heart rates not reported; this value is taken from control rats that were curarized but not trained (Fields, 1970a, Table 1).
[e] Initial heart rates for the increase and decrease groups were inadvertently reversed in the published paper (cf. Thornton, 1972, Figure 6.6).
[f] Succinylcholine.
[g] Peak inspiratory pressure was adjusted on-line to hold chest circumference constant.

during minor surgery 7–10 days earlier. This assembly also served as a terminus for subdermal electrodes that were implanted in order to measure heart rate. Artificial respiration was provided by a positive-pressure respirator (E and M Company V5KG), which operated at 70 cycles per minute with an inspiration–expiration ratio of 1:1 and a peak inspiratory pressure of approximately 12 cm of water (abbreviated herein as 70/1:1/12). The latter variable was adjusted for individual rats during the first 60 min of paralysis in an effort to produce a stable heart rate of between 380 and 480 beats per minute (bpm) with a 10–30 bpm peak-to-trough variability in the cardiotachometer record. After this initial adaptation period, respirator parameters were unaltered for the remainder of training. Continuous intraoral suction was used to prevent accumulation of fluids that may have otherwise been blown down the trachea by the force of positive-pressure ventilation. The rear feet of the rat were drawn down through the restraining platform and had silver chloride electrodes attached to them for measurement of the plantar skin potential. Skin-potential measurements were referred to sites on the tail that were situated anterior to shock electrodes that were also placed here. The restraining platform was warmed by a heating pad fixed at a medium setting in an effort to maintain body temperature and peripheral vasomotor tone. This apparatus could also be used to carry out experiments in the normal state. In this case, the head clamp and face mask were removed, and a collar was placed behind the rat to prevent chewing of electrodes attached to the feet and tail. In addition to the electrocardiogram, heart rate, rectal temperature, peak inspiratory pressure, circumferential chest movements, and skin-potential responding were recorded for all rats throughout the session.[1]

Approximately one hour following initial paralysis and after all the respiratory adjustments had been completed, a small laboratory computer (PDP-8/L) was engaged on-line and used subsequently to maintain a running memory of the rat's 100 most recent RR intervals. If the rat was to be trained to increase its heart rate, all intervals exceeding the 90th percentile of the distribution contained in memory were followed by tail shock when punishment training began. If, on the other hand, the rat was to be trained to decrease its heart rate, all intervals falling below the 10th percentile of the distribution contained in memory were punished when conditioning commenced. The occurrence of an RR interval in the appropriate tail of the distribution (a "criterion" beat) constituted a single training trial and was followed, during punishment training, by an unsignaled time-out period of 300

[1] Further details are appendicized at the end of the chapter.

msec during which no shocks were given. Shock (a capacitor discharge of 28-msec duration) was applied 1.2 msec following the occurrence of each criterion heartbeat. In the experiments reported in the present paper, each rat received 1000 trials of operant level, 3000 trials of conditioning, and 2000 trials of extinction in a single experimental session that lasted approximately four hours. Performance was assessed by an examination of the RR, PR, and PP intervals associated with the occurrence of each criterion heartbeat and with subsequent heartbeats occurring during the time-out period. These measurements were taken and stored by the computer, which printed out mean values for each cardiac interval in blocks of 25 trials throughout training. In addition, histograms containing all heartbeats emitted by the rat were compiled and printed out every 250 trials.

Several checks were run to verify the accuracy of the shaping procedure. In one of these checks, the upper beam of a dual-beam oscilloscope was triggered continuously by the EKG, while the lower beam was driven by a binary flip-flop whose state was altered by the computer whenever a P or R wave was detected. Inspection of the oscilloscopic display indicated that measurement of cardiac intervals was accurate to within the sampling rate of the computer (200 μsec). The lower beam was also superimposed upon the electrocardiogram throughout training to provide a visual check on possible changes in detection thresholds owing to alteration of the EKG or equipment malfunction. These displays were photographed during operant level and later during extinction and were compared for an evaluation of the stability of both the EKG and the method used to detect P and R waves. Changes in the electrocardiogram were judged to have occurred in only two of the total sample of 55 rats that completed heart-rate training. These changes were observed primarily in the shape of the P wave and appear to have had little effect on the measured value of the RR interval that was being conditioned. Shock intensity was measured oscilloscopically following the completion of extinction, and sensitivity of the rat to shock was verified by inspection of the skin-potential record.

Several assessments of the accuracy of the shaping procedure were also made possible by data analysis following completion of the experiment. These included (1) examination of the recovery functions in all three cardiac intervals associated with successive heartbeats during the time-out period; (2) calculation of the percentage of the rat's total responses that was followed by shock; (3) representation of the mean criterion RR interval in each block of 250 trials in terms of a standard score; and (4) calculation of correlations among the three cardiac intervals during various stages of conditioning. The first of

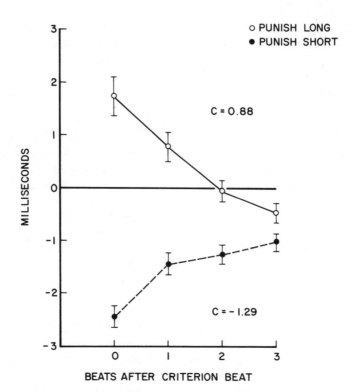

FIGURE 1.   Criterion RR intervals and three successive RR intervals thereafter. Data are taken from the last 250 trials of operant level. The average RR interval during these trials was subtracted from each heartbeat. The parameter C is the mean criterion interval in standard deviation units; the bars are ±1 standard error. The recovery functions are asymmetrical with respect to zero because distributions of RR intervals were positively skewed.

these four measures taken at the end of operant level is depicted in Figure 1 for all rats that completed operant conditioning. The recovery functions shown here for the RR interval were characteristic of those observed at all stages of training and serve to indicate that the computer was indeed detecting the appropriate tail of the RR interval distributions in each bidirectional group.

A total of 63 rats was paralyzed for five experiments utilizing this shaping procedure. Of these, 6 rats were subsequently discarded because of unstable heart rates that resulted in death (1 rat) or required adjustments to peak inspiratory pressure before the end of training; 2 others were discarded because of equipment failure. The remaining sample of 55 rats completed training without intervention by the experimenter in any aspect of the experimental procedure. Of these subjects, 45 were assigned to bidirectional groups on the basis of a coin toss after all adjustments had been completed. The remaining 10 rats were allocated to bidirectional groups in the various studies to equate sample size.

The initial and concluding status of the 55 subjects that successfully completed training is summarized briefly in Table 2. The average heart rate (438.6 bpm) and heart-rate variability (mean SD = 11.3 bpm) were calculated from distributions containing approximately 2500 consecutive heartbeats that were compiled during the last 250 trials of operant level, approximately 90 min after paralysis (Trial 1000, Table 2). Modal heart rates were slightly faster than mean heart rates for most rats, indicating that distributions of interbeat intervals were skewed. Measurements provided in the last three columns of Table 2 show how several variables had changed by the last 250 trials of extinction (Trial 6000), approximately 4 hours after injection. Inspection of these data reveals that mean heart-rate and skin-potential activity decreased significantly over training, as did the magnitude of circumferential chest movements (an indirect measure of tidal volume). Heart-rate variability and rectal temperature, on the other hand, increased slightly but significantly over the duration of paralysis. These findings are similar in several respects to those reported in

TABLE 2
Status Before and After Conditioning[a]

Variable	Trial 1000	Trial 6000	Difference	t
Mean heart rate	438.6	429.7	−8.9	−2.12[b]
Modal heart rate	441.9	432.9	−9.0	−2.15[b]
Maximum heart rate	500.0	541.0	—	—
Minimum heart rate	356.3	328.2	—	—
Mean heart-rate SD	11.3	14.9	3.6	2.01[b]
Skin-potential responding	23.5	18.7	−4.7	−3.49[c]
Skin-potential level	24.4	19.5	−4.9	−1.86[d]
Rectal temperature	37.1	37.3	0.2	2.65[b]
Peak inspiratory pressure	12.2	12.2	0.0	−0.31
Chest circumference	12.1	10.2	−1.9	−4.91[c]

[a] Computed from 55 rats that completed punishment training without intervention by the experimenter. Of these, 38 were paralyzed by succinylcholine, 11 by D-tubocurarine, and 6 by dimethyl tubocurarine. Drug groups are combined owing to a lack of significant differences among them. Bidirectional groups have also been combined. Data were taken from the last 250 trials of operant level (Trial 1000) and the last 250 trials of extinction (Trial 6000). Heart rate in beats/minute; skin-potential responding in responses/minute; skin-potential level in mV negative; temperature in °C; peak inspiratory pressure in cm H_2O; chest circumference in arbitrary units (mm).
[b] $p < .05$, two-tailed test.
[c] $p < .01$, two-tailed test.
[d] $p < .05$, one-tailed test.

earlier studies of operant conditioning in the curarized rat (Brener *et al.*, 1974; Miller and DiCara, 1967) and are considered later.

The results of five experiments using this basic method of training are summarized in Figure 2. The upper portion of each panel depicts changes in the mode of distributions containing all RR intervals emitted by the rat during successive blocks of 250 trials. The lower portion of each panel, on the other hand, shows how the duration of criterion heartbeats changed in each bidirectional group over the course of punishment training. The data were evaluated statistically by the application of *t* tests to indices of conditioning performance that were computed separately for each rat by the subtraction of performance during the last 250 trials of operant level from performance during the first 250 trials of extinction. This method is analogous to that used in previous research (Roberts, Lacroix, and Wright, 1974) and provides a measure of learning uncontaminated by the presence of shock. Analyses of variance that took more data into account were also carried out, but these did not alter conclusions with respect to learning and are therefore not reported.

The first experiment in this series was undertaken in an attempt to replicate a bidirectional difference in the direction of learning that was obtained in a preliminary study (Wright, 1974, Experiment 4), in which several parameters pertaining to maintenance and the shaping procedure were adjusted by the experimenter according to predetermined criteria over the course of operant conditioning. In contrast to that experiment, all aspects of the procedure were automated in the present study. Rats were paralyzed by succinylcholine and received 0.4-mA tail shock for all criterion heartbeats that occurred outside of the time-out periods. The results are shown in Panel A of Figure 2. Statistical analyses failed to reveal a significant bidirectional difference in conditioning indices based upon modal or criterion RR intervals. The bidirectional groups actually tended to diverge in the wrong direction over the course of conditioning. Rats that were punished for long RR intervals tended to emit longer criterion intervals toward the end of conditioning and during the early stages of extinction than did rats that were punished for short RR intervals.

The second experiment (Panel B, Figure 2) examined the effect of shock intensity on learning. Since subjects in the first experiment appeared if anything to change in the wrong direction over conditioning, we decided to see what would happen if the shock were made more aversive. In this experiment, shock intensity was increased to a value (2.8 mA) that will be shown later to support Pavlovian conditioning of skin-potential responding in the curarized rat. Once again,

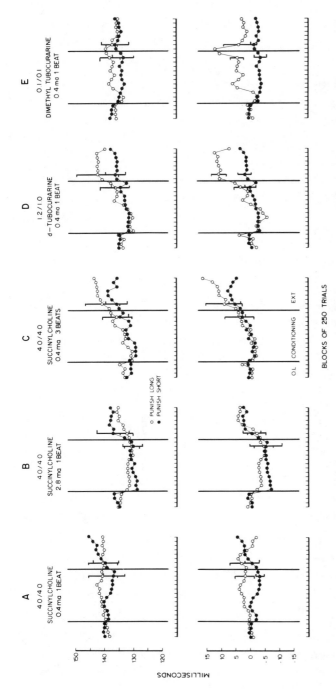

Figure 2.   Changes in the RR interval during operant heart-rate conditioning. Modes of distributions containing all RR intervals emitted by the rat are depicted in the upper row; changes in the mean criterion RR interval from operant level are shown in the lower row. The bars are ±1 standard error. The first number above each panel is the initial dosage (mg/kg); the second is the nominal intramuscular infusion (mg/kg/hr). Sample sizes (punish long/punish short) for Panels A–E are 9/9, 5/5, 5/6, and 3/3, respectively. RR intervals falling in the upper or lower 40% of the distribution contained in memory were tallied as criterion responses in Panel C, to maintain shock density at approximately 0.5 shocks/sec.

statistical analyses failed to provide any evidence of learning, although a larger unconditioned response to shock was observed when punishment training began.

Another possibility we considered was the following. It is conceivable that the neural process that is correlated with reinforcement when punishment is conditional upon single heartbeats, differs from the neural process that is correlated with reinforcement when shock is conditional upon the occurrence of three successive heartbeats beyond criterion. The latter procedure may be more successful in identifying just-reinforceable differences in heart rate. However, increasing the response unit to three successive beats beyond criterion did not lead to learning. This outcome is shown in Panel C in Figure 2, which summarizes the performance of rats that received 0.4-mA shock when they emitted three successive heartbeats in the appropriate tail of their RR-interval distributions.

The remaining experiments were undertaken to compare the performance of rats paralyzed by succinylcholine with the performance of rats paralyzed by either D-tubocurarine or dimethyl tubocurarine. These drugs were chosen because they are known to differ markedly in their blocking action at autonomic ganglia in dogs and cats (Howard, Gaebelein, Galosy, and Obrist, 1975) and possibly with respect to their central nervous system and histamine-releasing properties as well (Grob, 1967; Koelle, 1970). In each experiment, rats received 0.4-mA shock for single-criterion heartbeats falling outside of the time-out periods. The results are shown in Panels D and E of Figure 2, which may be compared to Panel A, where the same conditioning procedure was applied to rats paralyzd by succinylcholine. Inspection of these findings provides no evidence consistent with an interpretation of learning in any preparation. In each experiment, punishment for long RR intervals tended to produce longer criterion beats during extinction than did punishment for short RR intervals. This paradoxical effect was found to be reliable when t tests were applied to indices of conditioning performance based upon criterion beats for rats paralyzed by D-tubocurarine. However, the effect was not reliable when all five experiments were considered together. Comparison of Panels A, D, and E in Figure 2 does not encourage the view, suggested by Howard *et al.* (1974), that choice of paralyzing drug is critical to demonstration of operant heart-rate conditioning in the curarized rat.

The analyses of Figure 2 depicted the performance of all rats that completed punishment training without intervention by the experimenter in any aspect of the experimental procedure. One shortcoming of this practice, however, is that it overlooks previous reports that indicate that rats paralyzed by curare are heterogeneous with respect to cardiovascular impairment and cardiovascular state (Dworkin, 1973; Hahn, 1971, 1974a). The term cardiovascular *state* is taken here to refer generally to the composition of neurogenic and hormonal influences on cardiac action in the curarized rat. The term cardiovascular *impairment*, on the other hand, is intended to denote a specific cardiovascular state in which neurogenic control of the heart is profoundly diminished by pharmacological blockade of cardiac control fibers or is dominated by invariant homeostatic adjustments that are triggered by diminished cardiac output, radically altered blood gas composition, or other consequences of muscular paralysis and artificial respiration. It should be noted that alterations of cardiovascular state produced by the act of paralysis need not necessarily involve cardiovascular impairment as defined here. For example, it is possible that curarization may alter adrenal or beta-adrenergic contributions to heart-rate performance without leading to cardiovascular impairment, through elicitation of an acute stress response (Wilson and DiCara, 1975). Another possibility is that curarization may reduce the significance of baroreceptor feedback loops as a source of heart-rate variability by eliminating postural adjustments that affect cardiac output and blood pressure. Assessment of cardiovascular state with particular reference to the presence of cardiovascular impairment is a complex undertaking that requires more information than is provided by the present work (cf. Dworkin, 1973). However, as a first approximation, heart-rate responsiveness to shock coupled with spontaneous changes in heart-rate baseline unrelated to changes in respiratory function may be accepted as evidence that sources of impairment such as are present are insufficient to prevent expression of neurogenic or hormonal influences on cardiac action.

The next analysis was based upon this assumption and was carried out in the following way. Polygraph records for each rat were examined independently by two observers who assessed the record for breath-by-breath stability in respiratory pressure and chest circumference throughout training. Of the total sample of 55 rats, 49 were judged by both observers to have evidenced minimal variability in these parameters and to have encountered nothing more than occasional and transitory episodes of ventilatory obstruction throughout conditioning and extinction. This sample was reduced further by the exclusion of 4 rats that failed to evidence rectal temperatures exceeding 35°C throughout training and 2 subjects that became electrodermally unresponsive over the course of conditioning. From the remaining subjects, a sample of "responsive" rats was chosen by the selection of rats that displayed (1) unconditioned heart-rate responses to the introduction of shock with a visible acceleratory component and (2) spontaneous changes in heart rate exceeding approximately 10 bpm unrelated to respiratory function. Nine rats punished for short RR intervals and another nine punished for long intervals were judged by both observers to have fulfilled these requirements. The performance of these rats during operant conditioning is depicted in Figure 3. Representative cardiotachographic records, on the other hand, are shown in Figure 4, where records taken from rats that were judged unresponsive and from rats that were tested in an earlier experiment on classical conditioning in the normal state are also provided for purposes of comparison. Inspection of these data shows that although the heart-rate variability of responsive rats approached that of rats

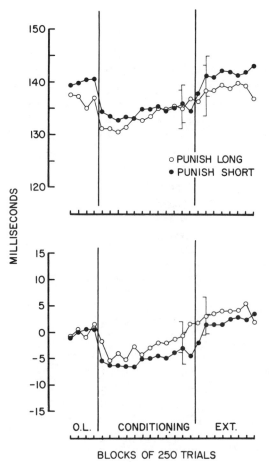

FIGURE 3. Performance of rats judged to have evidenced responsive heart rates. Distribution of rats across the five experimental conditions shown in Panels A through E of Figure 2 was (punish long/punish short) 1/3, 2/1, 2/2, 3/2, and 1/1, respectively. Performance is depicted as described in Figure 2.

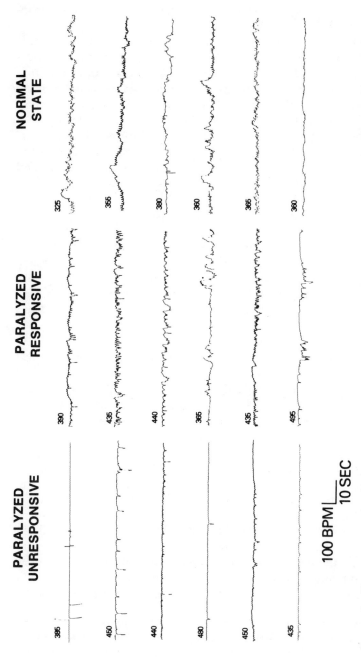

FIGURE 4. Heart-rate records of curarized rats judged to have been responsive or unresponsive are compared to records taken from partially restrained rats in the normal state. Each record is from a different rat. Epochs are taken approximately 4 hours after the start of paralysis (Trial 6000) or restraint and are representative of performance as a whole. Tonic heart rate is reported to the nearest five beats.

tested in the normal state, no evidence of operant heart-rate conditioning was obtained.

Further analyses were undertaken in an effort to identify possible
predictors of conditioning success. For this purpose, indices of conditioning performance based upon criterion RR intervals and computed
for each rat as described previously were plotted as a function of
putative determinants of learning (1) within each bidirectional group
in the five experiments separately; (2) within the subsample of
responsive rats judged to be relatively free of cardiovascular impairment; and (3) within bidirectional groups created by a pooling of the
results from all five experiments together. The predictors examined
pertained to cardiovascular impairment and state (for example, mean
initial heart rate and heart-rate variability), central nervous system
arousal (skin-potential level and response frequency), characteristics of
the subject (weight), and the shaping procedure (for example, temporal density of shock and the obtained percentile criterion). This
analysis failed to identify predictors of learning when scattergrams
were examined for each of the above groupings. In no case were
product–moment correlations depicting the relationship of each predictor to conditioning performance found to differ significantly from
zero.

A final analysis was conducted in the following way. The performance of each rat throughout training was depicted graphically by
a plotting of the mean criterion RR interval for successive blocks of 250
trials. An attempt was then made to select subjects that might
conceivably have learned, as evidenced by changes in the appropriate
direction during conditioning with a subsequent reversal in extinction. The purpose was to determine whether rats chosen on this basis
might have evidenced a pattern of characteristics predictive of performance, when no single variable sufficed. This analysis identified
eight rats that might have been considered to have learned.[2] The
properties of responding presented by these subjects were not remarkably different from the group as a whole, except for the fact that six of
the eight had previously been judged responsive by the criteria
outlined earlier. The latter result raises once again the prospect that
responsivity in the heart-rate record might have led to performances
reflective of learning. However, the interpretation that is to be given
to these observations is extremely problematical. Of the eight subjects

[2] Mean heart rate at Trial 1000 for this group was 435 bpm (range: 410–459 bpm), with
an average standard deviation of 11.53 bpm (range: 3.34–32.47 bpm). Mean change in
heart rate in the direction of training was 5.91% (range: 1.8–9.5%). All experimental
conditions except training under dimethyl tubocurarine were represented in the
sample.

identified by the present analysis, six also had been punished for emitting long RR intervals. The performance of these rats cannot be attributed unequivocally to operant conditioning, since the direction of the heart-rate changes was the same as the predominant uncondi-tioned response to shock. Furthermore, it should be noted that eight of the nine rats that were judged to have emitted responsive heart rates in the previous analysis evidenced changes in this response that were incompatible with learning, when punished for short RR inter-vals (Figure 3 above). Thus, although it is conceivable that learning played a role in some of the individual performances considered here, there is nothing in these data that requires the conclusion that learning had taken place. It should also be noted that the proportion of rats that evidenced heart-rate changes that might have been attributed speculatively to learning amounted to less than 15% of the total sample that completed operant conditioning.

It is apparent that the results of these experiments contrast sharply with the findings summarized previously in Table 1, in which operant conditioning was carried out in a preparation similar to that employed in the present work. They are particularly discrepant from the results of Fields (1970a,b) who reported that a similar shaping procedure could be used to operantly condition changes in the RR interval independently of the PR interval with a variety of attendant phenom-ena. For reasons mentioned earlier, the procedures employed in the two series of experiments were not strictly identical. Fields based beat-by-beat computation of the punishment criterion upon distribu-tions containing the last 512 consecutive heartbeats, rather than the last 100 heartbeats as was done in the present study. Another difference is that Fields did not employ a time-out period, as was done here. These differences very likely resulted in an increased temporal density of punishment and a tendency toward clustering of shock in Fields's (1970a,b) experiments, where the punishment criterion in effect at any given instant was less appropriate to the current heart rate than was the case in the present research. Other differences that are probably of greater importance to the issue of replication pertain to maintenance of the preparation before and during conditioning, but the nature of these is difficult to ascertain from the written protocol provided by Fields (1970a,b).

One possibility we did evaluate, however, is that some aspect of the procedure used to paralyze and maintain the rats in our study might have affected central neural functioning to the extent that no form of learning could reasonably have been expected to take place (cf. Roberts et al., 1974). Data bearing on this possibility are considered next.

B. Classical Conditioning in the Curarized State

The paralytic drugs commonly used in research in operant autonomic conditioning in the rat are quaternary compounds and do not
penetrate the blood–brain barrier (Koelle, 1970). There is, accordingly,
little basis on which to expect that a central nervous system (CNS)
state inimical to conditioning is induced by direct action of neuromuscular blocking agents on brain tissue. Nevertheless, intact neural
functioning cannot be assumed, insofar as the act of paralysis may
have consequences that indirectly affect neural systems that may be
necessary for learning. Several investigators have reported extensive
electrocortical synchronization following paralysis in dogs and cats,
even when factors that appear to favor the development of slow-wave
activities such as decreased blood pressure or hypocapnia appear well
controlled (Buchwald, Standish, Eldred, and Halas, 1964; Hodes,
1962). Hodes's (1962) report that cats evidencing electrocortical synchronization were also frequently unresponsive to a variety of alerting
stimuli despite apparently normal cardiovascular and respiratory signs
gives further reason to assess neurophysiological state in curarized
preparations.

Central nervous system electrical activity was not measured concurrently in the experiments on operant conditioning reported in the
previous section. However, we did examine EEG recordings and
evoked potentials in a small sample of rats paralyzed by the procedures described earlier. Evoked potentials were recorded from three
brain areas in each of seven rats, to produce a total of 21 recordings.
These data failed to reveal a clear effect of paralysis on evoked
potentials recorded from hippocampus, amygdala, preoptic nucleus,
ventromedial hypothalamus, or anterior neocortex in rats paralyzed
either by succinylcholine or D-tubocurarine. Evoked potentials recorded from these locations are, on the other hand, altered significantly by barbiturate anesthesia (Racine, personal communication,
1974). These observations are not definitive, but they suggest that
CNS electrical activity was reasonably well preserved in the preparations utilized in the present research.

The integrity of CNS functioning was examined further by
carrying out discriminative classical conditioning in the curarized rat.
The purpose of this effort was to establish whether rats paralyzed and
maintained by exactly the same procedures that were used in studies
of operant conditioning are able to learn anything at all. Subjects
received 18 positive and 18 negative conditioning trials in a single
experimental session that lasted as long (approximately 4 hours) as did
our experiments on operant conditioning. Conditioned stimuli (CSs)
consisted of 20-sec presentations of a clicker or a tone; positive trials

terminated with 2.8-mA tail shock, which was identical to that used in our second experiment on operant conditioning (Panel B, Figure 2). The results for each drug condition are shown in Panels A, B, and C of Figure 5, which depicts performance on the last block of six positive and six negative trials. Inspection of skin-potential performance, which is shown in the upper half of each panel, indicates clearly that rats paralyzed and maintained by the current methods were able to learn a simple Pavlovian discrimination. The differentiations evident in each drug condition were statistically reliable when considered separately ($t = 2.57, 3.03$, and 3.41 for D-tubocurarine, succinylcholine, and dimethyl tubocurarine, respectively; $p < 0.025$ or better in each case), with no differences in the magnitude of responding between drug groups ($F < 1$). The negativity of skin potential increased following presentation of CS+ in 26 of the 27 rats that were trained while paralyzed; 21 of the subjects evidenced larger changes to CS+ than to CS− in the last block of six test trials. These results replicate those reported for a slightly different curarized preparation in an earlier paper by Roberts *et al.* (1974) and show that our inability to obtain operant heart-rate conditioning in the curarized rat cannot be attributed to an effect of paralysis or artificial respiration that rendered any form of learning impossible.

The results with respect to heart rate, on the other hand, are different and are of interest for the questions they raise concerning cardiovascular function in the curarized rat. Although it is apparent from the electrodermal record that rats paralyzed by each drug have learned, inspection of the lower half of Panels A, B, and C in Figure 5 shows that their learning was poorly reflected in the cardiovascular system. There was little evidence of heart-rate conditioning in rats paralyzed by dimethyl tubocurarine or succinylcholine. The slight differentiation that was noticeable in rats paralyzed by D-tubocurarine was statistically reliable ($t = 1.95, p < .05$) but averaged less than 4 bpm. The heart-rate differentiations observed for individual rats in all drug conditions are depicted in Figure 6, where performance has been represented by a t statistic and is plotted in relation to the same measure computed for electrodermal responding. Inspection of these data shows that only 2 of the 27 rats that were tested evidenced cardiac changes of a magnitude and consistency suggestive of genuine heart-rate conditioning, when performance was evaluated on an individual basis. However, 13 subjects evidenced reliable differentiations with respect to skin potential, indicating that a substantial proportion of the sample had in fact learned the discrimination. The results presented here for classical heart-rate conditioning are rather strikingly reminiscent of those described earlier for operant conditioning of this response. At best, only a small minority of rats can be expected to

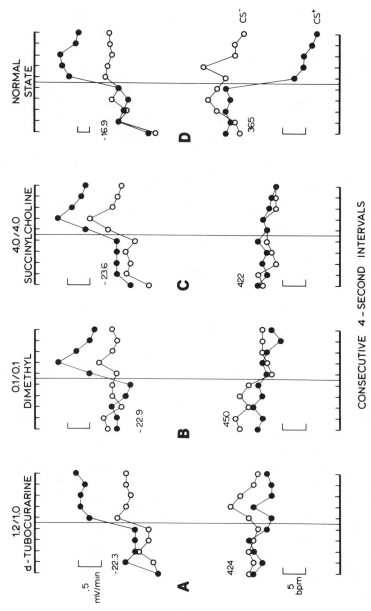

CONSECUTIVE 4 - SECOND INTERVALS

FIGURE 5. Discriminative classical conditioning in three curarized preparations and the normal state. The vertical line in each panel denotes onset of the CS. The top row depicts skin-potential performance; the bottom row is heart rate. The last block of 6 trials from a session of 42 trials is shown. The first block of 6 trials consisted of pretest trials on which the CSs (a clicker and a tone, counterbalanced across subjects) were presented without shock. The intertrial interval averaged three minutes. Sample sizes for Panels A–D were 9, 8, 10, and 8, respectively. Numbers to the left of the vertical lines are pre-CS means.

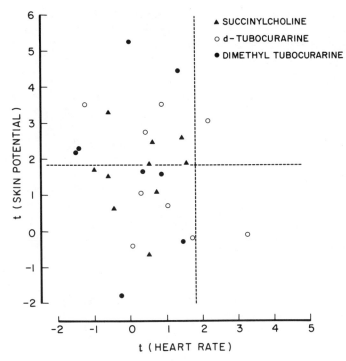

FIGURE 6. Individual performance during classical conditioning in the curarized rat. The skin-potential and heart-rate differentiations observed for each subject during the last block of six positive and six negative trials are depicted as t statistics. A positive value of t indicates that larger skin-potential responses and heart-rate decelerations were observed on positive trials. The broken lines depict $t_{.05}$ (one-tailed, uncorrected for multiple tests).

evidence cardiac changes suggestive of learning in the curarized state, when methods of paralysis and artificial respiration approximating those of the original curare literature are used.

A subsequent analysis was undertaken to determine whether performance during classical heart-rate conditioning could be predicted by an evaluation of responsivity in the heart-rate record, as was attempted for operant conditioning. A sort of the polygraph records employing the methods and criteria described earlier identified 8 subjects (29% of the total of 27, compared to 18/55 or 33% during operant conditioning) that were judged to have been responsive by both observers throughout training, when the results of the three drug conditions were combined. Representative cardiotachometer records for both responsive and unresponsive rats were similar to those depicted previously in Figure 4 for curarized subjects given operant conditioning. The skin-potential differentiations evidenced by the two groups during classical conditioning were found to be statistically reliable and did not differ significantly from one another. However, there was no evidence for a reliable change in heart rate from the pretrial baseline, or for heart-rate differentiation, in either group of subjects. As in operant conditioning, it was clear that cardiovascular learning could not be predicted by an assessment of responsiveness in the heart-rate record.

It is important to note that the relative insensitivity of heart rate to Pavlovian conditioning that is apparent in these experiments cannot be attributed simply to a peculiarity of the conditioning procedure that was used. This is shown by the fact that, as depicted in Panel D of Figure 5, heart-rate differentiations exceeding 15 bpm were obtained when exactly the same conditioning procedure was applied to partially restrained rats in the normal state. The skin-potential differentiations evidenced by rats in the normal state were not found to differ reliably from those evidenced under curare, when these performances were assessed by the computation of t statistics for individual rats as in Figure 6. However, the heart-rate performance of paralyzed rats was significantly poorer than the performance of rats trained in the normal state when differentiation was assessed in this way. It should further be noted that other investigators who have used methods of paralysis and artificial respiration similar to those of the present work have also encountered difficulty in demonstrating classical heart-rate conditioning in the curarized rat (Ray, 1972; Eissenberg, 1973; Gaebelein, Howard, Galosy, and Obrist, 1976; Pappas, DiCara, and Miller, 1972). These observations suggest that the procedures that were used to paralyze and respirate rats in previous experiments on both classical and operant heart-rate conditioning very likely produced a cardiovascular state that was inimical to the expression of learning in the cardiovascular system.[3]

[3] While it is clear that learning is poorly reflected in the cardiovascular system of rats maintained by the present procedures, it would be going too far to conclude that classical heart-rate conditioning was not evidenced at all under these circumstances. One rat in Figure 6 showed statistically significant differentiations with respect to both autonomic responses, suggesting that learning had taken place and was manifested in both response systems. It might also be noted that the t statistics depicted for heart-rate performance in this figure differ significantly from zero ($t_t = 2.04$, $p < 0.025$), suggesting that learning was expressed to at least a limited extent in the curarized state. However, skin-potential differentiations were significantly larger than heart-rate differentiations in curarized rats ($t_{SP\ vs\ HR} = 3.20$, $p < 0.01$), while the same comparison was not significant in the normal state, where both differentiations were substantial. It appears that electrodermal discrimination is better preserved in the face of paralysis, than is differentiation with respect to heart rate (Figure 5, above).

Considerable effort has been devoted recently to the study of factors that may interfere with the development of classical heart-rate conditioning in the curarized rat (Wilson and DiCara, 1975; Dworkin and Miller, 1977; Gaebelein *et al.*, 1976). This approach has been based upon the assumption that factors that are found to interfere with the progress of classical heart-rate conditioning under curare may also account for present difficulties in replicating earlier studies of operant heart-rate conditioning in this preparation. This effort is reviewed briefly in the next section of the chapter, where several considerations relevant to reinterpretation of the original operant conditioning studies are discussed.

III. The Case against Learning

Failure to replicate previous studies of operant heart-rate conditioning in the curarized rat has been reported in several laboratories in addition to our own. The details pertaining to several unsuccessful attempts that were undertaken elsewhere are summarized in Table 3, where two unsuccessful efforts to operantly condition intestinal motility are reported as well. In addition to the present experiments, these failures include an attempted replication by Dworkin (1973) of the original shock-avoidance study of DiCara and Miller (1968a) and attempted replications by Dworkin (1973) and by Ball and Lynch (cited in Dworkin, 1973) of Miller and DiCara's (1967) study in which large changes in heart rate were shaped by operant conditioning with brain-stimulation reward. Dworkin (1973) subsequently attempted to operantly condition both cardiac and intestinal activity using shock-avoidance procedures and improved methods of respiration, again without success. It should be noted that in addition to these and other formal attempts listed in the table (such as Middaugh, 1971), Brener *et al.* (1974) and Hahn (1974a,b) have acknowledged further unspecified difficulties in obtaining learning in the curarized rat, as have DiCara (1974), Gaebelein (personal communication, 1975), and Dworkin (1973; Dworkin and Miller, 1977). The effort expended in pursuit of replication has been both diverse and considerable.

The discrepancy between these efforts to operantly condition heart rate and earlier reports by Miller (1969), DiCara (1971), and Fields (1970a,b) is sharp and suggests consideration of the following two alternatives. First, one could hold to the view that the results of the original studies were a product of learning. In this case, some reason must be found to explain why heart rate has been so refractory to operant conditioning in subsequent work. Sources of difficulty may

TABLE 3
Unsuccessful Replications and Extensions

Reference	Response	Procedure[a]	Comment
Dworkin, 1973, page 32	Heart rate	Discrimination training with brain-stimulation reward	Attempted replication of Miller and DiCara (1967).
Ball and Lynch, cited in Dworkin, 1973, page 32	Heart rate	Discrimination training with brain-stimulation reward	Attempted replication of Miller and DiCara (1967).
Dworkin, 1973, page 32	Heart rate	Discriminated avoidance training	Attempted replication of DiCara and Miller (1968a).
Dworkin, 1973, Experiment 1	Intestinal contractions	Discriminated avoidance training ($N = 20$)	Attempted replication of Banuazizi (1968, 1972).
Goesling and Brener, 1972	Heart rate	Feedback procedure with tail-shock reinforcement ($N = 20$)	Rats were reinforced for activity or immobility in the normal state prior to heart-rate conditioning under curare; the effect of heart-rate conditioning under curare was not statistically significant.
Middaugh, Eissenberg, and Brener, 1975, Experiment 2	Heart rate	Discrimination training with brain-stimulation reward ($N = 10$)	No evidence of learning was obtained when a peak inspiratory pressure of 20 cm H_2O was used; however, learning was obtained when peak inspiratory pressure was reduced to 12 cm H_2O (Experiment 3).
Middaugh, 1971, Experiment 3	Heart rate	Feedback procedure with brain-stimulation reward ($N = 10$)	Training procedure was similar to that of Hothersall and Brener (1969); bidirectional difference in heart rate was not significant after 60 min of training, despite the use of a low peak inspiratory pressure (12 cm H_2O).

Dworkin, 1973, Experiment 2	Heart rate	Discriminated avoidance training (N = 30)	Used modified Harvard respirator and added 5% CO_2 to inspired air; initial heart rate was 383 bpm and variability improved, but learning was not obtained.
Dworkin, 1973, Experiment 3	Heart rate	Discriminated avoidance training (N = 20)	Used constant-volume respirator with 5% CO_2 added to inspired air; rats tracheotomized and intubated. Orienting response to S^D was observed, but learning was not obtained.
Dworkin, 1973, Experiment 4	Intestinal contractions	Discriminated avoidance training (N = 24)	Rats tracheotomized, three gas mixtures used. No evidence of learning. Successful performance was not predicted by blood gas composition.
Wright, 1974, Experiment 1 (see Roberts et al., 1974)	Heart rate	Nondiscriminated punishment training approximating percentile reinforcement (N = 24)	Bidirectional difference was found only when five electrodermally unresponsive rats were discarded; interpretation was clouded further by failure of groups to converge during 60 min of extinction.
Wright, 1974, Experiment 3	Heart rate	Nondiscriminated punishment training approximating percentile reinforcement (N = 16)	Peak inspiratory pressure was lowered to 14 cm H_2O and was adjusted to hold chest excursions constant; rats paralyzed by succinylcholine. No evidence of learning was obtained.
Roberts, 1978 (the present chapter)	Heart rate	Nondiscriminated punishment training with percentile reinforcement (N = 55)	Shaping procedure was similar to Fields (1970a,b). Performance was not related to shock intensity, punishment density, response unit, choice of paralyzing drug, or variability in the heart-rate record. However, preparations learned a Pavlovian discrimination with respect to skin potential.

[a] Sample size (bidirectional groups combined) is reported where available.

pertain to (1) some aspect of the procedures used to prepare and maintain rats in a curarized state and/or (2) some aspect of the operant shaping procedure. Alternatively, one might argue that learning did not contribute prominently to the results of the original experiments, as was once believed. In this instance, one must explain how the original findings were obtained. Possibilities include (1) inadequate control of variables pertaining to maintenance in the curarized state and/or (2) inadequacies associated with the shaping procedure. It should be stressed that this second alternative as developed here does not assert that operant conditioning of autonomic responses is impossible in the curarized state or that learning made no contribution whatsoever to the original findings. Rather, it holds that any contribution that derived from learning was proably modest and confounded with contributions that derived from a failure to control several variables that appear in retrospect to have had a substantial impact upon cardiac performance. Demonstration of bona fide learning effects requires a degree of control over these variables that was neither exercised in the original studies nor achieved in subsequent attempts to replicate.

The initial attempts to explain discrepant findings when the problem of replication first came to public attention in 1972 understandably focused on the first of these two alternatives (Dworkin, 1973; Miller and Dworkin, 1974). Consequently, a considerable effort was undertaken to identify procedural variables that might have been critical to the production of the desired effects. However, this position has been seriously undermined by several considerations and recent developments. Five of these considerations and developments, which will be reviewed briefly in this section, pertain to (1) procedural similarities between original studies and subsequent attempts to replicate; (2) similarity of the cardiovascular states evidenced in the two series of experiments; (3) lack of success in identifying variables critical to demonstration of a repeatable operant conditioning phenomenon in the curarized rat; (4) the apparent fragility of classical heart-rate conditioning under curare; and (5) recognition of several potential sources of error that might have generated the findings of the original operant conditioning studies.

A. Procedural Similarities

Three of the earliest, unsuccessful attempts referenced in Table 3 have been described by Dworkin (1973, p. 32) as "exact" replications of earlier experiments by Miller and DiCara (1967) and DiCara and

Miller (1968a) on operant heart-rate conditioning and of Banuazizi's (1972) experiment on intestinal contractions. It is reasonable to assume that the respiratory and pharmacological practices followed in these experiments duplicated as closely as possible those of the earlier studies. Subsequent efforts to replicate have either approximated this procedure (Wright, 1974, Experiment 1)—in some instances, with lowered inspiratory pressure to improve heart-rate responsivity (Wright, 1974, Experiment 3)—or have utilized new methods of respiration in an attempt to produce learning (Dworkin, 1973; Gaebelein, personal communication, 1975). There is also considerable overlap between the original studies and attempted replications with respect to the shaping procedures utilized in both series of experiments. Methods used in the attempted replications have included DiCara and Miller's discriminated shock-avoidance procedure (Dworkin, 1973); discriminative operant conditioning with brain stimulation reward (Dworkin, 1973; Ball and Lynch, cited in Dworkin, 1973, p. 32); the discriminated feedback procedure of Hothersall and Brener (Goesling and Brener, 1972; Middaugh, 1971); and the present computerized percentile reinforcement schedules, which approximate the nondiscriminative punishment procedures utilized by Fields (1970a,b). In each case, application of these procedures failed to produce an outcome compatible with learning.

B. Similarity of Cardiovascular State

It no longer appears possible to defend a learning interpretation of the original studies by arguing that rats paralyzed by the procedures employed in these experiments evidenced a cardiovascular state that was not achieved in subsequent attempts to replicate. The similarity of the procedures with respect to respiration and pharmacological techniques derives this argument of much of its force. Comparison of the properties of cardiovascular responding obtained in these studies also appears unfavorable to this view. The mean heart rate obtained during operant conditioning in the present research (438 bpm) fell well within the range of heart rates reported for the original studies (395–473 bpm, Table 1), as did the heart rates reported in attempted replications by Wright (1974) and Dworkin (1973). Comparison of the cardiotachometer tracings of Figure 4 of the present work to those depicted in unsuccessful replications by Dworkin (1973) and more successful efforts by Middaugh et al. (1975) and Thornton (Thornton, 1971; Thornton and Van-Toller, 1973b) also suggests that considerable overlap was achieved among these studies with respect to the range of heart-rate variability that was encountered. Although tracings are not available from the original DiCara and Miller studies, the report by these investigators that standard deviations in heart rate averaged less than 2 bpm when computed over 5-min segments of training, and that the rates evidenced by individual subjects were "remarkably regular" over the course of conditioning (Miller and DiCara, 1967, p. 14), suggests that the heart-rate records obtained in the original studies approximated those depicted for unresponsive rats in Figure 4 of the present chapter. The further report by Miller and DiCara (1967) that standard deviations in heart rate increased significantly over the course of paralysis was also replicated in the present research, even though learning was not obtained (Table 2, above). These observations do not rule out the possibility that cardiovascular states may have been different or more homogeneous in the earlier research, but they give adequate reason to suggest that the degree of overlap that was achieved between the two series of experiments with respect to heart-rate variability and other properties of cardiovascular activity was considerable. It is further relevant to note that efforts to predict learning by an examination of variability in the heart-rate record proved unsuccessful in both operant (Figure 3, above) and classical heart-rate conditioning, in the present research.

Recent assessments of blood gas composition in rats maintained by the DiCara and Miller respiratory technique also suggest a similarity of cardiovascular state in the original studies and attempted replications. The results of several studies indicate that arterial pCO_2 can be expected to approximate 34 mm Hg in the unanesthetized, uncurarized rat (Altland, Bruback, Parker, and Highman, 1967; Chapot, Barrault, Müller, and Dargnat, 1972; Eissenberg and Brener, 1976; Gliner et al., 1975; Hahn, Schwartz, and Sapper, 1975; Van Liew, 1968). However, blood gas determinations taken recently by Hahn et al. (1975) have shown that artificial respiration of the curarized rat with the technique and respirator settings of the original operant conditioning studies (E and M 5VKG respirator set to 70/1:1/20) reduces pCO_2 to approximately 25 mm Hg, producing a hypocarbic state. The pCO_2 determinations obtained by Hahn et al. (1975) agree well with those reported for the preparation of the original experiments by DiCara (1970) and suggest that the gas tensions that prevailed in these experiments were comparable to those achieved in several unsuccessful replications that employed the same respiratory parameters and ventilation procedure (see Dworkin, 1973; Wright, 1974). Continued maintenance under hypocarbic conditions could have serious consequences for physiological state insofar as the pCO_2 is an important determinant of oxygen exchange with the tissues, a higher pCO_2 favoring dissociation of oxygen from hemoglobin and higher oxygen turnover (Riley, 1966). However, while the available data are not entirely consistent (see below), most attempted replications in which efforts were undertaken to raise pCO_2 to normal levels by a variety of techniques (lowering peak inspiratory pressure, adding carbon dioxide to the inspired gas mixture, or manipulating respiratory parameters to control expired CO_2) have failed to obtain learning (Dworkin, 1973; Gaebelein, personal communication, 1975; Wright, 1974). These observations cannot be interpreted to mean that control of blood gas composition is unnecessary in experiments on operant conditioning in the curarized rat, since it is possible that an effect of this variable might have materialized in the aforementioned studies had other impediments to learning been removed. However, these observations do suggest that the overlap between the original studies and attempted replications with respect to blood gas composition was substantial and that production of learning requires more than simply a normalization of this important variable.

C. Failure to Identify Variables Critical to Learning

Also unfavorable to a learning interpretation of the original studies is the present lack of success in relating performance during operant conditioning to features of cardiovascular or CNS functioning that are predictive of learning, and in modifying preparation and shaping procedures so as to produce a repeatable operant conditioning phenomenon. Indices of cardiovascular and CNS state that were examined with regard to learning in the present research included heart rate and heart-rate variability, rectal temperature, properties of the EKG, and spontaneous skin-potential activity as a measure of CNS arousal. Other unsuccessful efforts have examined performance in relation to mean arterial pressure and blood gas composition (Dworkin, 1973). Several variables pertaining to the shaping procedure have also been explored in an effort to produce a repeatable learning effect. The scope of this effort is depicted to some extent in Table 3 and has included the study of type of reinforcement (tail shock versus brain-stimulation reward), magnitude of reinforcement, reinforcement density, stringency of the reinforcement criterion, presence of a discriminative stimulus, choice of response to be conditioned (heart rate versus intestinal activity), and definition of the response unit.

Efforts to obtain operant conditioning by manipulation of preparation variables have focused upon choice of paralyzing drug and respiratory technique (Brener *et al.*, 1974; Dworkin, 1973; Gaebelein, personal communication, 1975; the present research). The only report of success in relating performance during operant conditioning to one of these variables was that of Middaugh *et al.* (1975), in which curarized rats were given bidirectional heart-rate conditioning with a peak inspiratory pressure of either 20 or 12 cm of water, using brain stimulation as a reward. No evidence of learning was obtained at the higher peak inspiratory pressure, which produced an elevated and invariant heart rate (490 bpm at the start of training) similar to that depicted for unresponsive rats in Figure 4 of the present chapter. However, a bidirectional difference of approximately 40 bpm was obtained after 3 hours of training at the lower peak inspiratory pressure, which produced a lower initial heart rate (430 bpm) and increased heart-rate variability as well. Although it is possible that this result was a product of learning, this experiment itself does not appear to have been subjected to an attempted replication. It should further be noted that evidence compatible with learning was not obtained in other studies that employed a lower peak inspiratory pressure (Wright, 1974; Figures 2 and 3 above) or that adopted alternative measures in an effort to normalize cardiovascular state (Dworkin, 1973; Gaebelein, personal communication, 1975). Nor was learning predicted successfully by qualitative judgments with regard to responsivity and variability in cardiotachographic records in the present research. These observations lead one to question whether a simple reduction of peak inspiratory pressure is likely to establish a repeatable learning effect.

D. *Fragility of Classical Heart-Rate Conditioning under Curare*

As indicated in the previous section of the chapter, recent difficulties in obtaining operant heart-rate conditioning in the curarized rat have been paralleled by several unsuccessful efforts to obtain classical heart-rate conditioning in this preparation (Eissenberg, 1973; Gaebelein *et al.*, 1976; Ray, 1972; Figure 5, above). Failure to obtain classical heart-rate conditioning cannot be attributed to a failure to learn, since several subjects that failed to evidence heart-rate differentiation in the present research were nevertheless shown to have discriminated between positive and negative trials with respect to skin potential. Recent research on classical conditioning has suggested that the expression of learning in the cardiovascular system may be prevented in curarized rats by a combination of factors, including (1) possible blockade of peripheral autonomic ganglia by curariform drugs; (2) cardiovascular impairments deriving from inadequate artificial respiration; and (3) alteration of cardiovascular state by an adrenal-mediated stress response. The brief review of this work that follows raises the question of how a stable learning phenomenon could have been produced in the early studies of operant heart-rate conditioning, when so much appears to have been left uncontrolled.

1. Blockade of Autonomic Ganglia by Curariform Drugs

Although curariform drugs are used for their competitive and depolarizing effects at the myoneural junction, the pharmacological action of these drugs is not restricted to this site. Guyton and Reeder (1950) reported that cardiac deceleration produced by stimulation of the vagus nerve was abolished in dogs when D-tubocurarine was given in a dosage sufficient to block electromyographic responding (EMG) in the gastrocnemius muscle. Cardiac acceleration to sympathetic stimulation was also blocked by this drug, but only when it was infused at approximately 10 times the paralyzing dose. These effects were generally confirmed by Black (1971), who observed that discriminated changes in heart rate produced by prior operant conditioning in the partially curarized dog disappeared when drug dosage was increased to abolish EMG. More recently, Howard, Gaebelein, Galosy, and Obrist (1975) compared the effect of D-tubocurarine, dimethyl tubocurarine, and succinylcholine on heart-rate and blood-pressure responses to direct stimulation of the cardiac nerves in anesthetized cats. In each drug condition, dosage was titrated continuously to maintain EMG block in the sartorius muscle. Sympatholytic effects were not evidenced under any drug condition, nor were responses to vagal stimulation altered substantially by administration of succinylcholine or dimethyl tubocurarine. However, cardiovascular responses to stimulation of the vagus nerve were abolished by D-tubocurarine. The vagolytic action of the latter drug appeared sufficient to prevent the expression of learned changes in heart rate when discriminative classical conditioning was subsequently carried out in unanesthetized, paralyzed subjects. These observations led Howard et al. (1974, 1975) to suggest that ganglionic blockade may contribute substantially to the unresponsive cardiovascular state of rats paralyzed by D-tubocurarine.

The vagolytic action of D-tubocurarine does not appear to be as profound in rats, however, as in dogs and cats. Vertes (as described in Miller and Dworkin, 1974) found that dosages of D-tubocurarine up to 7 mg/kg in the rat (twice the maximum dosage used in most studies of operant heart-rate conditioning) did not appear to have a significant effect on cardiac responses to stimulation of the nucleus ambiguous, one source of the vagus nerve. Further evidence for retention of vagal restraint was provided by Roberts et al. (1974), who showed that heart rate increased sharply following atropinization in rats paralyzed by either 1.2 or 3.6 mg/kg D-tubocurarine. These observations indicate that substantial neurogenic control of the heart is retained when rats are paralyzed by dosages of D-tubocurarine that abolish EMG and are identical to or greater than those used in earlier studies of operant heart-rate conditioning (also see Thornton, 1971). However, the available evidence does not point unequivocally to the absence of ganglionic blocking effects in this species. Hahn (1974a) reported that although parasympathetic restraint was clearly retained in most rats paralyzed by 3 mg/kg D-tubocurarine, the cardiac response to direct stimulation of the unsevered vagus varied substantially from subject to subject, with a small number of rats evidencing nearly total nerve block, while others apparently became more sensitive to stimulation over the course of testing. These variable effects cannot be attributed unequivocally to the action of D-tubocurarine, since vagal afferents were stimulated by Hahn's procedure; furthermore, Nembutal anesthetic was infused in addition to curare. Nevertheless, Hahn's observations caution against concluding that ganglionic blocking effects are of no consequence when operant and classical conditioning are carried out in the curarized rat.

Bronchial congestion and diminished elasticity of the lungs and thorax are also well-documented effects of D-tubocurarine that appear to be secondary to the histamine-releasing properties of this drug (Howard et al., 1974; Safar and Bachman, 1956). Although these effects have been studied primarily in the dog rather than in rats, fluid congestion and reliable decrements in chest excursions are frequently encountered over the course of operant conditioning in the latter species (Eissenberg and Brener, 1976; Table 2, above). It is reasonable to suggest that these effects may interfere with proper gas exchange and contribute to cardiovascular unresponsiveness in a significant number of subjects when training is carried out in the curarized state.

2. Artificial Respiration

The problems involved in providing adequate ventilation in the paralyzed rat are numerous and have been discussed previously by Brener et al. (1974) and DiCara (1974) and more recently by Dworkin and Miller (1977). One set of problems has to do with ensuring the delivery of a constant volume of air to the lungs on each respiratory cycle. Perhaps the most serious obstacle to this goal occurs when the larynx and the trachea are displaced from their normal position above the soft palate by the force of positive-pressure ventilation, as described by Dworkin and Miller (1977). When this happens, a substantial portion of the inspired air delivered through the nostrils is shunted down the esophagus into the gut, thereby lowering effective tidal volume. This event is usually signaled by a precipitous decrease in heart rate or by rate instability, which may recover spontaneously at some later time as the junction between the larynx and the palate is restored. The problem may be aggravated further by an accumulation of mucus and saliva, which obstructs access to the bronchial tree and further impairs gas exchange. Recently, both Gaebelein and Howard (1974) and Dworkin (Dworkin and Miller, 1977) have attempted to obviate these problems by substituting an endotracheal tube for the face mask used in previous research on operant and classical conditioning. Dworkin's method employs a dual-lumen tube that separates the inspired and expired air, thereby allowing bronchial secretions to be withdrawn down the expiratory pressure gradient to prevent fluid congestion. The improved stability and responsivity of cardiovascular state reported by these investigators in recent studies of classical heart-rate conditioning (see below) probably stems in part from the increased stability of respiration inherent in this new and clever respiratory technique (Dworkin and Miller, 1977).

Another problem alluded to previously concerns maintenance of proper gas exchange in the paralyzed preparation. Recent efforts have been directed primarily to increasing the arterial pCO_2 in order to avoid possible interference with expression of learning by hypocarbic state. One approach that may be undertaken when the conventional E and M respirator is used is to reduce peak inspiratory pressure at the beginning of curarization and then subsequently adjust this variable over the course of training so as to hold circumferential chest movements constant (Eissenberg and Brener, 1976). Incrementing inspiratory pressure to control chest excursions may preserve tidal volume in the face of diminished lung compliance, thus preventing depletion of arterial pO_2, which may otherwise be expected to occur when a lower peak inspiratory pressure is used (DiCara, 1970; Hahn et al., 1975). However, this practice is undesirable in that it requires on-line adjustment of a parameter that is an extremely important determinant of heart rate (Middaugh et al., 1975). A better method of normalizing blood gas composition that has been adopted by Dworkin (1973) is to add carbon dioxide to the inspired gas mixture. This practice was adopted after it was shown that manipulation of the arterial pCO_2 by this method had a pronounced effect on heart rate in the curarized rat. Addition of approximately 3% CO_2 to the inspired air appears sufficient to raise pCO_2 to within normal limits and to produce a responsive heart rate averaging approximately 400 bpm in a 400-g rat (Dworkin, 1973).

Dworkin and Miller (1977) have recently combined the latter technique with other important technical improvements (including constant-volume respiration by a dual-lumen endotracheal tube and automatic titration of curare dosage to maintain muscle blockade) in experiments on classical heart-rate conditioning in which training was carried out in a single session of paralysis that lasted approximately five *days*. Although the time course of learning evidenced by individual rats in these experiments was quite variable, a large decelerative heart-rate response specific to the positive stimulus was reported to have developed in each of an unspecified number of subjects exposed to this procedure. In some cases, the response consistently approximated −100 bpm on positive trials. The success achieved by Dworkin and Miller (1977) in this work represents an important development and raises for the first time the prospect of carrying out conditioning experiments in a preparation in which blood gas parameters may not only be held within normal limits but may be manipulated as well. Preliminary investigation by these researchers has indicated that even small changes in the inspired gas mixture (for example, a decrease in carbon dioxide content from 4% to 3%) alters the magnitude of cardiac changes normally seen on positive conditioning trials (Dworkin, personal communication, 1974; Dworkin and Miller, 1977). This observation suggests the importance of controlling blood gas composition in experiments on learning in the curarized rat, although a quantitative assessment of the relationship between cardiac performance and blood gas variables is not yet available.

3. Stress Response

Another factor that may contribute to alteration of the cardiovascular state in the curarized rat derives from the stress imposed by this procedure. Evidence for the role of a stress response has been gathered recently by Wilson and DiCara (1975). These investigators first lightly etherized and then administered a single 2.5 mg/kg dose of D-tubocurarine to one group of rats on each of three consecutive days. A second group of subjects was simply etherized and returned to their home cages without being exposed to the stress of paralysis. Beginning on the fourth day, both groups were curarized and given Pavlovian conditioning on each of three consecutive days. Curare-preadapted rats developed a decelerative heart-rate response approximating 15 bpm on the second and third conditioning sessions under curare (the fifth and sixth sessions of paralysis), whereas subjects that were not preexposed to curarization showed no evidence of learning over three days of training. Wilson and DiCara interpreted their results to suggest that the cardiovascular consequences of an immobilization-induced stress reaction may have prevented the elaboration of a decelerative heart-rate response in subjects that were not preexposed to paralysis. In a subsequent study (Wilson, Simpson, DiCara, and Carroll, 1977), curarized rats that were subjected to prior adrenalectomy were observed to develop cardiac conditioned responses (CRs) within two or three sessions of classical conditioning, whereas nonadrenalectomized controls failed to learn even when conditioning was extended to five days. These data suggest that either habituation of an adrenal-mediated stress response or the development of a classically conditioned compensatory physiological state (Siegel, 1975) may be required for performance of cardiovascular changes during studies of classical and perhaps operant heart-rate conditioning in the curarized rat.

The pattern of autonomic activation produced by curarization in rats is generally consistent with this hypothesis. Although there are grounds for expecting a diminution of cardiac output consequent upon muscular paralysis (see Brener et al., 1974), recent assessment of this variable by Gliner et al. (1975) suggests that cardiac output may actually be elevated with respect to normal levels during the first 60 min of curarization (cf. Vizek and Albrecht, 1973). Increased cardiac output appears further to be a product not only of an acceleration of heart rate but also of an increase in contractile force, since stroke volume appears to be well preserved during the initial stages of paralysis despite a substantial increase in the rate of ventricular contraction (cf. Gliner et al., 1975; Vizek and Albrecht, 1973). This cardiovascular picture is indicative of an increase in sympathetic tone and could be mediated by enhanced beta-adrenergic outflow to the heart or by increased secretion of catecholamines by the adrenal medulla, or both.[4] Further evidence for a substantial increase in sympathetic arousal is given in Figure 5 of the present chapter, where it may be seen that the negativity of skin potential is elevated by curarization over levels observed in partially restrained rats trained in the normal state (-22.6 mV/min versus -16.9 mV/min, $t = 4.01$, $p <$ .01). Although increased catecholamine secretion by the adrenal med-

---

[4] Although the cardiac outputs reported by Gliner et al. (1975) for curarized rats exceed those reported for noncurarized subjects, Gliner (personal communication, 1976) has cautioned that interpretation of the available data is complicated by differences among studies with respect to method of measurement (thermal dilution versus the Fick technique) and by the considerable variability of cardiac output in the freely moving rat.

ulla could be expected to exert a tonic cardiovascular effect that might mask phasic changes in heart rate deriving from neurogenic control, this mechanism would not be expected to affect electrodermal differentiation since the postganglionic sudomotor fiber is cholinergic in the rat (Roberts *et al.*, 1974). It is possible that the heart-rate differentiations obtained recently by Dworkin and Miller (1977) resulted in part from technical improvements designed to minimize stress response (for example, cystectomy to prevent painful distention of the bladder), as well as from the extended duration of the training session, which provided an additional opportunity for stress reactions to habituate.

Nevertheless, there are data that question the inevitability and time course of the hypothesized stress reaction. Pappas and DiCara (1973) and DiCara, Braun, and Pappas (1970) reported decelerative heart-rate CRs approximating 20 bpm during a single session of classical conditioning that was carried out under paralysis, even though no special effort appears to have been undertaken to adapt the animals to stress prior to curarization. Another inconsistency is that although Wilson and DiCara (1975) found that classical heart-rate conditioning developed during a fourth conditioning session under curare in unadapted subjects, no evidence of learning was obtained in a subsequent study (Wilson *et al.*, 1977) after five days of conditioning in a comparable group, even though other requirements for learning (sufficient opportunity for adaptation to stress and receipt of an adequate number of conditioning trials) appear to have been met. Unfortunately, the basis for these discrepant observations is unclear. It is conceivable that some unreported feature of the pretraining procedure in the studies by Pappas and DiCara (1973) and DiCara *et al.* (1970) immunized rats against the deleterious effects of stress on cardiovascular state. It is also possible that the cardiovascular effects of stress are easily exacerbated by failure to adequately control other variables pertaining to respiration and pharmacological procedures, when classical conditioning is carried out in the curarized rat.

It is not possible at the present time to determine to what extent improved control over the ganglionic effects of D-tubocurarine, pulmonary gas exchange, or stress reactions contributed to the success Dworkin and Miller (1977) have recently achieved in studies of classical heart-rate conditioning in the curarized rat. Nor can it be assumed that factors that appear to be inimical to the expression of learning during classical conditioning of heart rate also impede performance during operant conditioning of this response, since the mechanisms of conditioning in the two cases may be different. Nevertheless, the likely dependence of classical heart-rate conditioning upon these factors raises the question of how a substantial learning phenomenon could have been obtained repeatedly in earlier experiments on operant conditioning of heart rate, which used methods of paralysis and artificial respiration that appear in retrospect to have provided inadequate control over several variables that influence the expression of learning in the cardiovascular system.

E. Sources of Error

If the results of the early curare studies are not to be attributed primarily to learning, as was originally believed, then one must explain how these results were obtained. The best that can be done by way of retrospective account is to consider briefly several sources of error that might have been involved.[5]

The importance of artificial respiration as a determinant of heart rate in the curarized rat is well known (Middaugh *et al.*, 1975) and has been depicted quantitatively by Dworkin (1973), who reported a regression of 14 bpm/cm H_2O between these variables. The practice adopted in the early DiCara and Miller experiments was to set the respirator to conventional parameters (70/1 : 1/20) for all rats and to hold these constant throughout training. Changes in performance misinterpretable as learning could not have derived from this practice, provided that even occasional deviations were prohibited. However, not all investigators appear to have used this method. Several researchers reporting positive findings (for example, Middaugh *et al.*, 1975; Slaughter, Hahn, and Rinaldi, 1970; Thornton, 1971; Wright, 1974, Experiment 4) adopted the practice of adjusting respiratory parameters (usually peak inspiratory pressure) during adaptation for each rat individually, in an effort to produce a responsive heart rate. Once this goal was achieved, ventilation was unaltered for the duration of the experiment. DiCara himself appears to have moved toward this practice in later work, where peak inspiratory pressures are lower (DiCara and Weiss, 1969; DiCara *et al.*, 1970) and it is recommended

---

[5] It should not be assumed that the experiments cited below are more vulnerable to questioning on methodological grounds than are studies that have not been discussed. Papers that provided extensive information were more likely to have been useful and to have been referenced than papers that reported fewer data. Several of the efforts discussed below (for example, Thornton, 1971) were remarkable for their scope and detail, even though the interpretation given to the outcome can be questioned. It might also be noted that a more comprehensive analysis of the curare literature than is provided here yielded little that was definitive with respect to the relative importance of the sources of error outlined in this section.

that this parameter be adjusted to compensate for body weight (DiCara, 1970). If this practice is followed, it is necessary that subjects be allocated randomly to bidirectional groups after respiratory parameters have been fixed, so as to avoid any possibility of confounding preconditioning respiratory procedure with direction of training. Dworkin (1973) has stressed the importance of this procedure, which was adopted in the present experiments and in earlier research by Wright (1974, Experiment 4). However, the extent to which this practice was followed in other studies is difficult to ascertain on the basis of published protocol.

Another potential source of error in the maintenance of curarized subjects derives from the procedures utilized to regulate body temperature. Wright (1974) reported a strong relationship between heart rate and rectal temperature in curarized rats. The between-subject regression of within-session changes in heart rate on within-session changes in temperature was substantial (27.1 bpm/°C) and highly significant, even though the changes in temperature that occurred over the course of training were quite small (mean absolute change = 0.56°C). The same regression computed for rats in the present research was 21.2 bpm/°C over a similar temperature range.[6] These regressions are strikingly congruent with a recent report by Cabanac and Serres (1976), who found that heart rate increased an average of 21.1 bpm/°C when rectal temperature was manipulated within individual curarized rats by alternate cooling and warming throughout a considerable temperature range (24–37°C). Many of the reports cited in Table 1 failed to indicate whether rectal temperature was measured or whether precautions were taken to guard against changes in heart rate as a consequence of temperature adjustments administered by the experimenter. Attempted replications by Dworkin (1973) and Wright (1974) controlled this variable, as did the experiments of the present chapter, in which all subjects were warmed by a commercial heating pad fixed at medium to maintain peripheral vasomotor tone. No deviation from this setting was allowed.

---

[6] This relationship was obtained in the present work, even though heart rate decreased significantly over the duration of paralysis while temperature increased (Table 2, above). This decrease indicates that temperature and heart rate are influenced significantly by variables that are to some extent specific to one or both responses. For example, temperature may have drifted upward slightly in the present research as a result of the use of a heating pad; heart rate, on the other hand, may have diminished owing to a reduction of tidal volume or sympathetic arousal (Table 2). Rats whose temperature increased the most as a result of passive heating presumably evidenced the lowest heart-rate decrements attributable to other factors.

Another possible source of error concerns the operant conditioning procedure itself. In practice, the details of the operant conditioning procedure are defined by criteria for *reinforcement* and *shaping*, which are administered to individual rats over the course of training. The criterion for reinforcement designates a value of the response (for example, an interbeat interval) beyond which reward or punishment is to be administered. In the original curare studies, this criterion was typically chosen to produce a temporal density reinforcement that was thought to be conducive to learning. The criterion for shaping, on the other hand, consists of a rule (or a set of rules) that states when and by how much the reinforcement criterion is to be changed as a result of improvement or deterioration in performance over the course of operant conditioning. The precision with which these criteria are applied to individual subjects is of special concern when operant conditioning is applied to response systems that display an intrinsic rhythmicity and are readily driven by noncontingent punishment and reward, as are most visceral response systems. In particular, two requirements must be met. First, the reinforcement and shaping criteria employed during training must effectively control and equate the pattern and density of reinforcement applied to the two bidirectional groups. Only when this is accomplished can differences between the groups be attributed unequivocally to operant conditioning. Second, criteria for reinforcement and shaping must be applied to individual rats without regard to the outcome of shaping over the course of operant conditioning. If this latter requirement is not met, it is conceivable that performance may be determined by complex interactions between the experimenter and the subject as described below, rather than by the operant contingency.

The extent to which the first requirement was satisfied was usually ascertained in the curare literature by an examination of the frequency and distribution of reinforcing events received by the two bidirectional groups. A detailed analysis of bidirectional differences in reinforcement was carried out by DiCara and Miller (1968a), who examined shock frequency and duration in relation to performance and direction of training. Performance during heart-rate conditioning was not related to either of these variables within either bidirectional group, nor did the groups differ with respect to the number of shocks or total duration of shock they received. However, different results were reported by Gliner *et al.* (1975), who used a shaping procedure similar to that of DiCara and Miller (1968a), and also by Wright (1974, Experiment 4), who used an unautomated version of the percentile reinforcement procedure that was employed in the present research. Both of these investigators found not only that rats that were trained to increase heart rate evidenced significantly higher heart rates following conditioning than did rats that were trained to decrease heart rate but that the former group received significantly more shock as well. Gliner *et al.* (1975) further reported that although performance was unrelated to reinforcement variables across rats in the increase group, the same was not true of rats in the decrease group, where it was found that subjects evidencing the best performance received significantly fewer shocks. This observation raises the possibility that the reinforcement and shaping criteria used by Gliner *et al.* (1975) may have generated a bidirectional difference in reinforcement density (and in heart rate) by selectively exempting from punishment those rats that evidenced tonic heart-rate trends compatible with the direction of training in the decrease group.

There are also conflicting reports with respect to whether rats trained to increase heart rate are likely to encounter different patterns of shock over the course of training, compared to rats trained to decrease heart rate. Statistically reliable differences in the temporal distribution of shock have been reported by Wright (1974, Experiment 4), Thornton (1971, Experiment 1), and Thornton and Van-Toller (1973b). In each study, the nature of these differences was that rats trained to decrease heart rate were more likely to have received uninterrupted trains of shock than were rats trained to increase heart rate, particularly during the early stages of operant conditioning. Thus, it is conceivable that the lower heart rates evidenced by decrease rats in these experiments may have been attributable to this consequence of the shaping procedure rather than to the operant contingency. For example, lower heart rates may have derived from states of helplessness or protective inhibition that were engendered by clustering of shock during operant conditioning (after Black, 1974b). Alternatively, lower heart rates may have been a consequence of the fact that decrease rats received relatively fewer of their shocks during the later stages of training compared to rats that were trained to increase heart rate (Thornton, 1971). The further report by Thornton and Van-Toller (1973b) that application of potassium chloride to the cortex abolished bidirectional differences in heart rate without eliminating differences in pattern of shock does not rule out these possibilities, since one could argue that an intact cortex (a possible site of cardiosomatic integration) is necessary if differences in the pattern of shock are to generate tonic and unconditioned cardiac changes in the curarized rat. It should be noted that the practices adopted with respect to the analysis of reinforcement variables in relation to performance and direction of training appear to have ranged from the relatively fastidious (Banuazizi, 1968; DiCara and Miller, 1968a; Gliner *et al.*, 1975; Thornton, 1971; Wright, 1974) to almost total neglect of the issue (Cabanac and Serres, 1976; Fields, 1970a,b).

The extent to which the second requirement of the conditioning procedure was fulfilled in the early curare studies is difficult to ascertain. The practice typically adopted to meet this requirement was to formulate criteria for reinforcement and shaping prior to training and to adhere to them as strictly as possible while conditioning was carried out (for example, see the description by DiCara and Miller, 1968a). However, this practice may not have been fully adequate. Comparison of the shaping criteria described by Miller and DiCara (1967) with the criteria described by DiCara and Stone (1970) reveals that different criteria were employed in these two studies, even though the conditioning procedure in each was presumably the same. The differences evident in these two papers may have derived from unsystematic adjustments that were made to the shaping criteria in an effort to accommodate individual rats that appeared not to shape by the criteria employed previously. In actual fact, the technology that was used to carry out operant conditioning in the early curare studies was generally such that measurement and precise control of the reinforcement and shaping criteria applied to individual subjects was not likely to have been a practical possibility.

It is instructive to consider examples of experimenter–subject interactions that may have resulted from an inability to adequately control this aspect of the conditioning procedure. One possibility is that an experimenter might have inadvertently employed less stringent reinforcement and shaping criteria during avoidance conditioning for those rats that evidenced temporal trends in heart rate that were consistent with the direction of training. That is to say, subjects that evidenced such trends may have been allowed to emit larger heart-rate responses in an inappropriate direction before reinforcement was applied, or to have avoided shock for a longer period of time before the reinforcement criterion was readjusted in accordance with the rules for shaping, than rats that evidenced heart-rate trends that were incompatible with the direction of training. Consequently, the latter subjects may have received significantly more shocks than the former subjects and may have manifested heart-rate changes that were determined largely by the noncontingent effects of the reinforcing stimulus. Another and very different possibility is that rats that evidenced unconditioned responses to shock in the direction of training may have inadvertently been subjected to more stringent reinforcement and shaping criteria and thus received more shock than rats that evidenced unconditioned responses of another form. These experimenter–subject interactions (or inadvertent biases) might have well gone undetected by analyses that examined the total number of reinforcements given to each bidirectional group or that examined differences in the temporal pattern of reinforcement between the two training conditions. They might not have been reflected in regressions of performance on reinforcement density either, if both biases were operative or if other undetected sources of error were simultaneously present. The opportunity for subtle and undetected bias originating from inconsistent application of reinforcement and shaping criteria to individual subjects is reduced by the automation of the conditioning procedure, as was done in the present experiments, where conditioning was carried out by a small laboratory computer. This practice does not guarantee that reinforcement will bear exactly the same relationship to responding in all rats within bidirectional groups, but it does ensure that the application of reinforcement and shaping criteria to individual subjects will not be influenced inadvertently by the experimenter's appreciation that a rat may or may not be performing as expected. The likelihood of biases deriving from this source would also be lessened by the employment of a fixed reinforcement criterion, as was done in Trowill's original study, in which very modest bidirectional differences were found (Trowill, 1967). However, once again the explanation of earlier positive results does not appear to lie exclusively with any single source of error, since Fields (1970a,b) reported results consistent with a learning interpretation when the conditioning procedure was computerized.

Recent reports of successful operant heart-rate conditioning in the curarized rat by several researchers can be questioned on the basis of several of the considerations raised above. The aforementioned differences in the number of shocks received by the bidirectional groups in experiments by Gliner et al. (1975) and Wright (1974, Experiment 4) preclude attributing these results unequivocally to operant conditioning, particularly when it is recognized that the unconditioned response to shock is usually (but not always) an increase in heart rate in the curarized rat. It will also be recalled that Wright (1974, Experiment 4) Thornton (1971, Experiment 1), and Thornton and Van-Toller (1973b) reported that rats trained to decrease heart rate were more likely to have received uninterrupted clusters of shocks than rats that were trained to increase heart rate. Once again bidirectional differences in heart rate cannot be attributed unambiguously to the operant contingency. The remaining reports by Middaugh et al. (1975) and Cabanac and Serres (1976) provide little information on maintenance and respiratory procedure or on the pattern and distribution of reinforcing events and are therefore difficult to evaluate. However, it should be apparent that the pitfalls in research on operant conditioning in curarized subjects are so numerous that occasional reports of learning in the absence of further data demonstrating that such reports are repeatable and unambiguously a product of the operant contingency are not likely to rekindle the hope of recovering the phenomena of the original curare experiments.[7]

IV. Status of the Original Experiments

It is apparent that the effort to replicate the results of the original curare experiments has failed. Furthermore, the diversity of this effort together with data attesting to the inadequacy of the original curare preparation provides adequate reason to conclude that continued pursuit of replication in the preparation of the original studies is not likely to prove worthwhile. Although it is not possible to determine precisely how the original findings were obtained, the foregoing considerations suggest that any contribution that derived from learning was exceedingly fragile and inadvertently confounded with contributions deriving from a failure to control several variables that must be judged in retrospect to have been primarily responsible for the

[7] Cabanac and Serres (1976) reported that the relationship of heart rate to temperature was altered in opposite directions when hypothermic rats were rewarded with peripheral heating for increases or decreases in heart rate. An effect of operant conditioning on this relationship was examined in the present research by division of within-subject changes in heart rate by the corresponding change in temperature (dHR/dT) for operant level and conditioning separately. The resulting ratios for conditioning were then plotted as a function of the ratios for operant level, with individual rats used as the unit of observation. Ratios averaged 33.1 bpm/°C and were significantly correlated across operant level and conditioning, as would be expected if these measures were partially sensitive to the dependency of heart rate on temperature. However, no evidence for a change in dHR/dT dependent upon direction of training was found. The reasons for the discrepancy between these observations and the report by Cabanac and Serres (1976) cannot be ascertained on the basis of the available data. However, it should be noted that the analysis carried out by these investigators did not take total performance into account but instead focused upon portions of the heart-rate record that appeared to have been homogeneous with respect to patterns of responding that were observed during operant conditioning. This procedure is attractive in that it takes into consideration the possibility that rats may display distinctive patterns of learned response that may be missed by more global analyses, but it is nevertheless fraught with serious hazard. The analysis of Cabanac and Serres (1976) would have been more convincing had the same response patterns been sought in both bidirectional groups, and preferably also in yoked controls. It would also have been desirable to establish the reliability of the scoring procedure, preferably through the use of observers who were blind with respect to direction of training.

production of these effects. It seems clear that conclusions pertaining to the plasticity of visceral function can no longer be based upon this body of work.

In one respect this conclusion appears to strain the limits of plausibility. In addition to DiCara, who collected the data of the early, seminal studies (DiCara and Miller, 1968a; Miller and DiCara, 1967), several other researchers reported positive results in early research on the curarized preparation (for example, Banuazizi, 1972; Hothersall and Brener (1969); Slaughter, Hahn, and Rinaldi (1970); Table 1 above). How could spurious results have been attributed to learning by so many investigators? One possibility that might be mentioned for the sake of completeness is that the original results may have been made to appear genuine by deliberate intent. However, few who have had first hand experience with the curare problem seriously entertain this view. The number and reputation of the principals involved weigh too heavily against it; furthermore, the potential sources of error in the curare preparation are so numerous that a thesis of deliberate deception is unnecessary. Instead, a second possibility seems more likely to be correct.

Briefly stated, this possibility is as follows. The curare experiments were undertaken with a specific objective in mind, namely, to demonstrate that cardiovascular activity could be operantly conditioned in the absence of somatomotor and respiratory correlates. Furthermore, the experimenters involved in the original work do not appear to have been dispassionate observers of the outcome. Rather, the objective was interpreted as critical to the status of visceral responses as operant responses, and it was strongly believed that positive results would be obtained (Miller, 1969). These expectations may have lead to a succession of procedural errors that eventuated in the production and misinterpretation of the original findings. Insufficient attention may have been paid to variables that influenced the response system that was being conditioned. Disturbing features of the data that in a more neutral climate might have aroused suspicion were overlooked. Analyses of preconditioning heart-rate trends or of bidirectional differences in reinforcement variables that might have further questioned a learning interpretation were insufficiently carried out. After the initial successes, priority was given to demonstration of operant conditioning of new responses and to the study of new shaping procedures, rather than to parametric study of the original phenomena that would have provided an opportunity to disconfirm the initial findings. Publication of the early successes may have raised expectations in other laboratories and created a general bias toward acceptance and reporting of positive rather than negative results. It was only when efforts were undertaken by new investigators to duplicate the procedures of the initial successes within the same laboratory that the problem of replication came to light and the process of reassessment began (Dworkin, 1973; Hahn, 1974b).

The history of the curare problem has not been one in which a few investigators have consistently obtained positive results while others have failed totally. Rather, the case seems to be that most researchers who have developed the problem for themselves have at some time or other obtained a result suggestive of learning. In our case, we obtained evidence compatible with a learning interpretation on three occasions. The first of these occasions was in 1971, before the problem of replication came to public attention. In this study, punishment training was employed in an attempt to suppress the curarized rat's spontaneous skin-potential response. A yoked-control procedure was used. To our surprise and delight, this experiment appeared at first to have worked. However, a subsequent effort at replication that was undertaken as part of a series of parametric studies designed to relate the phenomenon to determining variables failed to reproduce the original effect (see Roberts et al., 1974, for a summary of this work). I can recall vividly how excited we were with the initial results, which appeared to demonstrate operant conditioning of a response that had not previously been trained in the curarized rat. I also remember the disappointment that followed when the negative evidence began to accumulate. We were fortunate in this instance to have been able to identify retrospectively a probable cause of the original, misleading outcome. Briefly, we found that rats that had been assigned to the experimental group emitted significantly smaller skin-potential responses during the operant level period than did rats that were treated as yoked controls. Differences between the groups that developed over operant conditioning were therefore likely to have been caused by differential habituation rather than by operant conditioning. This inadvertent confounding of group assignment with response amplitude was not evident upon inspection of the polygraph records because amplifier sensitivity had been adjusted individually for each rat to produce skin-potential deflections of a constant amplitude. However, the error quickly became apparent when detailed analyses of response amplitude were carried out and when parametric work was attempted with the same conditioning procedure.

The second occasion on which results compatible with a learning interpretation were obtained was Wright's effort (1974, Experiment 1) to operantly condition heart rate in the curarized rat. A reliable difference in the direction of training was obtained in this study, provided that one examined only those rats that remained electrodermally responsive throughout the training session. However, we had by this time been sensitized by our experience with operant electrodermal conditioning and were unwilling to attribute this result to learning, for several reasons (see Roberts et al., 1974). The most important of these reasons was that no convergence of heart rate was observed between the bidirectional groups over one hour of extinction. Furthermore, detailed analyses of the distribution of shock showed that the largest heart-rate changes in the direction of training were obtained at the lowest shock densities in each bidirectional group. Although this result might have been interpreted to mean that the observed changes in heart rate were indeed a product of learning and that shock density was an important determinant of conditioning success, a more disturbing interpretation was that the experimenter inadvertently applied less stringent punishment criteria to those rats that displayed tonic heart-rate trends consistent with direction of training in each bidirectional group. A conservative stance with respect to interpretation of these data was also made easier by discovery that other investigators were encountering difficulties with operant conditioning in the curarized rat, as well.

The third occasion on which results compatible with learning interpretation were obtained in my laboratory was in the aforementioned experiment by Wright (1974, Experiment 4), in which punishment training was once again applied to heart rate. Unlike in the previous study, bidirectional differences in heart rate diminished to statistical insignificance over the course of 30 min of extinction in this experiment. Furthermore, changes in heart rate over the course of conditioning were negatively related to shock density within both bidirectional groups. However, the interpretation that is to be given to these results was clouded by the presence of significant differences in the amount and temporal distribution of shock received by the bidirectional groups. Furthermore, we could not rule out the possibility of undetected and perhaps unavoidable bias in the administration of the rather demanding shaping and respiratory procedures that were employed in this work. Our failure to replicate these results when all aspects of the experimental procedure were automated (Panel A, Figure 2) strongly suggests that the original findings were not a product of the operant contingency.

The experience with early success followed by repeated failure that is evidenced in the curare literature does not appear to be altogether uncommon in biological and behavioral research. Examples of difficulties encountered by other investigators have been cited by Miller and Dworkin (1974). Another instance has been described to me by Bennett Galef (personal communication, 1976), who reported the following experience in research on social transmission of avoidance behavior in the rat. Galef was interested in the possibility that naive rats could be trained to escape a previously neutral stimulus in the absence of explicit reinforcement, if they were allowed to interact with conspecifics that had previously been trained to escape the same cue. The hypothesis was entertained on the basis of field observations that suggested that social transmission may serve as one basis for the development of predator avoidance behavior. After extensive pilot work, a formal experiment was undertaken and provided results consistent with a social transmission hypothesis. Several subsequent studies incorporated various refinements and once again provided positive results. At this point, the phenomenon seemed sufficiently well documented to warrant preparation of a paper that was submitted and accepted for publication by a prominent scientific journal. Galef then undertook a series of experiments designed to assess the extent to which social interaction with demonstrator rats was necessary for transmission of avoidance behavior. This study failed to replicate the original effect. Three additional and painstaking efforts to replicate were also completely unsuccessful. At this point, the article describing the initial studies was withdrawn from publication and further work on the problem was abandoned:

> How could such a thing happen, a strong phenomenon disappearing in replication using the same subjects, apparatus, procedures, and experimenters? I suppose I shall never know but I have my suspicions. First, I think we wanted to find the effect a bit too much. We weren't really doing science in the sense of asking whether or not social transmission of an avoidance response exists, but rather trying to demonstrate its existence. Second, we tended to ignore apparently unimportant problems in the data and concentrated instead upon the main effect. For example, naive rats did just as well on the tenth test trial following training as on the first. We didn't worry enough about the absence of extinction. Also it was much easier for naive animals to learn from conspecifics than it was for us to train the demonstrators. We should have been suspicious. As I indicated I don't know to this day if the effect was real or not (others have told me they have replicated) and, if it wasn't, where we went wrong. However, I do know that I no longer have sufficient faith in the results of our initial five studies to publish them. (Galef, personal communication, 1976).

The history of operant autonomic conditioning in the curarized rat bears some resemblance to this report by Galef, and many who have worked on the problem will sympathize with these remarks. Experiments on operant autonomic conditioning in the curarized preparation are extraordinarily difficult to do well. The problem is complicated by the fact that the experimenter is obliged to manipulate several variables (pertaining to respiration, drug maintenance, application of reinforcement, and so on) that may have substantial and spurious effects on the response that is to be conditioned. The technology that is required for proper studies in this preparation is only now being developed and tested (Dworkin and Miller, 1977). Perhaps the most remarkable aspect of the curare experience is not that learning appeared to have been obtained in the early studies, but that the enthusiasm generated by these studies carried them into the published literature and raised strong expectations of success before subsequent efforts that should have replicated a robust learning phenomenon revealed the tenuous and misleading nature of the original findings.

V. Implications

The implications of the assessment of the curare literature that has been developed in this chapter fall into two categories. First, there are relatively mundane but nevertheless important implications pertaining to general research strategy. Automation of experimental procedures is highly desirable in studies of operant autonomic conditioning in both animal and human subjects and offers greater advantage than has generally been acknowledged (Lang, 1974). In addition to minimizing sources of error originating from the experimenter's behavior, automation facilitates subsequent replication by requiring that attention be paid to procedural details that may be important to learning and easily overlooked when more conventional methods are used. Parametric research within the same conditioning procedure also seems to be highly desirable at an early stage in a research program, not only because such work may identify important determinants of conditioning success but also because it provides opportunities to disconfirm the original findings. The curare experience also underscores the need for objectivity in the conduct of basic and applied biofeedback research. Several investigators have expressed their concern that biofeedback may be one area of scientific inquiry in which such an attitude is notably lacking (Black, 1972; Miller and Dworkin, 1974; Obrist, 1970; Schwartz, 1975).

Other implications of the present assessment pertain to substantive issues in biofeedback and self-regulation. In the introduction to this chapter, it was argued that the impact of the curare experiments derived largely from the implications that these experiments were believed to have for the mechanism of operant conditioning and for general conceptions of the plasticity of the autonomic nervous system. These experiments were widely credited with having established biofeedback research on a firm empirical basis (Blanchard and Scott, 1974) and were in some instances interpreted to indicate that basic questions concerning the mechanism of conditioning and the properties of visceral operants had been largely resolved (Katkin, 1971). However, the data pertaining to these issues are far from complete. A brief review of selected research relevant to questions of mechanism and plasticity suggests not only that much remains to be learned but that in some instances the conclusions that are supported by the available data are very different from those asserted by the curare literature.

A. The Mechanism of Operant Conditioning

Recent studies of operant heart-rate conditioning in the rat have shown that operantly conditioned changes in heart rate are associated with somatomotor correlates, when training is carried out in the normal state. In one of these studies, Black, Osborne, and Ristow (1977) began by adapting rats to an activity wheel for five daily sessions. A modified percentile-reinforcement procedure was subsequently used to train separate groups of animals to increase or decrease heart rate. Brain-stimulation reinforcement was available during discrete 100-sec trials signaled by presentation of a tone (S^D). The results of 10 days of training with this shaping procedure are shown in Figure 7. Inspection of the cardiac performance in the upper panel of the figure shows that subjects trained to increase heart rate evidenced accelerations approximating 20 bpm during S^D periods on the first training day. Subjects trained to decrease heart rate also evidenced discriminative control in the expected direction, but in this case, acquisition of the response was less rapid. In both groups, there was a tendency for performance to improve as a function of extended training. The somatomotor performance of the two groups is depicted in Figure 8, which presents the results of an analysis of activity patterns that were recorded by videotape on the last day of training. Inspection of the upper panel of the figure shows that the motor activities exhibited by rats in the two bidirectional groups were indistinguishable during periods of training in which the S^D was absent and reinforcement was not available. However, inspection of the lower panel of the figure shows that rats trained to increase heart rate shifted their activity patterns toward more vigorous behaviors (such as rearing) when the S^D was presented, whereas subjects in the decrease group engaged in less vigorous activities (such as movements of the head) in the presence of this cue. These findings show that the

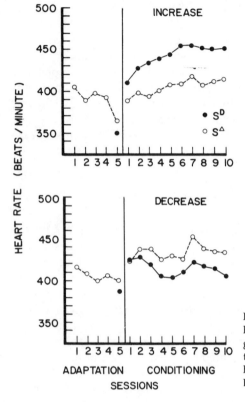

FIGURE 7. Operant conditioning of heart rate in the normal state. Separate groups of rats received brain-stimulation reward for emitting fast or slow heart rates, for 10 daily sessions. (From Black *et al.*, 1977.)

cardiac performance evidenced by the two training groups was associated with distinctive patterns of motor activity.[8]

Similar results have recently been obtained by Brener, Phillips, and Connally (1977), using a shock-avoidance procedure. As in the previous study, rats received five days of adaptation in an activity wheel. Separate groups were then trained to increase or decrease heart rate for 15 consecutive days. Discrimination training was employed in which a discriminative stimulus (illumination of the experimental chamber) was presented in alternate 8-min blocks. During the S^D, failure to emit criterion behavior was signaled by presentation of a

[8] In another study, Black *et al.* (1977) exposed a third group of rats to random reinforcement in the presence of the discriminative stimulus. This procedure did not affect heart rate over five days of training. This observation together with the stimulus control that is evident in both bidirectional groups in Figure 7 suggests that performance was determined by the operant contingency rather than by classical conditioning or other effects of the training procedure.

tone. A single shock was presented subsequently if the subjects emitted five consecutive response units consisting of five interbeat intervals that failed to meet criterion, after which the tone was turned off for a 10-sec time-out period. The heart-rate performance of rats trained by this procedure is depicted in the upper panel of Figure 9, where it is apparent that discriminative control of both increases and decreases in heart rate was obtained. Once again, discriminative control of heart-rate decreases developed more slowly than did control of increases. Brener *et al.* (1977) also recorded running behavior and oxygen consumption during operant conditioning. The latter variable was included in an effort to measure total somatomotor activation as accurately as possible. Inspection of the data provided in the remaining panels of Figure 9 leave little doubt that the perform-ance of heart-rate change was associated with correlated changes in both of these measures of somatomotor performance.

Other recent studies have examined whether the somatomotor correlates that are observed when heart rate is operantly conditioned

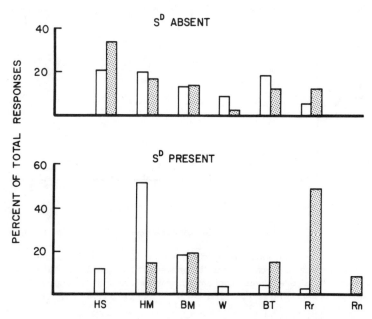

FIGURE 8.   Activity patterns evidenced by rats trained to increase (hatched bars) or decrease (open bars) heart rate, on the last day of training. Performance in the presence and the absence of the S^D is shown. HS = holding still; HM = head movement; BM = body movements; W = walking; BT = body turn; Rr = rearing; Rn = running. (From Black *et al.*, 1977.)

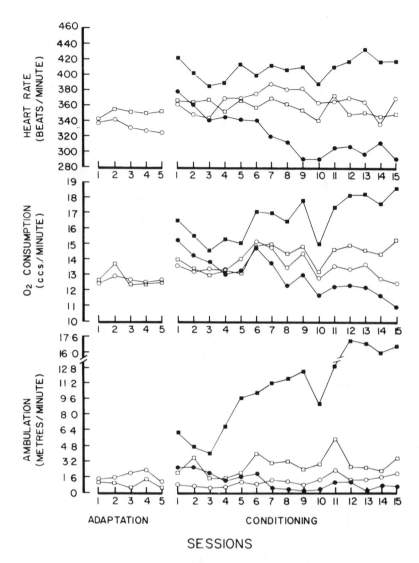

FIGURE 9. Operant conditioning of heart rate in the normal state. Rats were punished for emitting inappropriate heart rates in the presence of a discriminative stimulus, for 15 daily sessions. Heart rate, oxygen consumption, and ambulation are shown. ■ increase S^D; □ increase S^Δ; ● decrease S^D; ○ decrease S^Δ. (From Brener et al., 1977.)

are necessary for the performance of cardiac change. Black (1974a) attempted to dissociate somatomotor and cardiac responding through the use of a disjunctive conditioning procedure. In this procedure, rats received brain-stimulation reward whenever they emitted three successive criterion heartbeats in the presence of a discriminative stimulus; however, reinforcement was given only if the rats emitted criterion heartbeats while holding still. Each of two subjects exposed to this procedure successfully shifted its distributions of interbeat intervals toward faster heart rates while satisfying the somatomotor response requirement. However, an analysis of videotape records revealed that one of the subjects satisfied the criterion for reinforcement by engaging in what appeared to be deliberate, episodic movements that were executed with greater temporal precision than were the associated heart-rate changes, which typically took longer to return to baseline. Reinforcement occurred when instantaneous response states were asynchronous. The other subject did not appear to utilize this response strategy, but the possibility that undetected respiratory maneuvers or isometric muscle activity may have contributed to performance could not be ruled out on the basis of the data that were collected. A further observation of importance in this study was that although both rats subjected to the procedure shifted their interbeat intervals toward faster heart rates when they were holding still, in neither case were the heart rates evidenced in the absence of movement as fast as those evidenced while the subjects were engaging in motor activity. This observation suggests that imposition of somatomotor constraints limits the magnitude of cardiac changes that can be produced by operant conditioning in the rat.

Results supporting the same conclusion have been reported by Obrist *et al.* (1975) for human subjects. These investigators examined operant heart-rate conditioning as a function of the extent to which somatomotor and respiratory maneuvers were discouraged by explicit verbal instructions and respiratory pacing techniques. A discriminative shock-avoidance procedure was used. Subjects who were trained to increase heart rate were found to display faster heart rates and higher levels of somatomotor activity (gross body movement, EMG, ocular activity, and respiratory maneuvers) than subjects who were reinforced either randomly or for decreases in heart rate. Bidirectional differences in these measures were also found to depend upon the extent to which somatomotor and respiratory maneuvers were discouraged by the instructions the subjects received. The effect of this variable is shown in Figure 10, which depicts the heart-rate and EMG performance of subjects who were trained to increase heart rate under three levels of somatomotor and respiratory control. Also depicted here is the performance of subjects who received reinforcement randomly under conditions of maximum somatomotor constraint. Inspection of these data shows that limiting somatomotor and respiratory activity led to an attenuation of somatomotor and cardiac responding during operant heart-rate conditioning. However, application of constraints did not abolish learning altogether, since subjects

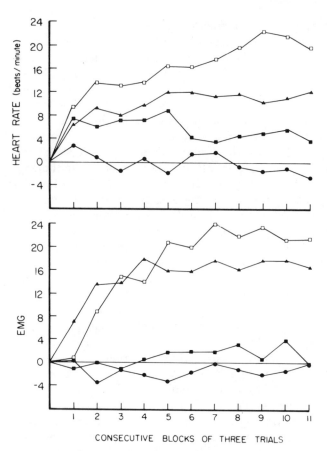

FIGURE 10.   Avoidance conditioning of heart rate in noncurarized human subjects. The effect of constraining somatomotor and respiratory maneuvers on heart-rate and electromyographic performance is shown. (Redrawn from Obrist *et al.*, 1975.) □ HR up—no control; ▲ HR up—minimum control; ■ HR up—maximum control; ● random—maximum control.

who were exposed to maximum somatomotor control nevertheless evidenced heart rates that were reliably faster than subjects who received random reinforcement under this condition (Obrist *et al.*, 1975).

The results reported in these studies of operant heart-rate conditioning in the normal state are consistent with an extensive body of evidence that indicates that cardiovascular efferents are closely integrated within somatomotor control mechanisms in the central nervous system (Smith, 1974). The attenuating effect on cardiac performance of imposing somatomotor and respiratory constraints, either by the use of disjunctive conditioning procedures (Black, 1974a) or by verbal instructions (Obrist et al., 1975), suggests further that the neural systems that integrate cardiovascular and somatomotor activity are deeply involved in the performance of cardiac change during operant conditioning. The persistence of motor correlates when operant heart-rate conditioning is carried out for as long as 15 days (as was done by Brener et al., in press) also suggests that fragmentation of cardiosomatic integration is not likely to be achieved merely by an extension of the duration of training in the absence of contingencies designed specifically to dissociate these two aspects of behavioral activity. A different result, on the other hand, was obtained by DiCara and Miller (1969b). These investigators reported that subjects given operant heart-rate conditioning under curare evidenced diverging heart-rate trends with converging somatomotor and respiratory activity when heart-rate conditioning was continued during a subsequent session in the normal state. These findings have been interpreted to suggest that there are conditions under which somatomotor and respiratory responses may not be necessary for the performance of heart-rate change (DiCara and Miller, 1969b; Goesling and Brener, 1972).

Unfortunately, the weight that should be given to DiCara and Miller's (1969b) report is a matter of sheer conjecture in view of the difficulties surrounding the curare literature. There is, however, a basis on which to suggest that dissociation of cardiac and somatic responding may be possible. Whereas heart-rate changes that are closely related to motor activity in human subjects appear to be determined by modulation of parasympathetic outflow (Freyschuss, 1970), changes in heart rate that derive from augmented sympathetic activation under conditions of severe stress appear to be independent of somatomotor arousal (Obrist, 1976). It is possible that control of the heart by the latter process may have been observed in the aforementioned study by Obrist et al. (1975), in which avoidance conditioning was utilized to establish operant control of heart rate. Futher inspection of the results of this study in Figure 10 shows that although subjects who were trained to increase heart rate under maximum somatomotor and respiratory limitation emitted significantly faster heart rates than did subjects who were reinforced randomly under this condition, a similar difference was not obtained with respect to EMG. It may also be noted that the cardiac accelerations displayed by subjects in the former group developed rapidly within the first three conditioning trials and were roughly equivalent in magnitude to accelerations that were observed in the remaining groups at this stage of training. It is tempting to suggest (as did Obrist et al.) that this initial acceleration of heart rate may have been produced by an augmentation of sympathetic control that was elicited by the subject's first encounters with shock and then sustained by the operant contingency. Heart-rate accelerations produced by this mechanism may not have been dependent upon simultaneous activation of somatomotor control systems.

Although it is possible that heart-rate changes produced by a sympathetic mechanism may not be related to somatomotor activation, it should nevertheless be noted that these changes do not necessarily represent novel alterations of cardiovascular organization that are produced by the operant conditioning procedure. That is to say, control of heart rate may not have been established by an uncoupling of cardiac activity from somatomotor influences, as the curare literature was widely interpreted to suggest. Rather, it is more likely that heart-rate changes that derive from this source are produced by activation of a different cardiovascular control mechanism. Excitation of this mechanism may also lead to changes in a variety of other response systems that serve to prepare the organism for vigorous activity, perhaps in the face of impending threat. The importance of such a mechanism in cardiovascular and behavioral regulation has long been recognized by psychophysiologists (Cannon, 1936), although the topography of activation produced by this system and the variables that control it have only recently become the subject of systematic inquiry in the biofeedback literature (Obrist et al., 1975; Obrist, 1976).

The data reviewed above are compatible with the more general proposition that operant autonomic conditioning succeeds by establishing control of neural systems within which visceral activity is normally integrated. When a visceral response is integrated with more than one distinct behavioral process, as is probably true of most visceral response systems, the process that is eventually controlled very likely depends upon details of the experimental procedure as well as upon the precise nature of the feedback contingency. In general, one would expect control by a given process to eventuate only to the extent that excitation of this process is compatible with the conditions of the experiment and to the extent that presentations of exteroceptive feedback are uniquely contiguous with variations in the visceral response that are determined by the neural process in question (Black, 1972; Roberts, 1977; Schwartz, 1974). Although the available data on operant heart-rate conditioning are generally consistent with these propositions, what is perhaps more notable is the lack of data pertaining to the applicability of these principles not only to cardiovascular function but to other visceral response systems as well. It would admittedly be unreasonable to attribute this lack of information entirely to the curare literature. Nevertheless, it is pertinent to recall that the specificity of reinforcement effects reported in this literature was widely interpreted to suggest that operant conditioning did not entail concomitant effects on other control systems (Katkin, 1971; Miller and Banuazizi, 1968; DiCara and Miller, 1969b). This conception of the mechanism of conditioning is not well supported by the data reviewed above, and it may have discouraged efforts to examine the effects of operant autonomic conditioning on other response systems and to analyze their relationship to the performance of visceral change.

B. Plasticity of Visceral Responding

A second set of questions that is basic to biofeedback research has to do with the properties that are evidenced by visceral responses when operant conditioning is carried out. At issue here is the question of the effectiveness of operant conditioning as a method for controlling visceral activity.

Two more specific questions may be distinguished. First, what can be accomplished by application of operant conditioning to a visceral response system? Several possibilities may be considered. For example, operant conditioning may establish the ability to control a response where such control did not previously exist (Cornsweet and Crane, 1973). Alternatively, operant conditioning may augment the degree of control that is possible, or it may modify the specificity (Schwartz, 1974) or precision (Schwartz, Young, and Volger, 1976) with which such control is expressed. Other possibilities concern the stimulus effects of operant autonomic conditioning. For example, discriminative operant conditioning may establish the ability to control the response in situations where such control was previously absent or unattainable.

The second question asks simply, what procedures are most effective in establishing operant control of the response? Are some criteria for reinforcement and shaping more effective than others? Does the magnitude of control depend upon variables such as the type of reinforcement, the nature of instructions given to subjects prior to training, or details pertaining to the feedback display? The answers to these questions are obviously relevant to assessment of the properties of cardiovascular and other visceral operants. The magnitude of cardiovascular control and the range of stimulus conditions under which such control is exercised may reasonably be assumed to depend

upon the procedures that are employed to establish control of responding to begin with.

One would have thought that after a decade of research on
operant autonomic conditioning, a considerable body of knowledge
pertaining to these questions would have been accumulated for
several response systems. However, it is surprising to note just how
little is known about these issues for most autonomic responses. Only
with respect to heart rate does the available literature appear to permit
tentative conclusions regarding properties of the response (for example, Brener, 1974; Roberts, 1977; Schwartz *et al.*, 1976) and optimal
conditioning procedures (for example, Black *et al.*, 1977; Blanchard and
Scott, 1974; Bouchard and Corson, 1976; Lang and Twentyman, 1974).
Even in this instance, much remains to be learned.

Data bearing on questions of plasticity are important not only
insofar as they are necessary for an appreciation of the modifiability of
visceral function. They are also relevant to an assessment of the
practicality and potential benefit of therapeutic applications. Consider, for example, the operant conditioning of erectile responses.
Recent work by Rosen and his colleagues (Rosen, 1973; Rosen,
Shapiro, and Schwartz, 1975) has suggested that both increases and
decreases in penile tumescence can be shaped through biofeedback
training. The data are clearest for decreases in this response, where it
has been shown that provision of feedback for increases in penile
tumescence together with verbal instructions to suppress erectile
behavior leads to significantly fewer erections when subjects listen to
erotic tape recordings than does provision of noncontingent feedback
or verbal instructions alone (Rosen, 1973). In view of these demonstrations, it is reasonable to ask whether therapies based upon operant
conditioning might be useful in the treatment of unconventional
sexual behavior (see Barlow, Agras, Abel, Blanchard, and Young,
1975). However, for clinical applications, it is important to know not
simply whether operant conditioning of penile tumescence is possible;
more importantly, one must establish the limits of this conditioning
process. Does suppression of erectile behavior to an inappropriate
sexual stimulus by operant conditioning extinguish quickly when
feedback is removed and the subject is no longer embarrassed by
public disclosure of his sexual response? Can stimulus control be
altered by discriminative operant conditioning in which an attempt is
made to produce sexual arousal to socially appropriate and previously
ineffective cues? Which conditioning arrangements facilitate these
behavioral modifications? For example, are some reinforcers (such as
presentation of a slide depicting the deviant but initially preferred
stimulus, as opposed to monetary reward or feedback alone) more

effective in establishing learned control than others? Is excitement of sexual arousal a prerequisite to the shaping process, and is it modified by it? Obviously, the utility of operant conditioning as a form of therapy for deviant sexual responsiveness depends upon answers to questions such as these (Barlow *et al.*, 1975).

Another example of a response system for which basic data are lacking concerns the peripheral vasculature. The possibility that substantial control of vasomotor activity can be established by operant conditioning has been suggested by recent studies in which subjects were instructed to change the temperature of one hand relative to some other site under conditions of exteroceptive feedback (for example, Keefe, 1975; A. H. Roberts *et al.*, 1975; also see Steptoe, Mathews, and Johnston, 1974). In one of these experiments (A. H. Roberts *et al.*, 1975), good performers achieved a temperature difference of approximately 5–6°C between the two hands on some training trials. However, the determinants and the properties of this response are poorly understood. It is not known, for example, whether provision of exteroceptive feedback is required for acquisition of control (Johnston, 1977) or whether control that is established during biofeedback training can be sustained on test trials on which exteroceptive feedback is removed. The physiological significance of the response is also unclear. The relationship of finger temperature to peripheral vasomotor activity is imprecise (Surwit *et al.*, 1976) and may be distorted in some instances by artifactual manipulation of the thermistor probe (Johnston, 1977). Most studies agree, however, that individual differences in the ability to control skin temperature are substantial. Recent reports by A. H. Roberts *et al.* (1975) and Lynch and his colleagues (Lynch, Hama, Kohn, and Miller, 1976) suggest that only a minority of subjects are able to develop substantial and stable control when given extended biofeedback training. This variability in performance in laboratory settings together with lack of knowledge about the physiological basis of the response gives adequate reason to be cautious about recent studies in which operant conditioning of finger temperature has been applied with considerable reported success in the treatment of migraine headache (Sargent, Green, and Walters, 1973; Turin and Johnson, 1976; Wickramasekera, 1973). Further data are needed to ascertain whether control of vasomotor responding is actually established during biofeedback therapy and to determine whether therapeutic improvement is related to the acquisition and performance of this learned skill as opposed to several other possible effects of the treatment procedure (Legewie, 1977).

It would again be unreasonable to attribute the present lack of data pertaining to the properties of visceral operants and determinants of conditioning entirely to the curare literature. To some extent, these gaps have been created by a desire to establish first that therapeutic benefits can be obtained by operant conditioning before more basic questions are attacked. However, the remarkable plasticity evident in the curare literature appears in retrospect to have encouraged neglect of basic issues by leading researchers to assume that substantial, highly specific, and transituational control of visceral responding can be established more readily by operant conditioning than may actually be the case. This literature also appears to have created a readiness to attribute therapeutic success to the acquisition and performance of visceral skills that may be unwarranted and premature. More effort needs to be devoted to the study of properties and determinants of visceral learning, not only for the purpose of designing effective treatment procedures but also for the purpose of evaluating the role that visceral learning plays in the production of therapeutic gain.

VI. CONCLUSION

The fact that the curare experiments have been widely cited in reviews of both basic (Harris and Brady, 1974) and applied (Blanchard and Scott, 1974) biofeedback research serves as one of several indications that these experiments have been believed to have established the phenomena of operant autonomic conditioning on a firm scientific basis. The assessment of these experiments that has been offered in this chapter gives reason to reflect briefly upon the adequacy of this basis in the absence of the curare literature.

Certainly, the issue of whether autonomic responses can be operantly conditioned is no longer a matter of serious dispute. There is also sufficient evidence to suggest that operant conditioning establishes control of visceral function by altering the activity of neural systems within which visceral responding is normally integrated. Although several reviewers have cautioned that the power of operant conditioning as a technique for treating visceral pathology appears to have been overstated in the past (Blanchard and Young, 1974; Legewie, 1977), there is evidence that suggests that some autonomic applications may be useful (for example, Engel and Bleecker, 1974; Engel, Nikoomanesh, and Schuster, 1974; Wickramasekera, 1973) and merit further study. Despite these significant accomplishments, however, one cannot help but be impressed by gaps in present knowledge pertaining to (1) properties of operantly conditioned autonomic responses; (2) optimal conditioning procedures; (3) mechanisms of conditioning; and (4) the basis and extent of therapeutic gains produced by biofeedback training.

The fact that so much remains to be researched should not be taken to mean that the answers are likely to prove exciting. On the contrary, there is reason to expect that continued study will show that the limits of visceral learning are considerably more constrained than was suggested by the curare experiments. Furthermore, it will not be surprising if in most instances the mechanisms involved in the performance of visceral operants turn out to be less remarkable than was assumed to be the case for the phenomena depicted in the curare literature. Nevertheless, continued study of these issues is likely to prove worthwhile. One product is certain to be a deeper understanding of the limits of visceral learning and of the organization of the autonomic nervous system. Another product will very likely be a better appreciation of the utility and limits of biofeedback training as a treatment for visceral pathology.

As a final consideration, one is led to ask whether the study of visceral learning is likely to profit from the continuing effort to demonstrate operant autonomic conditioning in the curarized rat (Dworkin and Miller, 1977). Clearly, the original justification for the use of paralysis is inadequate. Curarization does not control satisfactorily for the participation of somatomotor mechanisms in performance; instead, it is evident that central components of these mechanisms are capable of exerting a measurable influence on cardiovascular activity in the paralyzed state. That exclusion of somatomotor participation should be seen as a priority in biofeedback research can also be questioned, insofar as exclusion of somatomotor influences is not easily defended as a criterion for membership in an operant class. Nevertheless, it would be rash to conclude that continued study of learning in the curarized preparation cannot provide useful information about mechanisms of conditioning or the plasticity of visceral function. The use of a paralyzed animal offers certain advantages, provided that a satisfactory preparation can be devised. One of these is that operant conditioning may be applied to visceral activities that are not easily measured without artifact in the normal state. This feature may make possible systematic investigation of the determinants and limits of conditioning that may be impractical in human subjects or impossible in freely moving animals. Another advantage is that certain problems such as the analysis of neural circuits can be undertaken more readily in this preparation than in the normal state. Thus, it is possible that further study in the curarized rat (or some other more suitable species) may prove worthwhile. It should perhaps be stressed, however, that the status of operant autonomic conditioning as a veridical phenomenon does not depend in any critical sense upon a demonstration of learning under curariform paralysis, as was once believed. There also appears to be an adequate basis on which to conclude that the outcome of continued study in this preparation cannot be anticipated by an appeal to the original curare experiments. The phenomena reported in these experiments are unlikely to have been a product of learning and provide little, if any, information pertaining to the plasticity and organization of the autonomic nervous system.

APPENDIX

The subjects were male hooded rats descended from strains maintained by Quebec Breeding Farms, St. Eustache, Quebec. They weighed an average of 428 g (range, 300–520 g). Rats received extensive handling associated with weekly cage cleaning and with surgery that was carried out approximately 1 week prior to testing. They were also handled briefly and then placed in an open field for 2–3 min on each of the five days immediately preceding curarization. Food and water were removed from the home cage approximately 6 hr before testing.

Shock electrodes were zinc disks 1 cm in diameter and were placed 1 cm apart on the ventral surface of the distal third of the rat's tail. The tail was abraded lightly beneath each electrode to reduce the resistance of the corneum. The electrodes were coated with a commercial jelly (Beckman Electrode Paste) and then topped with a layer of pharmaceutical ointment (Unibase) containing 0.10 M NaCl to ensure good electrical contact with the skin and to minimize polarization. After application of the electrodes, the entire electrode site was covered with masking tape to prevent drying. Shock was a 28-msec capacitor discharge (100 μF charged to 150 V) through a series resistance totaling 48 or 378 Kohm. This arrangement produced a highly repeatable stimulus that averaged 2.87 ($\pm$ 0.16) mA or 0.46 ($\pm$ 0.05) mA across subjects, depending upon which series resistance was used. Measurements of skin potential during operant conditioning have shown that curarized rats remain sensitive to the lower of these two intensities of shock after having received up to 3000 stimulations over 90 min of training (Roberts *et al.*, 1974, Figure 17.5).

The lowest value of shock that consistently elicits a skin-potential response in the curarized rat appears to be about 0.2 mA.

Subjects received high intraperitoneal injections intended to produce rapid paralysis (after Brener et al., 1974). A disposable diaper was placed beneath the rat and then drawn loosely around the subject to conserve body heat after a Silastic strain gage had been looped around the thorax for measurement of chest circumference. Sterile ophthalmic solution (Isoptotears) was placed upon the eyes to prevent drying of the cornea. The rectum was manually evacuated before insertion of a thermistor probe for measurement of body temperature. Measurement of skin potential was accomplished as described by Roberts and Young (1971). Paralysis was maintained throughout the session by infusion of additional curariform drug in the thigh muscle of the left rear leg. The initial dosages and subsequent infusions were as reported in Figure 2. Subjects were placed inside a sound-attenuating chamber for the duration of training; recording was accomplished in an adjoining room.

Following these and other initializing procedures mentioned in the text, subjects were given approximately one hour of adaptation. During this time, peak inspiratory pressure was lowered in an effort to produce a stable heart rate averaging 380–480 bpm with evidence of spontaneous changes unrelated to the respiratory cycle. Rats were aspirated occasionally during this period (never afterward) if measurement of heart rate and respiratory function (peak inspiratory pressure and chest circumference) indicated that this was desirable. After all preparations had been completed, a coin was tossed to determine direction of training. Operant level was then begun.

Several supplementary and less systematic attempts at operant conditioning were carried out in addition to those described in the chapter. Brain-stimulation reward was substituted for shock reinforcement in a few rats, without apparent success; the PR interval was occasionally shaped instead of the RR interval, again without success. We also attempted to determine whether percentile reinforcement schedules could be used to establish control of heart rate in the normal state, before we carried out the experiments reported in the chapter. However, we were unable to complete this experiment, owing to severe EMG artifact that frequently masked the R wave when partially restrained rats were repeatedly shocked in the apparatus of the present research. Black et al. (1977) have subsequently shown that percentile reinforcement schedules can be employed to establish control of heart rate in the normal state, when subjects are given operant conditioning with brain-stimulation reward in an activity wheel.

REFERENCES

ADAMS, D. B., BACCELLI, G., MANCIA, G., AND ZANCHETTI, A. Relation of cardiovascular changes in fighting to emotion and exercise. *Journal of Physiology*, 1971, *212*, 321–335.

ALLEMAN, H. D., AND PLATT, J. R. Differential reinforcement of interresponse times with controlled probability of reinforcement per response. *Learning and Motivation*, 1973, *4*, 40–73.

ALTLAND, P. D., BRUBACK, H. F., PARKER, M. G., AND HIGHMAN, B. Blood gases and acid-base values of unanesthetized rats exposed to hypoxia. *American Journal of Physiology*, 1967, *212*, 142–148.

BANUAZIZI, A. Modification of an autonomic response by instrumental learning. Unpublished doctoral dissertation, Yale University, 1968.

BANUAZIZI, A. Discriminative shock-avoidance learning of an autonomic response under curare. *Journal of Comparative and Physiological Psychology*, 1972, *81*, 336–346.

BARLOW, D. H., AGRAS, W. S., ABEL, G. G., BLANCHARD, E. B., AND YOUNG, L. D. Biofeedback and reinforcement to increase heterosexual arousal in homosexuals. *Behaviour Research and Therapy*, 1975, *13*, 45–50.

BLACK, A. H. Transfer following operant conditioning in the curarized dog. *Science*, 1967, *155*, 201–203.

BLACK, A. H. Autonomic aversive conditioning in infrahuman subjects. In F. R. Brush (Ed.), *Aversive conditioning and learning*. New York: Academic Press, 1971.

BLACK, A. H. The operant conditioning of neural electrical activity. In G. H. Bower (Ed.), *The psychology of learning and motivation*, Vol. 6. New York: Academic Press, 1972.

BLACK, A. H. Operant autonomic conditioning: The analysis of response mechanisms. In P. A. Obrist, A. H. Black, J. Brener, and L. V. DiCara (Eds.), *Cardiovascular psychophysiology: Current issues in response mechanisms, biofeedback, and methodology*. Chicago: Aldine, 1974a.

BLACK, A. H. Summary: Failure of replication in the curarized rat. In P. A. Obrist, A. H. Black, J. Brener, and L. V. DiCara (Eds.), *Cardiovascular psychophysiology: Current issues in response mechanisms, biofeedback, and methodology*. Chicago: Aldine, 1974b.

BLACK, A. H., OSBORNE, B., AND RISTOW, W. C. A note on the operant conditioning of autonomic responses. In H. Davis and H. M. B. Hurwitz (Eds.), *Operant–Pavlovian interactions*. Hillsdale, N.J.: Erlbaum, 1977.

BLACK, A. H., YOUNG, G. A., AND BATENCHUCK, C. Avoidance training of hippocampal theta waves in flaxedilized dogs and its relation to skeletal movement. *Journal of Comparative and Physiological Psychology*, 1970, *70*, 15–24.

BLANCHARD, E. B., AND SCOTT, R. W. Behavioral tactics for clinical cardiac control. In K. S. Calhoun, H. E. Adams, and K. M. Mitchell (Eds.), *Innovative treatment methods in psychophysiology*. New York: Wiley, 1974.

BLANCHARD, E. B., AND YOUNG, L. D. Self-control of cardiac functioning: A promise as yet unfulfilled. *Psychological Bulletin*, 1973, *79*, 143–162.

BLANCHARD, E. B., AND YOUNG, L. D. Clinical applications of biofeedback training: A review of evidence. *Archives of General Psychiatry*, 1974, *30*, 573–589.

BOUCHARD, C., AND CORSON, J. A. Heart rate regulation with success and failure signals. *Psychophysiology*, 1976, *13*, 69–74.

BRENER, J. Factors influencing the specificity of voluntary cardiovascular control. In L. V. DiCara (Ed.), *The limbic and autonomic nervous systems: Advances in research*. New York: Plenum, 1974.

Brener, J., Eissenberg, E., and Middaugh, S. Respiratory and somatomotor factors associated with operant conditioning of cardiovascular responses in curarized rats. In P. A. Obrist, A. H. Black, J. Brener, and L. V. DiCara (Eds.), *Cardiovascular psychophysiology: Current issues in response mechanisms, biofeedback, and methodology.* Chicago: Aldine, 1974.

Brener, J., Phillips, K., and Connally, S. R. Oxygen consumption and ambulation during operant conditioning of heart rate increases and decreases in rats. *Psychophysiology,* 1977, *14,* 483–491.

Buchwald, J. S., Standish, M., Eldred, E., and Halas, E. S. Contribution of muscle spindle circuits to learning as suggested by training under flaxedil. *Electroencephalography and Clinical Neurophysiology,* 1964, *16,* 582–594.

Cabanac, J., and Serres, P. Peripheral heat as a reward for heart rate response in the curarized rat. *Journal of Comparative and Physiological Psychology,* 1976, *90,* 435–441.

Cannon, W. B. *Bodily changes in pain, hunger, fear, and rage* (2d ed.). New York: Appleton-Century, 1936.

Chapot, G., Brrault, N., Muller, M., and Dargnat, N. Comparative study of Pa_{CO_2} in several homeothermic species. *American Journal of Physiology,* 1972, *223,* 1354–1357.

Cornsweet, T. N., and Crane, H. D. Training the visual accommodation system. *Vision Research,* 1973, *13,* 713–715.

Culp, W. C., and Edelberg, R. Regional specificity in the electrodermal reflex. *Perceptual and Motor Skills,* 1966, *23,* 623–627.

DiCara, L. V. Analysis of arterial blood gases in the curarized, artificially respirated rat. *Behavioral Research Methods & Instrumentation,* 1970, *2,* 67–69.

DiCara, L. V. Learning of cardiovascular responses: A review and a description of physiological and biochemical consequences. *Transactions of the New York Academy of Sciences,* 1971, *33,* 411–422.

DiCara, L. V. Some critical methodological variables involved in visceral learning. In P. A. Obrist, A. H. Black, J. Brener, and L. V. DiCara (Eds.), *Cardiovascular psychophysiology: Current issues in response mechanisms, biofeedback, and methodology.* Chicago: Aldine, 1974.

DiCara, L. V., Braun, J. J., and Pappas, B. A. Classical conditioning and instrumental learning of cardiac and gastrointestinal responses following removal of neocortex in the rat. *Journal of Comparative and Physiological Psychology,* 1970, *73,* 208–216.

DiCara, L. V., and Miller, N. E. Changes in heart rate instrumentally learned by curarized rats as avoidance responses. *Journal of Comparative and Physiological Psychology,* 1968a, *65,* 8–12.

DiCara, L. V., and Miller, N. E. Instrumental learning of vasomotor responses by rats: Learning to respond differentially in the two ears. *Science,* 1968b, *159,* 1485–1486.

DiCara, L. V., and Miller, N. E. Long term retention of instrumentally learned heart-rate changes in the curarized rat. *Communications in Behavioral Biology,* 1968c, *2,* 19–23.

DiCara, L. V., and Miller, N. E. Heart-rate learning in the non-curarized state, transfer to the curarized state, and subsequent retraining in the non-curarized state. *Physiology and Behaviour,* 1969a, *4,* 621–624.

DiCara, L. V., and Miller, N. E. Transfer of instrumentally learned heart-rate changes from curarized to non-curarized state. *Journal of Comparative and Physiological Psychology,* 1969b, *68,* 159–162.

DiCara, L. V., and Stone, E. A. Effect of instrumental heart-rate training on rat cardiac and brain catecholamines. *Psychosomatic Medicine,* 1970, *32,* 359–368.

DiCara, L. V., and Weiss, J. M. Effect of heart-rate learning under curare on subsequent non-curarized avoidance learning. *Journal of Comparative and Physiological Psychology*, 1969, *69*, 368–374.

Dworkin, B. R. An effort to replicate visceral learning in curarized rats. Unpublished doctoral dissertation, Rockefeller University, 1973.

Dworkin, B. R., and Miller, N. E. Visceral learning in the curarized rat. In G. E. Schwartz and J. Beatty (Eds.), *Biofeedback: Theory and research*. New York: Academic Press, 1977.

Edelberg, R. The relationship between the galvanic skin response, vasoconstriction, and tactile sensitivity. *Journal of Experimental Psychology*, 1961, *62*, 187–195.

Edelberg, R. Mechanisms of electrodermal adaptations for locomotion, manipulation, or defense. In E. Steller and J. M. Sprague (Eds.), *Progress in physiological psychology*, Vol. 5. New York: Academic Press, 1973.

Eissenberg, E. The curarized rat and heart rate conditioning: A consideration of respiration parameters and neuromuscular blocking agents in a classical conditioning paradigm. Unpublished doctoral dissertation, University of Tennessee, 1973.

Eissenberg, E., and Brener, J. Intermittent positive pressure and the curarized rat: Implications for cardiovascular conditioning. *Physiology and Behavior*, 1976, *16*, 735–743.

Ellison, G. D., and Zanchetti, A. Specific appearance of sympathetic cholinergic vasodilatation in muscles during conditioned movements. *Nature*, 1971, *232*, 124–125.

Engel, B. T., and Bleecker, E. R. Application of operant conditioning techniques to the control of the cardiac arrhythmias. In P. A. Obrist, A. H. Black, J. Brener, and L. V. DiCara (Eds.), *Cardiovascular psychophysiology: Current issues in response mechanisms, biofeedback, and methodology*. Chicago: Aldine, 1974.

Engel, B. T., Nikoomanesh, P., and Schuster, M. M. Operant conditioning of rectosphincteric responses in the treatment of fecal incontinence. *New England Journal of Medicine*, 1974, *290*, 646–649.

Fields, C. I. Instrumental conditioning of cardiac behavior. Unpublished doctoral dissertation, Rockefeller University, 1970a.

Fields, C. I. Instrumental conditioning of the rat cardiac control systems. *Proceedings of the National Academy of Sciences*, 1970b, *65*, 293–299.

Freyschuss, U. Cardiovascular adjustment to somatomotor activation: The elicitation of increments in heart rate, aortic pressure and venomotor tone with the initiation of muscle contraction. *Acta Physiologica Scandanavica*, 1970 (Suppl. 342), 1–63.

Gaebelein, C. J., and Howard, J. L. An improved respiratory system for curarized rats. *Behavior Research Methods and Instrumentation*, 1974, *6*, 427–429.

Gaebelein, C. J., Howard, J. L., Galosy, R. A., and Obrist, P. A. Classical aversive conditioning of heart rate in curarized rats at different blood gas levels. *The Pavlovian Journal of Biological Science*, 1976, *11*, 76–85.

Gliner, J. A., Horvath, S. M., and Wolfe, R. R. Operant conditioning of heart rate in curarized rats: Hemodynamic changes. *American Journal of Physiology*, 1975, *228*, 870–874.

Goesling, W. S., and Brener, J. Effects of activity and immobility conditioning upon subsequent heart-rate conditioning in curarized rats. *Journal of Comparative and Physiological Psychology*, 1972, *81*, 311–317.

Grob, D. Neuromuscular blocking drugs. In W. S. Root and F. G. Hoffman (Eds.), *Physiological pharmacology*, Vol. 3. *The nervous system—Part C: Autonomic nervous system drugs*. New York: Academic Press, 1967.

GUYTON, A. C., AND REEDER, R. C. Quantitative studies on the autonomic actions of curare. *Journal of Pharmacology and Experimental Therapeutics*, 1950, *98*, 188–193.

HAHN, W. W. Apparatus and technique for work with the curarized rat. *Psychophysiology*, 1971, *7*, 283–286.

HAHN, W. W. The learning of autonomic responses by curarized animals. In P. A. Obrist, A. H. Black, J. Brener, and L. V. DiCara (Eds.), *Cardiovascular psychophysiology: Current issues in response mechanisms, biofeedback, and methodology*. Chicago: Aldine, 1974a.

HAHN, W. W. A look at the recent history and current developments in laboratory studies of autonomic conditioning. Presented at a symposium entitled "Self-regulation of cardiovascular function: Psychophysiological perspectives," Annual meetings of the Biofeedback Research Society, Colorado Springs, February 1974b.

HAHN, W. W., SCHWARTZ, M. L., AND SAPPER, H. V. The effects of D-tubocurarine chloride and respiratory settings on heart rate and blood gas composition in the albino rat. *Psychophysiology*, 1975, *12*, 331–338.

HARRIS, A. H., AND BRADY, J. V. Animal learning: Visceral and autonomic conditioning. *Annual Review of Psychology*, 1974, *25*, 107–133.

HODES, R. Electrocortical synchronization resulting from reduced proprioceptive drive caused by neuromuscular blocking agents. *Electroencephalography and Clinical Neurophysiology*, 1962, *14*, 220–232.

HOTHERSALL, D., AND BRENER, J. Operant conditioning of changes in heart rate in curarized rats. *Journal of Comparative and Physiological Psychology*, 1969, *68*, 338–342.

HOWARD, J. L., GAEBELEIN, C. J., GALOSY, R. A., AND OBRIST, P. A. Neuromuscular blocking drugs and heart rate changes after direct nerve stimulation and during classical conditioning in cats. *Journal of Comparative and Physiological Psychology*, 1975, *88*, 868–877.

HOWARD, J. L., GALOSY, R. A., GAEBELEIN, C. J., AND OBRIST, P. A. Some problems in the use of neuromuscular blockade. In P. A. Obrist, A. H. Black, J. Brener, and L. V. DiCara (Eds.), *Cardiovascular psychophysiology: Current issues in response mechanisms, biofeedback, and methodology*. Chicago: Aldine, 1974.

JOHNSTON, D. Biofeedback, verbal instruction and the motor skills analogy. In J. Beatty and H. Legewie (Eds.), *Biofeedback and behavior*. New York: Plenum, 1977.

KATKIN, E. S. *Instrumental autonomic conditioning*. New York: General Learning Press, 1971.

KATKIN, E. S., AND MURRAY, E. N. Instrumental conditioning of autonomically mediated behavior: Theoretical and methodological issues. *Psychological Bulletin*, 1968, *70*, 52–68.

KEEFE, F. J. Conditioning changes in differential skin temperature. *Perceptual and Motor Skills*, 1975, *40*, 283–288.

KIMBLE, G. A. *Hilgard and Marquis' conditioning and learning*. New York: Appleton-Century-Crofts, 1961.

KOELLE, G. B. Neuromuscular blocking agents. In L. S. Goodman and A. Gilman (Eds.), *Pharmacological basis of therapeutics*. New York: Macmillan, 1970.

KOSLOVSKAYA, I. B., VERTES, R. P., AND MILLER, N. E. Instrumental learning without proprioceptive feedback. *Physiology and Behavior*, 1973, *10*, 101–107.

KUCH, D. O., AND PLATT, J. R. Reinforcement rate and interresponse time differentiation. *Journal of the Experimental Analysis of Behavior*, 1976, *26*, 471–486.

LACROIX, J. M., AND ROBERTS, L. E. Determinants of learned electrodermal and cardiac control: A comparative study. *Psychophysiology*, 1976, *13*, 175.

LANG, P. J. Learned control of human heart rate in a computer directed environment. In

P. A. Obrist, A. H. Black, J. Brener, and L. V. DiCara (Eds.), *Cardiovascular psychophysiology: Current issues in response mechanisms, biofeedback, and methodology*. Chicago: Aldine, 1974.

LANG, P. J., AND TWENTYMAN, C. T. Learning to control heart rate: Binary vs analogue feedback. *Psychophysiology*, 1974, *11*, 616–629.

LEGEWIE, H. Clinical implications of biofeedback. In J. Beatty and H. Legewie (Eds.), *Biofeedback and behavior*. New York: Plenum, 1977.

LYNCH, W. C., HAMA, H., KOHN, S., AND MILLER, N. E. Instrumental control of peripheral vasomotor responses in children. *Psychophysiology*, 1976, *13*, 219–221.

MIDDAUGH, S. Operant conditioning of heart rate: The curarized rat as a subject. Unpublished doctoral dissertation, University of Tennessee, 1971.

MIDDAUGH, S., EISSENBERG, E., AND BRENER, J. The effect of artificial ventilation on cardiovascular status and on heart rate conditioning in the curarized rat. *Psychophysiology*, 1975, *12*, 520–526.

MILLER, N. E. Learning of visceral and glandular responses. *Science*, 1969, *163*, 434–445.

MILLER, N. E., AND BANUAZIZI, A. Instrumental learning by curarized rats of a specific visceral response, intestinal or cardiac. *Journal of Comparative and Physiological Psychology*, 1968, *65*, 1–7.

MILLER, N. E., AND DiCARA, L. V. Instrumental learning of heart rate changes in curarized rats: Shaping, and specificity to discriminative stimulus. *Journal of Comparative and Physiological Psychology*, 1967, *63*, 12–19.

MILLER, N. E., DiCARA, L. V., SOLOMON, H., WEISS, H. M., AND DWORKIN, B. Learned modifications of autonomic functions: A review and some new data. *Supplement I to Circulation Research*, 1970, *27*, 3–11.

MILLER, N. E., DiCARA, L. V., AND WOLF, G. Homeostasis and reward: T-maze learning induced by manipulating antidiuretic hormone. *American Journal of Physiology*, 1968, *215*, 684–686.

MILLER, N. E., AND DWORKIN, B. R. Visceral learning: Recent difficulties with curarized rats and significant problems for human research. In P. A. Obrist, A. H. Black, J. Brener, and L. V. DiCara (Eds.), *Cardiovascular psychophysiology: Current issues in response mechanisms, biofeedback, and methodology*. Chicago: Aldine, 1974.

OBRIST, P. A. The operant modification of cardiovascular activity: A biological perspective. Presented at a symposium entitled "A critical evaluation of the operant modification of visceral events." Annual meetings of the Society for Psychophysiological Research, New Orleans, 1970.

OBRIST, P. A. The cardiovascular-behavioral interaction—as it appears today. *Psychophysiology*, 1976, *13*, 95–107.

OBRIST, P. A., BLACK, A. H., BRENER, J., AND DiCARA, L. V. (Eds.), *Cardiovascular psychophysiology: Current issues in response mechanisms, biofeedback, and methodology*. Chicago: Aldine, 1974.

OBRIST, P. A., GALOSY, R. A., LAWLER, J. E., GAEBELEIN, C. J., HOWARD, J. L., AND SHANKS, E. M. Operant conditioning of heart rate: Somatic correlates. *Psychophysiology*, 1975, *12*, 445–455.

OBRIST, P. A., WEBB, R. A., SUTTERER, J. B., AND HOWARD, J. L. The cardiac-somatic relationship: Some reformulations. *Psychophysiology*, 1970, *6*, 569–587.

PAPPAS, B. A., AND DiCARA, L. V. Neonatal sympathectomy by 6-hydroxydopamine: Cardiovascular responses in the paralyzed rat. *Physiology and Behavior*, 1973, *10*, 549–553.

PAPPAS, B. A., DiCARA, L. V., AND MILLER, N. E. Acute sympathectomy by 6-hydroxydopamine in the adult rat: Effects on cardiovascular conditioning and fear retention. *Journal of Comparative and Physiological Psychology*, 1972, *79*, 230–236.

Pickering, T. G., Brucker, B., Frankel, H. L., Mathias, C. J., Dworkin, B. R., and Miller, N. E. Mechanisms of learned voluntary control of blood pressure in patients with generalized body paralysis. In J. Beatty and H. Legewie (Eds.), *Biofeedback and behavior*. New York: Plenum, 1977.

Platt, J. R. Percentile reinforcement: Paradigms for experimental analysis of response shaping. In G. H. Bower (Ed.) *Psychology of learning and motivation: Advances in research and theory*, Vol. 7. New York: Academic Press, 1973.

Ray, R. Use of conditional reflex to assess the temporal characteristics of curarization effects on heart rate responding. *Conditional Reflex*, 1972, 7, 19–32.

Riley, R. L. Gas exchange and transportation. In T. C. Ruch and H. D. Patton (Eds.), *Physiology and biophysics*. Philadelphia: Saunders, 1966.

Roberts, A. H., Schuler, J., Bacon, J., Zimmerman, R. L., and Patterson, R. Individual differences and autonomic control: Absorption, hypnotic susceptibility, and the unilateral control of skin temperature. *Journal of Abnormal Psychology*, 1975, 84, 272–279.

Roberts, L. E. Comparative and psychophysiology of the electrodermal and cardiac control systems. In P. A. Obrist, A. H. Black, J. Brener, and L. V. DiCara (Eds.), *Cardiovascular psychophysiology: Current issues in response mechanisms, biofeedback, and methodology*. Chicago: Aldine, 1974.

Roberts, L. E. The role of exteroceptive feedback in learned electrodermal and cardiac control: Some attractions of and problems with discrimination theory. In J. Beatty and H. Legewie (Eds.), *Biofeedback and behavior*. New York: Plenum Press, 1977.

Roberts, L. E., Lacroix, J. M., and Wright, M. Comparative studies of operant electrodermal and heart rate conditioning in curarized rats. In P. A. Obrist, A. H. Black, J. Brener, and L. V. DiCara (Eds.), *Cardiovascular psychophysiology: Current issues in response mechanisms, biofeedback, and methodology*. Chicago: Aldine, 1974.

Roberts, L. E., and Young, R. Electrodermal responses are independent of movement during aversive conditioning in rats, but heart rate is not. *Journal of Comparative and Physiological Psychology*, 1971, 77, 495–512.

Rosen, R. C. Suppression of penile tumescence by instrumental conditioning. *Psychosomatic Medicine*, 1973, 35, 509–514.

Rosen, R. C., Shapiro, D., and Schwartz, G. E. Voluntary control of penile tumescence. *Psychosomatic Medicine*, 1975, 37, 479–483.

Safar, P., and Bachman, L. Compliance of the lungs and thorax in dogs under the influence of muscle relaxants. *Anesthesiology*, 1956, 17, 334–346.

Sargent, J. D., Green, E. E., and Walters, E. D. Preliminary report on the use of autogenic feedback training in the treatment of migraine and tension headaches. *Psychosomatic Medicine*, 1973, 35, 129–135.

Schwartz, G. E. Toward a theory of voluntary control of response patterns in the cardiovascular system. In P. A. Obrist, A. H. Black, J. Brener, and L. V. DiCara (Eds.), *Cardiovascular psychophysiology: Current issues in response mechanisms, biofeedback, and methodology*. Chicago: Aldine, 1974.

Schwartz, G. E. Biofeedback, self-regulation, and the patterning of physiological processes. *American Scientist*, 1975, 63, 314–324.

Schwartz, G. E., Young, L. D., and Volger, J. Heart rate regulation as skill learning: Strength–endurance versus cardiac reaction time. *Psychophysiology*, 1976, 13, 472–478.

Siegel, S. Evidence from rats that morphine tolerance is a learned response. *Journal of Comparative and Physiological Psychology*, 1975, 89, 498–506.

Slaughter, J., Hahn, W., and Rinaldi, P. Instrumental conditioning of heart rate in the curarized rat with varied amounts of pretraining. *Journal of Comparative and Physiological Psychology*, 1970, 72, 356–359.

SMITH, K. E. Conditioning as an artifact. In G. A. Kimble (Ed.), *Foundations of conditioning and learning*. New York: Appleton-Century-Crofts, 1967.

SMITH, O. A. Reflex and central mechanisms involved in the control of the heart and circulation. *Annual Review of Physiology*, 1974, *36*, 93–123.

STEPTOE, A., MATHEWS, A., AND JOHNSTON, D. The learned control of differential temperature in the human earlobes: Preliminary study. *Biological Psychology*, 1974, *1*, 237–242.

SURWIT, R. S., AND SHAPIRO, D. Biofeedback and meditation in the treatment of borderline hypertension. In J. Beatty and H. Legewie (Eds.), *Biofeedback and behavior*. New York: Plenum, 1977.

SURWIT, R. S., SHAPIRO, D., AND FELD, J. L. Digital temperature regulation and associated cardiovascular changes. *Psychophysiology*, 1976, *13*, 242–248.

THORNTON, E. W. Operant heart-rate conditioning in the curarized rat. Unpublished doctoral dissertation, University of Durham, England, 1971.

THORNTON, E. W., AND VAN-TOLLER, C. Effect of immunosympathectomy on operant heart rate conditioning in the curarized rat. *Physiology and Behavior*, 1973a, *10*, 197–201.

THORNTON, E. W., AND VAN-TOLLER, C. Operant conditioning of heart-rate changes in the functionally decorticate curarized rat. *Physiology and Behavior*, 1973b, *10*, 983–988.

TROWILL, J. A. Instrumental conditioning of the heart rate in the curarized rat. *Journal of Comparative and Physiological Psychology*, 1967, *63*, 7–11.

TURIN, A., AND JOHNSON, G. Biofeedback therapy for migraine headaches. *Archives of General Psychiatry*, 1976, *33*, 517–519.

VAN LIEW, H. D. Oxygen and carbon dioxide tensions in tissue and blood of normal and acidotic rats. *Journal of Applied Physiology*, 1968, *25*, 575–580.

VIZEK, M., AND ALBRECHT, I. Development of cardiac output in male rats. *Physiologia Bohemoslovaca*, 1973, *22*, 573–580.

WEBSTER, J. B. An experimental analysis of response differentiation. Unpublished doctoral dissertation, McMaster University, 1976.

WICKRAMASEKERA, I. E. Temperature feedback for the control of migraine. *Journal of Behavior Therapy and Experimental Psychiatry*, 1973, *4*, 343–345.

WILSON, J. R., AND DICARA, L. V. Effects of previous curare-immobilization on Pavlovian conditioned heart decelerations in the curarized rat. *Physiology and Behavior*, 1975, *14*, 259–264.

WILSON, J. R., SIMPSON, C. W., DICARA, L. V., AND CARROLL, B. J. Adrenalectomy-produced facilitation of Pavlovian conditioned cardiodecelerations in immobilized rats. *Psychophysiology*, 1977, *14*, 172–181.

WRIGHT, M. L. Operant conditioning of heart rate in the paralyzed rat. Unpublished master's thesis, McMaster University, 1974.

ZEINER, A. R., AND POLLAK, M. H. Bidirectional changes in digital skin temperature using biofeedback in a cold room. Paper presented to the annual meetings of the Society for Psychophysiological Research, San Diego, 1976.

8 Acquired Control of Peripheral Vascular Responses

WESLEY C. LYNCH AND UWE SCHURI

I. INTRODUCTION: SCOPE AND ISSUES

The present chapter addresses the question of whether or not experience can lead to a modification of peripheral vascular function. Under normal circumstances, the vascular system of most mammals is regulated by automatic mechanisms. At issue here is whether individuals can learn to modify this automatic regulation.

The experimental investigation of acquired vascular control has extended over most of the present century. Early studies begun in Pavlov's laboratory around 1918 (Bykov, 1957) took advantage of the newly developed methods of classical conditioning. Somewhat later, workers in this country extended the use of Pavlovian techniques to questions about underlying mechanisms. More recently, interest has developed in the application of operant conditioning (instrumental learning) procedures to the study of autonomic control. In 1938, Skinner became the first to apply operant methods to vascular responses. In the past 10 years, investigation of acquired vascular control has been stimulated further by a widespread interest in biofeedback. Early studies suggested that biofeedback was a particularly effective method for training subjects to regulate autonomically mediated responses.

This long-standing interest in vascular self-control has had two major sources: (1) the advantages of the peripheral vascular system as a model for the study of autonomic learning and (2) the hope that successful vascular self-control would provide a new therapy for peripheral vascular disease. As a model, the vascular system has the

WESLEY C. LYNCH · Rockefeller University, New York, New York. Present address: John B. Pierce Foundation Laboratory, 290 Congress Avenue, New Haven, Connecticut. UWE SCHURI · Rockefeller University, New York, New York. Present address: Max-Planck-Institut für Psychiatrie, München, West Germany. Financial support for this work was provided by the Spencer Foundation.

advantages that its physiological control is fairly well understood, that it is responsive to many stimuli, and that its activity varies over a wide normal range without danger to the organism. Moreover, several techniques exist for its quantitative study, and its bilateral symmetry provides an intrinsic control for those interested in response specificity.

The body of the present chapter consists of three sections. The first reviews the basic anatomy and physiology of the peripheral vasomotor system. Emphasis is placed on particular variables that may inadvertently affect vascular responses, making the results of psychological studies difficult to assess. The second and third sections review selected literature concerning classical conditioning and instrumental learning of vasomotor responses. Emphasis in these sections is on questions relevant to a general understanding of the acquired control of autonomic responses. The scope of the review is otherwise limited to research highlighting selected issues. In particular, a number of studies reported at recent meetings have been omitted because of methodological weaknesses and lack of peer review. Most of the biofeedback literature dealing exclusively with therapeutic applications has been omitted for similar reasons. A particular shortcoming in this area has been the lack of placebo controls (for a discussion, see Miller and Dworkin, 1974). The interested reader may find this clinical literature reviewed by Taub (1977).

Several important issues in the study of autonomic learning have already been addressed by investigations of the vasomotor system. The question of whether or not vasomotor learning is possible has been studied extensively, but only recently have investigators attempted to control for alternative explanations. In classical conditioning studies, for instance, results may be due to pseudoconditioning or adaptation, whereas in studies of instrumental learning, one may ask whether learning is truly instrumental or the result of prior classical conditioning or innate responses. A related question concerns the mechanisms responsible for acquired control. For example, given that learning is truly instrumental, how do reinforcement contingencies have their effects? Is learning applied directly to autonomic responses (direct mediation) or indirectly via somatic mediators? Available studies of instrumental learning have evaluated such factors as the involvement of skeletal muscles and respiration, the importance of amount of training, sensitivity of feedback, and subject age. Others have examined the ability of subjects to learn highly specific vasomotor responses. Classical conditioning studies have been concerned with questions about the type of effective unconditioned stimulus, the nature of the thermal environment necessary for learning, the role of subject awareness of CS–US (conditioned stimulus–unconditioned stimulus) contingencies, and the specificity and differentiation of conditionable responses.

One final comment is required regarding terminology. We have chosen to use the term *acquired control* in preference to the terms *self-control* or *self-regulation* wherever feasible in the following pages. We have done this to avoid the connotation that control emanates solely from within the organism and to emphasize instead that responses are regulated by their association with certain external consequences (e.g., feedback, rewards, or unconditional stimuli). All three terms are used in this latter sense. The terms *biofeedback, operant conditioning,* and *instrumental learning* (or performance) are also used interchangeably. Whereas *biofeedback* places emphasis on sensory consequences in determining control, *instrumental learning* and *operant conditioning* go somewhat further to suggest that other variables may also be important for learning, such as past experience and motivation.

II. ANATOMY AND FUNCTION OF THE PERIPHERAL VASOMOTOR SYSTEM

The purpose of this section is to provide an overview of the anatomy and normal function of the peripheral vascular system. Psychophysiologists should be aware of what kinds of stimuli can influence vascular function so that the results of their experiments can be properly interpreted. Details of methods used to study vasomotion are not reviewed here, although they are important and their relationships should be understood by anyone undertaking the study of peripheral circulation. For a discussion of methods, the reader is referred to Lader (1967), Weinman (1967), and Prouty and Hardy (1950). Cook (1974) has recently reviewed data concerning interpretation of the plethysmographic response. Burton (1954) has provided an excellent discussion of the relationships among various measures of circulatory activity.

The use of skin temperature measurement to assess peripheral blood flow does deserve brief mention here because many studies of acquired vascular control have used skin temperature for this purpose. Thauer (1965) has made it clear that this relationship is complex. Blood flow and temperature are not linearly related. At low flow rates, sizable temperature changes follow very small changes in blood flow. On the other hand, when flow rate is high, skin temperature may change very little even with relatively great changes in blood flow. Furthermore, temperature can be used as a measure of blood flow only when environmental temperature and skin-to-environment heat flow are kept constant. Ideally, these conditions are satisfied in studies of acquired control. Burton (1954) has made an additional point regarding the limitations of the use of skin temperature: "The great disadvantage of skin temperature measurements is the large thermal lag involved, so that where there is a brief though drastic change in the circulation, skin temperature gives a most inadequate and wrongly-timed indication of that change. For changes that are relatively constant for several minutes, however, skin temperature can give valuable indications of peripheral circulation" (p. 13). The source of this thermal lag is the inertia of the skin, which may vary considerably among individuals. Another contributing factor is the thermal lag of recording devices, such as thermistors of large mass.

A. Basic Anatomy and Physiology

The term *peripheral circulation* is meant to include the cutaneous circulation and those parts of the muscular circulation of the limbs that have traditionally been studied by volume plethysmography. According to this definition, the peripheral circulation includes two distinct regions, the skin and the skeletal muscle. There are two good reasons why these circulations should be considered as distinct. First, each plays a distinctive role in the normal regulation of body function. Second, the means by which control is exerted is somewhat different for each region. The primary function of the muscle circulation is to supply essential nutrients to the working muscle and to remove waste products and heat resulting from this work, while the skin circulation has the primary role of dissipating and conserving body heat in order to maintain a constant internal temperature. This constant temperature is required to ensure that cellular metabolic functions are carried out effectively. In designing psychological studies, it is important to keep in mind the distinction between these circulatory regions and their primary physiological roles. Furthermore, one should be aware that the responses of different skin areas are not always the same even though these areas may be close together. Thus, reactions of the palm of the hand, the dorsum of the hand, and the forearm may all vary independently under certain conditions (Abramson, 1967).

The complete circulation consists of a pump (the heart) and connecting vessels for the transport of blood to and from the tissues (arteries, arterioles, capillaries, venules, and veins). The functions of the circulation are numerous, but among the most important are those already mentioned: supplying nutrients and oxygen and removing waste products, carbon dioxide, and heat from cells and regulating the overall heat content of the body. To achieve these functions, several control systems have developed in man and other mammals that have the purpose of regulating the two primary circulatory variables: vascular *pressure* and volume *blood flow*. The means by which pressure and blood flow are regulated constitutes the study of cardiovascular control systems. Control systems may be described as feedback loops (reflexes, when controlled neurally) that are sensitive to some form of peripheral or central stimulation, are integrated by a local or central (neural) process, and have as outputs one or more cardiovascular effects. By far the most significant control systems affecting peripheral circulation are those that modulate the level of tonic activity in the resistance vessels (small arteries and arterioles) of skin and muscle. These are largely integrated in the CNS (central nervous system) at the level of the medulla oblongata, although neural levels both above and below this bulbar area can affect vascular tone independently or via modulation of the medullary output.

While a change in vascular tone instigated by a cardiovascular reflex may have a range of effects *in vivo*, the most common outcome (other influences remaining relatively constant) is a change in vascular resistance leading to a change in blood flow. In general, flow is decreased by an increase in vascular tone and increased by a reduction in tonic influences. This is true of both skin and muscle circulation, although muscle also has an active mechanism for vasodilation.

In addition to reflex control of circulation, there are local influences that may become important under certain conditions. Most significant of these, particularly in muscle, is the buildup of the metabolites of cellular energy exchange. Metabolites generally increase muscle blood flow and thereby act, through a process of negative feedback, to decrease the buildup. In skin, a similar effect upon heat exchange is initiated by the local effect of sweating. The sweat glands, when stimulated neurally, produce certain chemicals that, in turn, stimulate vasodilation and thereby increase blood flow. This increased blood flow both supplements the heat loss due to sweating and supplies needed water. The connection between sweating and blood flow, however, is sometimes severed by "emotional or psychic" influences. These may become particularly important in psychophysiological studies. In cases of so-called emotional sweating, the blood vessels of the skin may remain fully constricted while profuse sweating occurs. In such instances, sweating is most often localized on the palms of the hands, the soles of the feet, and the forehead in man.

The skin circulation is principally controlled by the constriction and dilation of arterioles (resistance vessels). However, skin blood flow can also be regulated (in certain regions) by a direct passage of blood through special vessels that communicate between the arterioles and venules. These vessels, known as *arterial–venous anastomoses,* or A–V shunts, are seen in thermoregulatory regions in several mammals. The rabbit's ear has served as a model for the study of A–V shunts; in man, they are located predominantly around the fingernail beds and on the palms of the hands. A–V shunts have a muscular wall and respond in a manner similar to the arterioles. However, they are able to produce greater variations in blood flow than the arterioles and thus appear to play an important role in thermoregulation. By rapidly increasing or decreasing blood flow by large amounts, these vessels provide for highly effective control of heat loss from the skin.

B. *Psychophysiologically Relevant Influences*

In addition to the general control of peripheral circulation outlined above, certain specific facts are important to the proper design and interpretation of biofeedback, instrumental learning, or classical conditioning studies. Available literature indicates a remarkable lack of appreciation of some of these facts.

Since most recent studies of acquired control have been restricted to the vasomotor responses of human digits, the subsequent discussion is mainly limited to this region. In most cases, however, the comments made also apply to the resting forearm, which has been studied extensively by workers interested in classical conditioning (Bykov, 1957; Figar, 1965). Some complications may arise because of the muscular circulation of the forearm and because the skin of this area has both vasoconstrictor and vasodilator nerve supply. If the forearm circulation is to be studied, special precautions should be taken, especially to eliminate the circulatory effects of muscle tension and relaxation.

1. *Normal Skin Temperature and Its Variation*

Because of the large number of factors that may affect finger temperature, it is virtually impossible or at least impractical to establish norms. Nevertheless, two facts seem well established: (1) the greatest variations in skin temperature occur in the extremities, particularly the hands and feet in man and the ears in rabbits (Greenfield, 1963), and (2) the difference in temperature between comparable areas on two sides of the body is normally extremely small (Allen, Barker, and Hines, 1946).

The temperature and motion of air in the surrounding environment is the most significant factor influencing skin temperature in the extremities of a healthy, resting adult. In air held at "standard" temperature and humidity (26°C and 40% relative humidity), the temperature of the fingers ordinarily lies within the range 32°–35°C. In general, as the ambient temperature varies from 22°–25°C, hand skin temperature ranges from 30°–35°C (Rothman, 1954). Of course, these are only average values, and an otherwise normal individual may fall outside of this range.

In studies of biofeedback or learning, the bilateral symmetry of temperature is particularly important. Clinically, assymetrical temperatures greater than 2°C provide excellent evidence of impaired circulation on one side (Allen *et al.*, 1946). Likewise, in studies of the effect of psychological variables, exclusive of general mediating factors (e.g., in studies of instrumental vasomotor learning), a lateralized change of temperature larger than 2°C provides excellent evidence of specific effects. (Maslach, Marshall, and Zimbardo, 1972, have reported such large lateralized effects of hypnosis, and Roberts, Schuler, Bacon, Zimmerman, and Patterson, 1975, have reported similar effects of operant conditioning combined with biofeedback.)

2. Respiratory Effects on Cutaneous Circulation

Sharpey-Schafer (1965) has pointed out that intrathoracic pressure changes produced by respiration result in alterations in circulation lasting for only a few seconds. However, certain maneuvers such as a sudden deep breath (Bolton, Carmichael, and Stürup, 1936), sustained changes in respiration rate (Engel and Chism, 1967), or voluntary hyperventilation (Richards, 1965) may produce longer lasting effects. Among the important respiratory maneuvers that may influence temperature in psychophysiological studies are the Valsalva maneuver, coughs, deep inspirations, positive pressure respiration, changes in respiration rate, and voluntary hyperventilation.

The Valsalva maneuver consists of a "sudden sustained rise in intrathoracic pressure" that results first in a decrease in the effective filling pressure of the right heart and is followed in about 6 sec by a reflex vasoconstriction that acts to compensate and increase venous return to the heart (Sharpey-Schafer, 1965). An effect similar to that produced by Valsalva results from coughing. The reflex constriction results in a reduction in peripheral pulse volume. Whether a sustained Valsalva can affect skin temperature in the hands is apparently not known.

A short-lasting stimulus that has a more significant and longer lasting effect on peripheral circulation is a single deep inspiration. This maneuver causes constriction of hand vessels (Bolton *et al.*, 1936), which is mediated by a spinal reflex (Gilliatt, 1948) having an unspecified afferent branch. According to Sharpey-Schafer (1965), "hand bloodflow shows a sharp decrease with the gasp and may not regain control levels for more than a minute" (p. 1183). Thus, there is sufficient time for a substantial decrease in skin temperature as well.

Hyperventilation (forced breathing) produces a lowering of blood levels of CO_2 and a resulting reflex response in the periphery. According to Sharpey-Schafer (1965), this reflex consists of constriction in skin and dilation in muscle vessels. (However, Richards, 1965, noted that not all workers have been able to demonstrate an increase in muscle blood flow.) The effects of sustained hyperventilation on peripheral circulation have been reviewed by Brown (1953), who noted that a reduction in blood flow and pulse amplitude in the skin is universally found whether measurements are made by calorimetric, plethysmographic, or direct observation methods.

Engel and Chism (1967) have studied the effect of slight but sustained changes in respiratory rate on finger pulse volume in eight subjects. When 11–29% rate changes were sustained for 10 min, finger pulse volume decreased regardless of whether respiration rate increased or decreased. However, the direction of rate change did influence the latency of vasoconstriction. Slow breathing produced vasoconstriction within 1 min, fast breathing produced its effect only after 4 min. Associated with the pulse volume changes, these investigators also found slight reductions in skin temperature. Unfortunately, no data were presented to eliminate the possibility that these results were influenced by changes in respiratory volume. Recently, Shean and Strange (1971) reported that any change in ongoing respiration produced rapid (4–8 sec) vasoconstriction, with deep breathing producing the greatest effect. Stern and Anschel (1968) have shown that sustained deep breathing can reduce pulse volume by as much as 35%.

3. *Effects of Exercise, Muscle Tension, and Posture on Cutaneous Circulation*

Muscular contraction has two distinct effects on peripheral circulation. Within the muscle, contraction instigates an increase in sympathetic discharge, a rise in blood pressure, an increase in temperature and an increase in metabolite concentration (Barcroft, 1963). In nonactive areas, including other muscles, viscera, and skin, a compensatory vasoconstriction occurs (Robinson, 1968, p. 539) in proportion to the severity of activity in other muscles, which serves to aid the heart in regulating blood flow in proportion to the needs of all tissues. McDowall (1956) stated, "The increase in resistance in some parts prevents any part of the increase in cardiac output being applied to them and, indeed, slightly reduces the flow through them" (p. 209). Neural impulses that would otherwise produce constriction in the active muscle as well are overpowered by the opposition of dilation influences arising predominantly from the metabolites of activity.

Independent of the circulatory effects of moving from one position to another, a particular posture itself may affect circulation. This is particularly true in the limbs, where slight unilateral changes in posture may produce significant changes in heat dissipation (Greenfield, 1963). Particularly important, in this regard, is the level of the limbs relative to the heart. Roddie (1955) has shown that in a seated subject, when one hand is raised above heart level, heat elimination in that hand is reduced, while if the same hand is positioned below heart level, the rate of heat elimination is increased. Both of these effects were seen with changes in hand position of about 10 cm. Such an effect suggests that in studies of lateralized circulatory responses, the limbs should be positioned symmetrically and should be maintained in position throughout any evaluation period. Goetz (1950) has demonstrated what appears to be generally true of limb posture, namely, that raising the limb above horizontal produces an increase in pulse volume and lowering the limb reduces pulse volume.

In addition to the direct effects of muscular tension and posture, certain indirect factors may influence peripheral circulation. Ganong (1971) noted that muscle blood flow may increase in anticipation of actual movement. This increase, in turn, might be accompanied by reduced circulation through skin vessels, although such an effect has apparently not been demonstrated. Furthermore, changes in limb position inevitably increase heat loss from the skin surface due to the relative motion of the air during movement (convection). Similarly, when a new position is assumed, radiation may be increased or decreased depending on the nature of nearby objects. An example is the case of increased heat loss when a hand is placed near the arm of a chair or of decreased heat loss (or actual heat gain) when the hand is placed near a warmer part of the body, such as the thigh. Likewise, it is true that radiation from the hands can be influenced if they are cupped or if the fingers are extended and separated.

4. Effects of Environment on Peripheral Circulation

Temperature and relative humidity are the two primary environmental determinants of variations in peripheral circulation. Of these, temperature is by far the most important, with the effect of humidity becoming significant mainly at air temperatures above that of the body core (Abramson, 1967).

It would be most appropriate within the context of the present paper to discuss the effects of relatively small changes in environmental temperature and humidity within a relatively "normal" temperature and humidity range. Unfortunately, most investigations of environmental effects have been concerned with extreme variations. For this reason, many generalizations about the physiological effects of environment on peripheral circulation must be interpreted with caution when small variations in the "normal" range are observed or are manipulated intentionally.

The direct application of heat or cold to the body surface leads, respectively, to an increase or a decrease in blood flow through surface vessels of the skin. The effect on blood flow is most pronounced in the most distal parts of the extremities, especially the fingertips and toes, and is gradually less pronounced proximally. Only in the case of extreme heating do the leg and forearm begin to increase their blood flow appreciably (Abramson, 1967). The fact that distal extremities are the areas most responsive to environment is by no means an accident of nature. A relatively large part of the body's total surface area is represented by the extremities, and the greatest blood flow per unit volume of tissue occurs in the distal phalanges of the fingers, decreasing progressively more proximally.

Although it is generally true that heat increases and cold decreases peripheral circulation, this relationship is not fixed. Recently, Lovallo and Zeiner (1975) reported the interesting finding that a cold pressor (ice water) may lead to either an increase or a decrease in digital blood volume depending on the level of initial vascular tonus. Adaptation to a cold (12°C) environment produced an increase in blood volume, whereas adaptation to the warm (32°C) environment produced a decrease.

When one area of the body is heated or cooled, other parts may react by changing in the same direction. Theoretically, any area capable of a vasomotor response may take part in such an indirect reaction. However, not all areas are equally reactive and "the magnitude of the reaction depends upon the size of the skin region which is heated or cooled" (Thauer, 1965, p. 1930). Moreover, "on cooling or heating a finger or hand, reactions take place in the other fingers of the same hand and in the opposite hand" (Thauer, 1965, p. 1929). Thauer (1965) referred to this response as a "consensual reaction." In addition to cooling and heating a specific skin area, indirect reactions can result from the intake of hot or cold foods. In this case, peripheral circulation is adjusted so as to maintain thermal equilibrium. Hot foods cause peripheral vasodilation, cold foods cause constriction.

Within the range of normal room temperature, humidity plays little or no role in heat dissipation. However, if air temperature is high, a change in humidity can have a profound effect, causing an increase in heat loss by evaporation as humidity falls or a decrease in heat loss and a rise in body temperature as humidity rises (Abramson, 1967).

C. Summary

A wide array of variables can influence the peripheral circulation. In general, these variables produce their effects by stimulating a regulatory system that has the normal function of maintaining the integrity of the organism's internal environment. Among the more important factors that must be considered in psychophysiological experiments are the normal values and ranges of variation in skin temperature or blood flow and the modifying effects of respiration, exercise, muscle tension, posture, environmental temperature, and humidity. From the psychophysiologist's viewpoint, two facts should be kept in mind: (1) these variables must be accounted for so that the effects of psychological manipulations are not confounded by them, and (2) variations in a particular component of the circulation resulting from such manipulations will normally be limited to those that do not disrupt regulatory control for any extended period of time, since such disruption would ultimately lead to physical harm of the organism.

III. CLASSICAL CONDITIONING OF VASOMOTOR RESPONSES

A. Is Vasomotor Classical Conditioning Possible?

The study of vasomotor classical conditioning was apparently begun by Tsitovich in Pavlov's laboratory about 1918 (Bykov, 1957). Somewhat later, such studies were extended by Bykov and his associates, Rogov (1929, see Rogov, 1951) and Pshonik (1936, see Pshonik, 1952). In addition to providing initial evidence for such conditioning, these workers used both hot and cold stimuli as USs and found that a variety of neutral stimuli could become associated with the effects of these thermal events, that vasoconstriction was more readily conditioned than vasodilation, that differential conditioning was possible, and that conditioning required 20–30 CS–US pairings in their situation. Furthermore, Bykov (1957) suggested that such conditioning might form the etiological basis for certain vascular diseases.

More recently, there have been several studies reported in the American literature dealing with such diverse questions as the role of vasomotor conditioning in semantic processes and the therapeutic application of peripheral vasomotor conditioning to vascular disease. In most cases, these studies have employed aversive rather than thermal USs and have otherwise extended the range of parameters investigated while remaining largely within the basic framework outlined by their Russian predecessors.

Menzies (1937, 1941) was the first in this country to study vasomotor conditioning. Using a thermopile, he recorded temperature changes in the hand and found that subjects acquired a vasoconstriction (temperature decrease) response when the CS consisted of either a light pattern or a compound stimulus consisting of light and the subject's own vocalization. Furthermore, he showed that such conditioning was possible when the US was a cold stimulus applied to the opposite hand and that conditioning was stable in 20–40 CS–US presentations. Shortly after Menzies's studies, Roessler and Brogden (1943) provided evidence for differential vasomotor conditioning in two subjects selected for responses to a shock US. Using a hand plethysmograph, they first showed that four subjects, selected on the basis of their vasomotor reactivity, were able to learn a vasoconstriction response to a compound auditory–verbal CS. Later, two of these four also learned a differentiation between different vocal CSs and still later between these same CSs repeated subvocally. Another early study (Gottschalk, 1946) showed that subjects were able to decrease both finger blood volume and pulse volume. The fact that only 4 of 10 subjects were successful suggested that there were individual differences in learning ability. Gottschalk observed that subjects having more labile vascular systems were somewhat superior.

Beginning with Shmavonian (1959), however, a number of workers interested in vascular conditioning raised questions about the interpretation of these early studies. Shmavonian questioned whether they were free from muscular and respiratory "artifacts" and whether the techniques for measuring vasomotion and the nature of the thermal environment were adequate for conditioning. More recently, investigators such as Stoltz (1965), Fromer (1963), and Gale and Stern (1968) have sought to determine whether early demonstrations represented true conditioning or some form of pseudoconditioning or sensitization. Stoltz (1965), in particular, found no difference between a conditioning group and two pseudoconditioning control groups. Gale and Stern (1968), on the other hand, demonstrated successful differential conditioning in excess of responses achieved by either of two sensitization control groups. With regard to the question of appropriate controls, some results by Furedy and associates are of interest. In a series of studies (for a review, see Furedy, 1974), they provided further demonstrations of differential vasomotor conditioning. Several experiments addressed to the role of CS–US contingencies in differential autonomic conditioning included a "truly random" control (random presentation of CS– and US) as demanded by Rescorla (1967) and a traditional "explicitly unpaired" control condition. The data showed that responses to CS+ exceeded those to CS–; there was no difference between control groups in response to CS–.

Furedy's results and those by Gale and Stern (1968) demonstrate that US presentation alone (sensitization), as well as "explicitly unpaired" and "truly random" control conditions (pseudoconditioning), is less effective than consistent pairing of CS+ and US in establishing a reliable vasomotor response. Thus, it is clear that vasomotor classical conditioning is possible, but it remains uncertain what variables might mediate this conditioning. In fact, we are far from understanding exactly how such conditioning is achieved. What, for instance, is the role of somatic or cognitive factors? Are the vasomotor responses the result of generalized emotional conditioning?

B. How Is Vasomotor Classical Conditioning Achieved?

While the earliest studies took an uncritical view of how vasomotor conditioning was achieved, several more recent studies have analyzed this question in detail. In particular, interest has been focused on the possibility that conditioned vasomotor responses are secondary to skeletal or respiratory responses that have specific vascular consequences. As an alternative, it has been suggested that vasomotor activity merely represents one component of a learned pattern of autonomic responses that results from generalized emotional conditioning.

The question of respiratory or skeletal mediation has received little direct attention despite its acknowledged importance. Shmavonian (1959) first reviewed the detailed issues in the introduction to his "methodological" study, but his own controls were inadequate. While he monitored respiration rate, he made no attempt to pace respiration and, in fact, reported considerable variability in respiration rate, which he stated showed "no tendency toward conditioning" (p. 318). His statement, however, was not substantiated statistically. Furthermore, he made no attempt to measure or control respiration depth, although Bolton et al. (1936), several years earlier, had demonstrated the importance of this variable in producing a long-lasting vasoconstrictive effect. Stoltz (1965), who paced respiration in her subjects, was unable to demonstrate conditioning when she compared an experimental group with pseudoconditioning controls. She concluded that earlier results "may be artifactual, produced by failure to control for breathing, pseudoconditioning or both" (p. 182). The role of respiration in vasomotor conditioning is yet to be resolved.

Aside from the question of whether vasomotor conditioning is mediated directly by the autonomic nervous system or indirectly by some intervening response, there is the question of whether vascular reactions are specifically conditioned or are part of a more general emotional reaction pattern. A related question is whether nonemotional (although effective) USs can maintain a conditioned vasomotor response.

At present, there is apparently no clear evidence regarding the specificity of vasomotor conditioning. Shmavonian (1959) recorded heart rate during such conditioning and found no correlation with vasomotor responses. He noted, however, that he had previously failed to achieve discrete vascular conditioning with (nonemotional) thermal stimuli and concluded that the lack of correlation between heart rate and vasomotion did not rule out the possibility that vascular conditioning is part of a "pattern response" to an emotional US. In an earlier study, Harwood (1953) had failed to condition vasoconstriction using a mild electric shock US and concluded that a situation involving "greater urgency" was required before such conditioning could be demonstrated. In a study that is rare among those in the recent American literature, Stoltz (1965) attempted conditioning using a US other than shock. Despite the fact that the 95-dB buzzer employed was considered aversive by several subjects, Stoltz failed to demonstrate conditioning in excess of responses apparent in a pseudoconditioning control group. Work by Gale and Stern (1968) also suggests the importance of an "urgent" US. Although able to demonstrate true conditioning in excess of responses shown by sensitization control groups, these investigators reported an "adaptation" of pulse amplitude in all groups that persisted throughout training. Thus, despite the fact the CS–US pairing slowed the rate at which the vascular orienting response diminished over trials, it nevertheless approached zero in all groups. Possibly, with sufficient training, the true conditioning group might have reached a nonzero asymptote. Also, Miller (personal communication, 1977) has noted that successful conditioning may require more widely distributed trials (1–3/day) than have commonly been employed (20–60/hr). Thus, while it is by no means certain that vascular conditioning is impossible with an emotionally neutral US, recent evidence suggests that such stimuli are less effective than strong noxious stimuli.

One final group of studies relevant to the question of how vascular conditioning is mediated evaluated the role of cognitive factors. Shean (1968) first pointed out that stimulus awareness may play a central role in the establishment of vascular conditioned responses. In four groups of subjects, the level of awareness of CS–US contingencies was varied during aversive conditioning and extinction. It was found that only in those groups aware of contingencies was conditioning of vasoconstriction apparent; furthermore, in those aware that the shock US would no longer be presented, extinction often occurred in a single extinction trial. Baer and Fuhrer (1970) verified these results in a study employing differential trace conditioning. Of 20 conditioned subjects, 11 were rated as able to verbalize contingencies and 9 were rated as unable to verbalize on the basis of postconditioning interviews. When the digital vasomotor (pulse volume) responses of each group to CS+ and CS− were compared, a significant differentiation was apparent only in the "verbalizers." Raskin (1969) also noted parenthetically in discussing his results on semantic conditioning of GSR and finger vasomotion that, "the few Ss who were unable to identify any of the CS words showed no indication of conditioning" (p. 75). He concluded that implicit verbalizations may, therefore, mediate the production of conditioned responses.

The above evidence strongly suggests that awareness of reinforcement contingency may be necessary for successful vascular classical conditioning. More remarkable, however, is the possibility that such awareness may be *sufficient* for "conditioning" and/or "extinction." In the study by Shean (1968), for example, instructions that shocks would no longer be given resulted in immediate "extinction" of the vascular response. To explain the role of awareness in human differential autonomic classical conditioning, Dawson and Furedy (1976) proposed a "necessary-gate" hypothesis, according to which awareness of the CS–US relationship is necessary but not sufficient, with awareness having a gate but not an analogue effect on conditioning. The latter implies an all-or-nothing operation, so that there is no continuous increase in conditioning with increasing awareness. However, this hypothesis needs to be substantiated by further data on the vasomotor response system, and as Dawson and Furedy (1976) have noted, it has to be determined whether this hypothesis holds for single-cue conditioning as well as for differential conditioning. An analysis of the relationship between awareness and learning in logical terms may also prove to be necessary before the role of awareness is clearly appreciated (e.g., Spielberger and DeNike, 1966). Possibly, awareness affects conditioning by way of its effect on motivation.

C. What Is the Role of the Thermoregulatory State in Vascular Classical Conditioning?

Studies of man (Shmavonian, 1959; Teichner and Levine, 1968) and rabbit (Teichner, Beals, and Giambalvo, 1973) have demonstrated an interdependence of thermoregulatory and conditioned vasomotor responses. In his classic study, Shmavonian found that while conditioning of vasoconstriction was possible in a hand maintained at neutral or moderately cold temperature, no conditioning was apparent when the hand was kept in an extremely cold environment. He suggested that Harwood's (1953) failure to replicate earlier results was due to the low temperatures at which training was carried out. Teichner and his associates have further clarified the importance of environmental temperature in vasomotor conditioning studies. In human subjects, Teichner and Levine (1968) found that individuals given CS-shock conditioning trials during cold exposure developed a conditioned response of vasodilation, while individuals adapted to a hot environment developed vasoconstriction responses during conditioning trials. In an extension of this finding, vascular responses of the ears of rabbits were studied. It was found that whereas animals conditioned in an apparently thermoneutral environment (18–24°C) developed vasoconstriction as the predominant reaction, animals conditioned in warmer or colder environments tended to develop vasodilation reactions. Furthermore, the response elicited following conditioning was specific not to the conditioning environment but to the thermal environment present at the time of testing.

It is apparent from these results that the proper control of the thermal environment will contribute to a reduction in variability of results among laboratories. Furthermore, it seems reasonable to suppose that a more detailed study of the effect of environmental conditions on vascular conditioned responses may lead to a clearer understanding of how such responses are mediated. As Teichner et al. (1973) pointed out, "what is conditioned is not a specific qualitative event, but rather a tendency for change, the direction of which depends upon the state of the physiological system at the time that the response is elicited" (p. 243).

D. Conclusion

The review of vasomotor classical conditioning studies leads to the conclusion that while such conditioning is clearly possible, it is uncertain by what mechanism it operates. Subjective awareness of contingencies, the need for emotional or "urgent" unconditioned stimuli, and the effect of variations in the thermal environment all suggest that what is conditioned is not the peripheral vasomotor response *per se* but some antecedent "central" response that may have peripheral vascular effects as only one manifestation.

IV. Instrumental Control of Vasomotor Responses

A. Is Instrumental Vasomotor Learning Possible?

Before we review evidence on the instrumental control of vascular responses, a few comments should be made concerning two different lines of work that are relevant to the question of the feasibility of operant vasomotor learning. One group of investigators, including the present authors, have been mainly interested in the demonstration of vasomotor learning *without somatic mediation.* Their studies have included controls for muscular tension and respiratory responses that were regarded as "artifacts." With regard to the question asked in this section, they have distinguished between the demonstration of instrumental control in general (which may involve somatic mediation) and the demonstration of instrumental control without intervening somatic responses. We shall refer to the latter as "direct" control, meaning that control is exerted directly over the autonomic nervous system and does not *depend* on somatic responses, although these *may* occur. A factor that should be kept in mind in the reading of this section is that not all investigators have been equally concerned about controlling for such somatic "artifacts." Some workers have not considered somatic mediation as artifactual at all.

In one sense, vasomotor responses that occur as a result of hyperventilation or extreme muscular exertion are of more interest to pulmonary or exercise physiologists than to psychologists. However, it is certainly of interest to psychologists if, for example, conditioning affects the autonomic nervous system *exclusively* through its effects on respiration or muscle tension. While it may or may not be true that the autonomic nervous system is directly amenable to modification according to the contingencies of reinforcement (feedback), it certainly is true that progress toward understanding how vasomotor control is achieved will be more rapid if psychologists remain aware of the various possibilities.

1. Reinforcement of Nonspecific Responses

Until about 1965, instrumental or operant control of peripheral vascular responses was considered impossible. As Miller (1969) pointed out, there was a strong traditional bias against the possibility of instrumental autonomic conditioning. In fact, the autonomic-somatic distinction reflected the conviction that *autonomic* effector actions were truly *autonomous*. Skinner (1938) was apparently the first to seriously consider reinforcing emitted vascular responses. Paradoxically, the negative results of an experiment designed to reward vasoconstriction, by his colleague E. B. Delabarre, may have delayed further attempts to condition vascular responses for nearly three decades.

As late as 1968, Katkin and Murray could cite only three additional reports of instrumental vasomotor conditioning. Of these, two were brief reports from a single laboratory (Snyder and Noble, 1965, 1966); the other was a report of avoidance learning (Lisina, 1965), which the authors interpreted as being mediated by skeletal or respiratory responses. An early study by Kimmel and Kimmel (1967) was apparently overlooked by Katkin and Murray; nevertheless, it is fair to conclude that most work in this area has occurred in the past 10 years.

The first report of successful instrumental vasomotor conditioning in this country (Snyder and Noble, 1965, 1966) appeared in print in 1968. In this study, spontaneous vasoconstriction responses were recorded as short-duration reductions in finger blood volume. Subjects were provided with a visual cue that indicated each time that a criterion vasoconstriction occurred. Following a baseline period during which the criterion was established, subjects were instructed to turn on the visual (feedback) cue as frequently as possible. Responses associated with skeletal muscular events were not reinforced by cue presentation. When compared with a control group receiving noncontingent feedback, these subjects showed a significant increase in the frequency of vasoconstriction responses. Two recent experiments by Stern and Pavloski (1974) support these results. In both studies, efforts were made to rule out skeletal artifacts, although a questionnaire suggested that bodily movement might have been involved in successful performance.

Numerous other studies have elaborated on this general theme. Kimmel and Kimmel (1967), in a seldom-cited study, found that when unelicited vasoconstrictions were reinforced by visual feedback, the vasoconstriction frequency increased by about 15% over resting levels in a contingent group but by only 5% in a noncontingent group. While the GSR also increased in frequency in the contingent group, the change was smaller and more variable, suggesting some specificity of the effects of reinforcement even in a short 20-min training period.

Some of the most impressive data on vasomotor learning have been published by Taub and his associates. In contrast to the above-cited authors, Taub used temperature instead of the plethysmographic response as an index of vasomotion. By recording skin temperature on the dorsum of the hand and providing either continuous or discrete-step visual feedback, Taub has trained subjects to regulate skin temperature instrumentally. In a group of subjects first discussed by Taub and Emurian (1972), and more recently appearing in published form (Taub and Emurian, 1976), 19 of 21 individuals learned increases or decreases in hand temperature in four to six training sessions of 15 min each. A feedback light was provided that increased or decreased in brightness with corresponding changes in temperature. For the 21 subjects, a mean temperature change in the correct direction of 1.2°C (2.2°F) was recorded during Sessions 4 through 6, which included 51 individual runs. The largest temperature change recorded was 3.6°C (6.5°F). More recent work with these and other subjects has been summarized by Taub (1977). Among his most impressive findings are that (1) most subjects learn with as little as one hour of practice; (2) many subjects can increase or decrease temperature at "will" and can transfer the body locus of temperature change with little decrement in performance once training is complete; (3) feedback is needed only during the early stages of training; (4) with extended practice, the locus of control is gradually reduced to the location of the transducer responsible for feedback; (5) retention is nearly perfect after four to five months without practice; (6) control of variations in temperature as great as 9.86°C (17.75°F) are possible; and (7) despite the apparent robustness of these effects, an impersonal, skeptical, or uncertain attitude on the part of the experimenter can almost completely nullify the effects of training! This last point is illustrated by a replication of the original study, in which only 2 of 22 subjects were able to learn temperature control.

An initial experiment in our laboratory designed to replicate the procedures of Taub and Emurian (1972) was also largely a failure. In this study, five volunteers were given training that included establishing baseline stability before beginning practice, following each minute of practice with a 10-sec rest period, and providing visual feedback (a

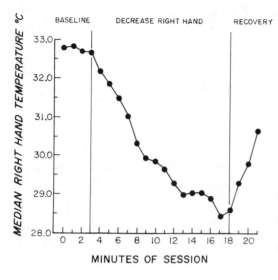

FIGURE 1. Median temperature of the fingertip of one untrained individual for 18 test sessions. During each session instructions were to relax for 3 min (baseline), to decrease right-hand temperature for the next 15 min, and to relax for the final 3 min (recovery).

meter movement) for changes in temperature. Each subject was given nine daily 15-min practice sessions with instructions to either increase (three subjects) or decrease (two subjects) the temperature of the index fingertip of one hand. After these nine sessions, the direction of temperature change was reversed. Four of the five subjects showed reliable decreases from baseline temperature during the initial nine sessions (regardless of instructions), which persisted following reversal. The one subject who was able to increase temperature from baseline during the initial two sessions asked to be dismissed because of dissatisfaction with her performance. Although the tendency to decrease temperature was greater during "decrease" than during "increase" sessions, these preliminary results were considerably different than Taub's.

Discussions with Taub and other workers suggested that our difficulties might depend on subject selection procedures. We reasoned that some unknown bias might have caused others to select particularly talented subjects or us to select untalented ones. On the basis of this notion, we devised a procedure to screen prospective subjects. Approximately 100 student volunteers were recruited from introductory biology and psychology classes at a nearby university. A portable electronic thermometer was used to record finger skin temperature and provide visual feedback from a meter sensitive to 0.05°C. Each individual sat quietly for a 3-min stability period, followed by a 5-min attempt at finger cooling. Of 14 subjects who succeeded at this task on the first try, 3 were able to repeat the decrease during a second test and also reversed this decrease on command. When brought to our laboratory for further study, only 1 of the 3 was able to demonstrate skin temperature control repeatedly.

The stability of this subject's control of skin temperature is indicated by results in Figure 1, which shows the median response for 18 practice sessions of 15 min each. During each session, the instruction to "decrease" was followed by a gradual drop in temperature averaging 4.2°C. The stability of temperature prior to the decrease and its subsequent recovery demonstrate the instrumental nature of the response. Clearly, some individuals can "voluntarily" regulate skin temperature even without prior training. This subject succeeded in cooling his finger on every occasion tested, regardless of distractions caused by observers or equipment used for monitoring other physiological activity. Close observations and electromyographic (EMG) recordings revealed no movements, and pneumograph recordings showed no systematic changes in respiration frequency or volume. Furthermore, recordings of digital blood velocity, by the use of a Doppler flow detector (see Miller, 1975), indicated that a sharp reduction of pulse volume and blood flow occurred prior to temperature decreases. In contrast to this remarkable ability, we were discouraged to find that further learning and transfer were nearly absent. An analysis of the magnitude of temperature decrease over sessions showed no trend toward improvement. Moreover, attempts to train finger warming were also unsuccessful.

Extensive practice proved moderately successful with one individual in this early phase of our work. Figure 2 shows the results from

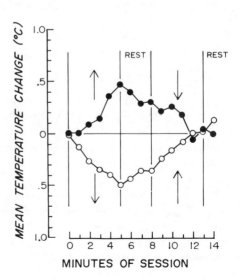

FIGURE 2. Mean temperature change of the fingertip in one individual given extensive prior training. Filled circles show data for eight test sessions following training when instructions were to increase (↑) then decrease (↓) finger temperature. Open circles show data from seven sessions when these directions were reversed. Rest intervals followed each 5-min practice period.

this subject, who received more than 30 daily practice sessions prior to collection of these data. During each session a 3-min baseline stability period was followed by a 5-min practice period, during which the subject attempted to change the temperature of one finger either upward or downward (arrows). A 3-min rest interval was followed by a second practice period, during which the direction was reversed. Temperature feedback was provided by a meter and a variable frequency tone. Whether instructions were to increase or decrease temperature during the first period was decided on a random basis. Figure 2 shows the mean temperature change for seven test days when instructions were to decrease and then increase temperature and eight test days when instructions were to increase and then decrease temperature. As can be seen, a temperature change of 0.5°C in each direction was achieved regardless of direction. While these data were very encouraging in light of our own earlier results, they were quite unimpressive when compared to reports from Taub's laboratory. Taub and Emurian (1972) reported changes of 1.2°C in either direction in most subjects given only four 15-min practice sessions.

A recent article by Surwit, Shapiro, and Feld (1976) indicates that other investigators have also had difficulties demonstrating bidirectional learning. By reinforcing digital skin temperature changes via feedback and monetary rewards, these workers trained 8 subjects to voluntarily vasoconstrict and 16 subjects to vasodilate. The training started after two baseline days and lasted either five or nine sessions. Summarizing their data, the authors concluded "that simply leaving subjects alone during long baseline periods seems to be as effective as feedback training in producing vasodilation" (p. 247). On the other hand, their subjects were able to voluntarily control digital vasoconstriction as indicated by decreasing hand temperature over trials within sessions. There was no evidence for an across-sessions training effect.

The results reviewed so far raise the question of how specific the reported vasomotor changes (if obtained) may become. Surwit *et al.* (1976) reported that although their "increase" and "decrease" groups showed significantly different temperatures, feedback did not result in group differences in heart rate or respiration rate. In the Kimmel and Kimmel (1967) study, on the other hand, both the GSR and the plethysmographic responses (reinforced) showed differential effects in a very short training period. It is especially interesting to compare those vasomotor changes on which the reinforcement was contingent with vasomotor changes in other locations. Again, the data are conflicting; Taub (1977) reported that with extended practice, the locus of control was gradually reduced to the location of the transducer responsible for feedback. In contrast, Surwit *et al.* (1976) measured bilateral changes of hand temperature despite the fact that feedback was given from only one hand.

2. Reinforcement of Differential Changes

Even though vasomotor responses may not become specific to the location of feedback, this does not mean that specific responses cannot be achieved. Several recent studies have been designed specifically to examine the question of response specificity. In these experiments, reinforcement was contingent upon differences of vasomotor activity from two locations. Such studies are especially important with regard to the question of *direct* vasomotor learning because they provide control for general mediating factors such as respiration. Using this paradigm, Roberts and his associates have reported remarkable effects resulting from the use of feedback plus hypnosis (Roberts, Kewman, and MacDonald, 1973) or feedback alone (Roberts, Schuler, Bacon, Zimmerman, and Patterson, 1975).

In the first of these studies, earlier work demonstrating one-hand (Hadfield, Oxon, and Edin, 1920) or two-hand differential changes in skin temperature (Maslach, Marshall, and Zimbardo, 1972) during hypnosis was extended by the addition of auditory feedback of the temperature difference between both hands. Of six subjects receiving from five to nine 1-hr training sessions, four showed statistically reliable differential temperature changes in the instructed direction. Temperature differences averaged about 1.5°C during the last three training sessions.

In a more recent study, Roberts *et al.* (1975) dispensed with hypnosis but retained the auditory feedback. Each of 14 subjects received 16 training sessions in which two-hand temperature differences were reinforced by auditory feedback. The results of this experiment were similar to those reported earlier (Roberts *et al.*, 1973).

The point of departure for studies such as those just described was a remarkable study of paralyzed rats reported in 1968 by DiCara and Miller. Two groups of six rats each were trained to independently vary the vasomotor responses of their ears. Both groups were paralyzed during training by D-tubocurarine and received reward for success from electrical stimulation of the medial forebrain bundle (the "reward center"). One group was rewarded for dilation of the left and constriction of the right ear, the other for the reverse direction. In a single training session lasting about 150 min, both groups learned to make appropriate and statistically reliable differential responses. Furthermore, the changes in the ears were not correlated with differential vasomotion in the paws, and both groups showed comparable changes in heart rate, core temperature, and tail blood volume. Unfortunately, no independent replication of this important study has yet been reported. It may be significant that Miller and his associates have had difficulties replicating similar experiments with curarized rats in which heart-rate and intestinal motility were rewarded (Miller and Dworkin, 1974).

A study similar to that by DiCara and Miller, employing human subjects, has recently been reported by Steptoe, Mathews, and Johnston (1974). Individuals were trained to control differences in temperature between their earlobes with the aid of auditory and visual feedback. Eight subjects took part in six training periods, the task being to warm one ear relative to the other without movement or muscle tension. Movement and facial muscle tension were monitored by closed-circuit TV and by EMG recording. While the magnitude of temperature changes was relatively small (0.3°C), reliable differences in the correct direction were nevertheless apparent by the final session. Movement and EMG activity were uncorrelated with success, although tension on one side of the face was associated with an incorrect vasoconstriction of that side in the first training periods.

A number of studies carried out in our laboratory from 1974 onward were concerned with the problem of differential temperature control. Blood flow of the fingertip (as reflected by temperature) was most commonly measured because of its variability and ease of recording. Experiments with individuals of different ages were designed to replicate the methods (and ideally the results) of Roberts and his co-workers.

In the first of these experiments, four subjects were trained by a procedure similar to that used by Roberts *et al.* (1973); however, our subjects were not hypnotized and they received visual and auditory feedback. Like Roberts, we gave specific feedback for temperature differences between the two hands, alternated the direction of this difference over three 8-min practice sessions each day, and provided directional auditory feedback and contingent money rewards. The auditory feedback device was built as an exact replica of the one employed by Roberts. Despite the similarities of procedure, we found no significant control of differential skin temperature, even though our subjects received four times as much training as did Roberts's.

Following a brief visit to the University of Minnesota Laboratory of Professor Roberts, another experiment was conducted according to the procedure described by Roberts *et al.* (1975). Eight subjects were given eight feedback training sessions, each consisting of three 8-min practice periods. Both visual and auditory feedback were provided for changes in the temperature difference between the two hands, and the direction of the required change was reversed at the end of each 8-min period. To our consternation, this experiment, like the previous one, was a virtual failure! Whereas Roberts *et al.* (1975) had reported a mean successful performance for all 14 of their subjects of 0.82°C by the eighth training session, our *best* individual subject produced a change of only 0.63°C during her *best* session! Computing our data by a method identical to that used by Roberts, the eighth session score for all eight subjects was 0.16°C. Our success at demonstrating differential temperature control was clearly limited.

For several reasons, which will be discussed later, we thought that children might be better vasomotor learners. In an experiment with four children aged 4 to 11 years (Lynch, Hama, Kohn, and Miller, 1976), three subjects were able to learn highly specific responses. When given feedback for temperature differences and a contingent money reward for success, these children were also able to demonstrate reliable control of the temperature difference between their two hands. One subject eventually learned to control the temperature difference between two fingers on one hand.

Taken altogether, work over the past 10 years demonstrates beyond any doubt that instrumental vasomotor learning is possible. It is even possible to learn highly specific responses, which suggests that vasomotor learning may be possible without generalized somatic mediation. Data reported from different laboratories, however, are highly variable with regard to the number of learners and the magnitude and direction of changes. Both Taub and Roberts (personal communication, 1974) have had some trouble repeating their own earlier results. Surwit *et al.* (1976) and our group (Lynch, Hama, Kohn, and Miller, 1974) have found fewer learners and generally have had more difficulty training vasodilation than vasoconstriction. Thus, there remains the question of what variables are responsible for these differences.

B. Significant Variables in Instrumental Vasomotor Learning

During the three years of our work on instrumental control, one of our main goals was to determine the most effective conditions for promoting vasomotor learning. The fact that nearly all of our early results were much less impressive than those that we were trying to replicate motivated us to search for critical variables that had been overlooked. Published reports from the laboratories of Taub and Roberts provided few clues about such variables, so that we received much of our early detailed information about their procedures through personal communications and visits to their respective laboratories. As a result, by the fall of 1974, we instituted several changes in procedure that we hoped would improve our results. Our discussions suggested that the *attitude of the experimenter* and the *atmosphere of the experimental room* were important factors. To deal with these, we moved to a new laboratory and modified aspects of our equipment and methods.

Whereas previously the experiment was run in a room housing the recording equipment and the experimenter, our new laboratory included a spacious and quiet room isolated from the equipment and the experimenter (except for closed-circuit TV). In all subsequent experiments, the subjects reclined on a comfortable bed with their heads raised slightly. The room was temperature-regulated and was kept dimly lit. Music of the subject's choice was available at all times between training periods. A new visual feedback display replaced the one we had been using. It was suggested that the *type or sensitivity of feedback* might be another important determinant of our results. A digital voltmeter allowed us to provide feedback for temperature changes as slight as 0.01°C, whereas previously changes no smaller than 0.05°C were discriminable. Finally, a new research assistant joined our group who was specifically selected to meet certain criteria suggested by Taub (see Taub, 1977, regarding the "person factor"). She was warm and friendly with subjects and always expressed confidence in their abilities to succeed; she remained informal but was always very efficient in her duties. Unfortunately, these changes did not improve our results.

We also tested the importance of *feedback sensitivity*. Four subjects assigned to each of three groups received feedback at one of three sensitivities. The low-sensitivity group got digital visual feedback discriminable to 0.1°C, which was accompanied by an auditory frequency change of 44 Hz. Medium- and high-sensitivity groups got feedback that was twice or four times this sensitive. In addition to the measurement of skin temperature differences between the two hands, the *subjective motivation* of each group was also evaluated. Subjects were asked to rate their motivation before and after sessions on 7-point scales by answering several questions, such as: "How much do you feel like participating today?" (before each session). Each group was given six daily practice sessions like those in the preceding study. Again, the task was to control the temperature difference between the two hands. For each session, the subjects received a fixed fee of one dollar plus a contingent reward for success of 25 cents/degree/min.

Figure 3 shows the group mean change in temperature differences for all groups, positive values representing correct changes. As can be seen, none of the three groups acquired significant instrumental control of differential skin temperature. Furthermore, statistical analysis of the individual performance revealed no individual who was able to regulate skin temperature. An interesting finding based on the rating scale data was that motivation in all three groups declined over training sessions. This result suggests that it may be important to promote learning in early training sessions in order to avoid the adverse effects of declining motivation.

In subsequent studies, we investigated the usefulness of the *escape–avoidance paradigm* for teaching subjects to control reductions in finger pulse amplitude in hopes that once a vasomotor reaction was elicited, it might be sustained by feedback. We initially found that in the absence of feedback, a stimulus that was described as signaling impending shock reliably elicited a pulse amplitude decrease despite the fact that shock never occurred. In a further study, one group of four subjects received a visual (oscilloscope) display of pulse amplitude and instructions to try to enhance the reduction in pulse amplitude elicited by the shock signal. A second group of four received similar instructions but simply observed an unmodulated sine wave display (no feedback). Each group participated in eight sessions of 10 practice trials each (80 trials). Both the feedback and the no-feedback groups produced significant reductions in pulse ampli-

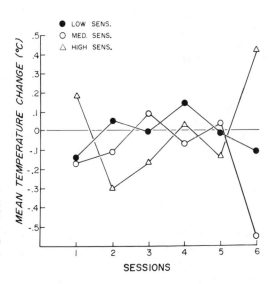

FIGURE 3. Mean change in the temperature difference between two hands for three groups of four subjects. Each group received feedback, for temperature differences, at one of three sensitivities (see text for details).

tude over the 10 sessions, according to a sign test ($p = .004$); there was no difference between groups. Apparently feedback did not enhance the ability to reduce pulse amplitude.

As mentioned earlier, our studies of children were begun because we believed that they might be better vasomotor learners than adults. They are known to be superior at learning some motor skills and language, they are rather easily motivated to learn, and they tend to attempt the solution to a new problem without questioning its feasibility. We reasoned that such factors as lack of motivation or belief in the feasibility of vasomotor learning might have hindered the performance of our adult subjects.

In an initial experiment, six children ranging in age from 3 to 11 years were given feedback training to increase and decrease the temperature of one hand. Feedback was provided by the movement of a meter needle. All subjects received six 15-min sessions in which they attempted to decrease the temperature of one finger, followed by six sessions of increase training. In remarkable contrast to the adults, all six children were able to increase finger temperature, and four of them were able to decrease temperature. Tests of the three best subjects showed no correlation between changes in respiration and temperature. In a subsequent study (Lynch, Hama, Kohn, and Miller, 1976), three other children ranging from 9 to 11 years were able to learn highly specific responses (see p. 39).

These preliminary studies suggested the need for a more direct *comparison of children and adults.* If we could demonstrate a reliable difference between adults and children, it might provide clues about how instrumental vasomotor control was achieved. In order to follow up our earlier work with children, we carried out an extensive study of 16 individuals. Since this work has not previously been published, a detailed description of it is presented here. Our main purpose was to examine the role of age in the acquisition of specific instrumental control of the temperature difference between the two hands. In addition, we wanted to evaluate further the significance of extended training and to analyze, in greater detail, the individual abilities of those subjects who were especially proficient.

1. Method

Subjects were eight children and eight of their parents. Parent-child pairs were selected as a partial control for background, social class, and so forth. The parent group consisted of seven females and one male ranging in age from 30 to 42 years (mean 36.1). The children were five females and three males ranging from 10 to 12 years (mean

10.9). The experimental room and the equipment were the same as those already mentioned. Communication with the subject was via intercom; however, the subject was observed constantly over closed-circuit TV. Room temperature was 24 ± 1°C. Skin temperature of the middle finger of each hand and respiration were recorded continuously during each session. Feedback for the difference in temperature between the two hands was both visual and auditory. In addition, a counter provided a running indication of earned money. This counter was driven at a rate of 20 cents/degree/min when the correct response was made.

Prior to the first session, instructions were given concerning the task, the nature of the feedback, and the method of payment. Each subsequent session consisted of a 5-min baseline, two 8-min trials, and a 5-min recovery. During the baseline period, the subject was instructed to relax and was given the option of listening to music. Following the baseline period, the first trial began immediately, the task being to warm one hand and cool the other. After 8 min the direction of the temperature change was reversed, and practice continued for another 8 min. The hand warmed first was randomly selected, with the stipulation that each hand was first an equal number of times. All 16 subjects initially completed 8 sessions run on alternate weekdays. An additional 4 sessions were completed after a one-month hiatus, bringing the total number of sessions to 12.

2. Results

In order to determine whether children and adults differed significantly in their ability to control skin temperature, we performed a two-way analysis of variance (Winer, 1971, p. 302). Data consisted of a general mean score (G-mean) computed for each subject and each session. We obtained the score by determining the change in temperature difference from the beginning to the end of each 8-min trial and then computing a mean for both trials of that session. The change within each trial consisted of the mean temperature difference during the last 5 min of practice minus the difference during the last baseline minute. A G-mean was positive if the overall change was correct and negative if it was incorrect.

3. Group Data

Figure 4 shows the mean temperature change for the two groups across sessions. There was a significant group difference ($p < .025$), and as the figure indicates, the difference was due to the superior

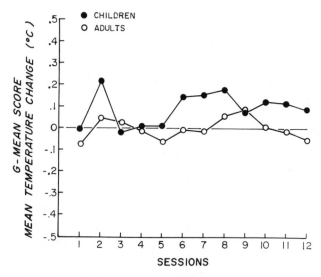

Figure 4. Mean change in the temperature difference between two hands for two groups of eight subjects each. Filled circles represent data for children; open circles show data for their parents—"adults" (see text for details).

ability of the children. While the G-mean scores for the adults remained consistently near or below zero, those for the children were generally in the correct direction.

The lack of a significant sessions effect or a group x sessions interaction indicated that the ability of neither group changed over sessions. This conclusion was verified further by an analysis of data for the individual sessions of each group. T tests comparing the change in each session with a hypothetical mean change of zero showed that only the children were successful as a group during only 3 of the 12 sessions (2, 6, and 7:$p < .05$).

4. Individual Performance

In order to test the reliability of individual temperature changes over sessions, t tests were carried out in which the mean change was compared to a hypothetical mean of zero. Among the eight children, three showed significant positive deviations ($p < .02$), whereas only one adult deviated significantly from zero. In the latter case the direction of the deviation was incorrect ($p < .02$).

Subject A.G. So that we could determine whether reliable performance could be maintained during further training, one especially talented child (A.G., a female, aged 10) received 3 additional sessions.

The results of an analysis of her performance over all 15 sessions indicated highly reliable temperature changes in the instructed direction ($p < 0.002$).

The exceptional talent of subject A.G. was precisely what we had hoped to find so that we could carefully analyze performance. No movements were apparent from TV observation, and although respiration was irregular during practice periods, it did not vary according to the direction of temperature change. To aid in our analysis, a small one-way mirror was installed in the wall of the experimental room near the subject's left side; later, EMG activity was recorded from both arms. During Sessions 16 and 17, A.G. was merely observed while performing as usual. No attempt was made to modify the training conditions other than to allow adaptation to the one-way mirror. The experimenter observing the subject watched closely for slight movements that might suggest muscle tensing. Such observation revealed that A.G. was, in fact, making isometric muscle contractions of the shoulder and trunk muscles ipsilateral to the cooler hand. This movement had not been detected by observation over closed-circuit TV. Beginning with Session 18, therefore, a record of the EMG activity in the *deltoid* muscle (shoulder) of each arm was obtained. And, beginning with Session 20, instructions were given on alternate sessions that were designed to inhibit the use of somatic muscles.

The result of these instructions (and verbal shaping when needed) was to gradually eliminate EMG activity. These reductions were accompanied by proportional decreases in the subject's ability to control differential temperature. Although on some trials a nearly complete suppression of *deltoid* EMG was accompanied by continued (but greatly reduced) control of skin temperature, the possibility that muscles of the trunk or some other region may have been active could not be ruled out.

Our analysis of subject A.G. led us to the conclusion that *isometric exercise* was a significant means of reducing skin temperature (which in her case produced temperature differences between the two hands). One final experiment examined the cardiovascular effects of exercise more generally. Since this work has recently been published elsewhere (Lynch, Schuri, and D'Anna, 1976), we do not review it in detail here except to say that relatively moderate exercise had significant effects. Both pulse amplitude and skin temperature of the left hand were reduced during exercises as slight as 10% of maximum voluntary contraction with the right hand or 30% of maximum with the right leg. It is unlikely that exercises such as these would be detected in most studies of cardiovascular self-control. This fact dictates the need for extremely careful evaluation of somatic activity if one's goal is to demonstrate direct autonomic control of cardiovascular responses.

C. Conclusion

The critical variables and conditions that can promote instrumental vasomotor learning are not yet clearly established, and a close replication of the methods reported in the available literature does not ensure a replication of results. In many of the experiments reviewed, more insight has been obtained into those factors that are insignificant (or at least much less important than originally assumed) than into those that are critical.

A particular concern for ruling out somatic "artifacts" may have accounted for the fact that experiments from our laboratory yielded so few talented individuals. Some investigators, particularly those interested in therapy, have made little or no attempt to control for somatic involvement. Others have been less cautious about controlling slight movements or the very subtle isometric exercises that we eventually found could be so influential.

Our comparison of children and adults and our subsequent studies of isometric exercise illustrate the technical difficulties arising from attempts to establish *direct* vasomotor control. (By *direct control*, we mean control that is exerted directly over the autonomic nervous system and not via intervening mediators.) While it may, in fact, be impossible to establish such direct control, the benefits in new knowledge and in therapeutic potential make the effort of further research well worth the cost.

But effort and a hope that direct control is possible are not sufficient. One must be constantly aware that factors other than direct autonomic learning may account for positive results. Additional knowledge about what other variables and conditions may be important is essential. Our progress will be more rapid if emphasis is placed on discovering relationships among variables rather than on seeking particular results.

To establish the possibility of direct vasomotor control we need more data. Among the facts that would greatly increase our confidence that direct instrumental control is possible would be: (1) demonstrations of reliable learning by a large number of individuals; (2) evidence of very large magnitude responses in a few individuals; (3) further examples of specific regulation of the direction and locus of response, such as those reported by Taub and Emurian (1972) and Roberts *et al.* (1975); and (4) doing all of the above when somatic responses are rigorously controlled and/or monitored. Present evidence suggests that these data may not be forthcoming for some time.

Meanwhile, what can be done? Among the more profitable lines that might be pursued are the following: (1) detailed study of the relationships between vascular responses and other responses, both visceral and skeletal; (2) further investigation of the patterns of vascular response to various kinds of introceptive and extroceptive stimuli; (3) evaluation of the sources of individual differences among subjects both in their reactions to stimuli and in their abilities to learn vascular control; and (4) examination of the degree to which the ability to regulate one autonomic response (e.g., skin resistance) determines the ability to regulate another (e.g., vasomotor).

Finally, one must be aware that direct autonomic control is only one means of regulating vascular activity. Particularly important are the ways that somatic responses may affect autonomic responses. Miller has noted that somatic activity can have its effects by direct mechanical stimulation either of the visceral organ (in our case, the vascular system) or of the recording device used to measure its activity, or it can have its effect by stimulating the receptive field for the visceral reflex, for example, when a deep inspiration initiates peripheral vasoconstriction. Obviously, a great deal is yet to be done.

V. Discussion

The preceding review has shown that individuals can learn to control peripheral vascular responses. What remains uncertain is how control is achieved. Despite extensive research, the training conditions necessary for learning have not yet been specified. Even under apparently comparable conditions, results vary among (and sometimes within) laboratories. Variables that deserve further study include the type of US (or feedback) employed, the subject's expectations of success, the source of his motivation to succeed, the relative difficulty of learning increases versus decreases in blood flow, and the role of isometric exercise in the performance of specifically localized responses.

In addition to conditions of training, some differences in results may be due to variations in the goals and expectations of different workers. In our laboratory, for example, the main question we sought to answer was whether or not individuals could acquire *direct* control of vasomotor responses. To answer this question, we obviously had to hold constant other factors that might lead to indirect control. Because respiration and exercise can affect vascular function (see Section II), it was necessary to control these "artifactual" responses. Other workers have had different interests and expectations. Assuming that direct control was well established, their interests have gone beyond questions of feasibility to questions about the magnitude and differentia-

bility of responses, individual differences among subjects, the therapeutic benefits of training, and so forth. There was little concern (at
least initially) about whether or not learning was possible. Workers in
various laboratories asked different questions and expected different
answers.

In the past three years, serious questions have arisen about the
possibility of eliminating somatic artifacts or, in Obrist's terminology,
the possibility of "uncoupling" somatic and autonomic responses
(Obrist, Howard, Lawler, Galosy, Meyers, and Gaebelein, 1974).
Dworkin and Miller (1976) have discussed several ways that autonomic
and somatic responses might be coupled. Their analysis suggests that
the demonstration of direct autonomic control (in the sense of control
without a necessary contribution from the somatic muscles themselves) will, at best, be a technically difficult task. Moreover, until it
becomes clear that autonomic responses *can* be acquired without
mediation via peripheral skeletal muscles, it makes little sense to ask
higher-order questions. If, for example, vascular control is achieved by
lateralized isometric exercise, it makes little sense to study the effect of
amount of training. Simple instructions concerning the best muscles to
use might produce superior control.

A primary goal of psychophysiology is to elucidate the relationships between psychological and physiological events. These may be
relatively simple relationships, as when an aversive stimulus produces
an acceleration of the heart, or they may be quite complex, as when
the recall of a traumatic childhood experience leads to a diffuse pattern
of central and peripheral reactions. The study of autonomic self-
regulation aims to determine whether and how experience (within the
constraints of physiology) allows the individual organism to acquire
control of an otherwise automatic bodily function. The methods of
instrumental learning, classical conditioning, and biofeedback are
useful tools for achieving this purpose. But like any particular methods, these paradigms carry with them certain assumptions about what
variables (both antecedent and consequent) are most likely to be
critical in the final analysis. For instance, biofeedback implies that
knowledge of results is important for establishment of self-control,
whereas operant conditioning emphasizes the importance of response–reinforcement relationships. These implications guide the
conduct of experiments and ultimately determine what data are
collected; each paradigm places a limit on the relationships investigated. Biofeedback and learning paradigms, which have guided the
research reviewed in this paper, are apparently inappropriate to the
analysis of certain important determinants of vascular control. Investigations formulated in the operant conditioning paradigm, for in-

stance, are not ideally suited to an analysis of the roles of subject awareness, isometric exercise, or the interactions between subject and experimenter.

What we are suggesting is that certain of the problems that have slowed progress toward understanding autonomic self-regulation (e.g., replication difficulties) may have resulted from a failure of investigators to appreciate the intrinsic limitations of specific paradigms for observing certain potentially important relationships. Future progress may be facilitated if investigators remain flexible in the methods they use, allowing their course of investigation to be guided less by *a priori* assumptions about how control *should* be achieved and more by the intrinsic capacity of one experimental outcome to suggest subsequent strategies and methods.

ACKNOWLEDGMENT

We wish to express our thanks to Professor Neal E. Miller for his support and guidance of the research reported here.

REFERENCES

ABRAMSON, D. I. *Circulation in the extremities.* New York: Academic Press, 1967.

ALLEN, E. V., BARKER, N. W., AND HINES, E. A. (Eds.). *Peripheral vascular diseases.* Philadelphia: Saunders, 1946.

BAER, P. E., AND FUHRER, M. J. Cognitive processes in the differential trace conditioning of electrodermal and vasomotor activity. *Journal of Experimental Psychology,* 1970, *84,* 176–178.

BARCROFT, H. Circulation in skeletal muscle. In W. F. Hamilton and P. Dow (Eds.), *Handbook of Physiology, Sec. 2: Circulation, Vol. 2.* Washington: American Physiological Society, 1963. Pp. 1353–1385.

BOLTON, B., CARMICHAEL, E. A., AND STÜRUP, G. Vaso-constriction following deep inspiration. *Journal of Physiology, London,* 1936, *86,* 83–94.

BROWN, E. B., JR. Physiological effects of hyperventilation. *Physiological Review,* 1953, *33,* 445–471.

BURTON, A. C. A critical survey of methods available for the measurement of human peripheral bloodflow. In *Ciba Foundation Symposium.* London: Churchill Ltd., 1954. Pp. 3–22.

BYKOV, K. M. *The cerebral cortex and the internal organs.* Translated and edited by W. H. Gantt. New York: Chemical Publications, 1957.

COOK, M. R. Physiology of peripheral vascular changes. In P. A. Obrist, A. H. Black, J. Brener and L. V. DiCara (Eds.), *Cardiovascular psychophysiology.* Chicago: Aldine Co., 1974. Pp. 60–84.

DAWSON, M. E., AND FUREDY, J. J. The role of awareness in human differential autonomic classical conditioning: The necessary-gate hypothesis. *Psychophysiology,* 1976, *13,* 50–53.

DiCARA, L. V., AND MILLER, N. E. Instrumental learning of vasomotor responses by rats: Learning to respond differentially in the two ears. *Science*, 1968, *159*, 1485–1486.

DWORKIN, B. R., AND MILLER, N. E. Visceral learning in the curarized rat. In G. E. Schwartz and J. Beatty (Eds.) *Biofeedback: Theory and research*. New York: Academic Press, 1977.

ENGEL, B. T., AND CHISM, R. A. Effect of increases and decreases in breathing rate on heart rate and finger pulse volume. *Psychophysiology*, 1967, *4*, 83–89.

FIGAR, S. Conditional circulatory responses in men and animals. In W. F. Hamilton and P. Dow (Eds.) *Handbook of Physiology, Sec. 2: Circulation*. Washington: American Physiological Society, 1965. Pp. 1991–2035.

FROMER, R. Conditioned vasomotor responses in the rabbit. *Journal of Comparative and Physiological Psychology*, 1963, *56*, 1050–1055.

FUREDY, J. J. Experimental assessments of the importance of controlling for contingency factors in human classical differential electrodermal and plethysmographic conditioning. *Psychophysiology*, 1974, *11*, 308–320.

GALE, E. N., AND STERN, J. A. Classical conditioning of the peripheral vasomotor orienting response. *Psychophysiology*, 1968, *4*, 342–348.

GANONG, W. F. *Review of medical physiology*. Los Altos, Calif.: Lange Medical Publications, 1971.

GILLIATT, R. W. Vaso-constriction in the finger after deep inspiration. *Journal of Physiology, London*, 1948, *107*, 76–88.

GOETZ, R. H. Effect of changes in posture on peripheral circulation with special reference to skin temperature readings and the plethysmogram. *Circulation*, 1950, *1*, 56–75.

GOTTSCHALK, L. A. A study of conditioned vasomotor responses in ten human subjects. *Psychosomatic Medicine*, 1946, *8*, 16–27.

GREENFIELD, A. D. M. The circulation through the skin. In W. F. Hamilton and P. Dow (Eds.), *Handbook of Physiology, Sec. 2: Circulation, Vol. 2*. Washington: American Physiological Society, 1963. Pp. 1325–1351.

HADFIELD, J. A., OXON, M. A., AND EDIN, M. B. The influence of suggestion on body temperature. *The Lancet*, 1920, *2*, 68–69.

HARWOOD, C. W. Vasomotor conditioning in human subjects. Unpublished Ph.D. thesis, University of Washington, 1953.

KATKIN, E. S., AND MURRAY, E. N. Instrumental conditioning of autonomically mediated behavior: Theoretical and methodological issues. *Psychological Bulletin*, 1968, *70*, 52–68.

KIMMEL, H. D., AND KIMMEL, E. Inter-effector influences in operant autonomic conditioning. *Psychonomic Sciences*, 1967, *9*, 191–192.

LADER, M. H. Pneumatic plethysmography. In P. H. Venables and I. Martin (Eds.), *A manual of psychophysiological methods*, Vol. 29. New York: Wiley, 1967. Pp. 693–752.

LISIN, M. I. The role of orientation in the transformation of involuntary reactions into voluntary ones. In L. G. Voronin, A. N. Leont'ev, A. R. Luria, E. N. Sokolov, and O. S. Vinogradova (Eds.), *Orienting reflex and exploratory behavior*. Washington: American Institute of Biological Sciences, 1965.

LOVALLO, W., AND ZEINER, A. R. Some factors influencing the vasomotor response to cold pressor stimulation. *Psychophysiology*, 1975, *12*, 499–505.

LYNCH, W. C., HAMA, H., KOHN, S., AND MILLER, N. E. Instrumental learning of vasomotor responses: A progress report. Paper presented at 1974 meeting of Biofeedback Research Society.

LYNCH, W. C., HAMA, H., KOHN, S., AND MILLER, N. E. Instrumental control of peripheral vasomotor responses in children. *Psychophysiology*, 1976, *13*, 219–221.

LYNCH, W. C., SCHURI, U., AND D'ANNA, J. Effects of isometric muscle tension on vasomotor activity and heart rate. *Psychophysiology*, 1976, *13*, 222–230.

MASLACH, C., MARSHALL, G., AND ZIMBARDO, P. G. Hypnotic control of peripheral skin temperature: A case report. *Psychophysiology*, 1972, *9*, 600–605.

MCDOWALL, R. J. S. *The control of the circulation of blood. (Suppl. Vol.).* London: Dawson, 1956.

MENZIES, R. Conditioned vasomotor responses in human subjects. *Journal of Psychology*, 1937, *4*, 75–120.

MENZIES, R. Further studies of conditioned vasomotor responses in human subjects. *Journal of Experimental Psychology*, 1941, *29*, 457–482.

MILLER, N. E. Learning of visceral and glandular responses. *Science*, 1969, *163*, 434–445.

MILLER, N. E. Applications of learning and biofeedback to psychiatry and medicine. In A. M. Freedman, H. I. Kaplan, and B. J. Sadock (Eds.), *Comprehensive Textbook of Psychiatry*. Baltimore: Williams & Wilkins, 1975. Pp. 349–365.

MILLER, N. E., AND DWORKIN, B. R. Visceral learning: Recent difficulties with curarized rats and significant problems for human research. In P. A. Obrist, A. H. Black, J. Brener, and L. V. DiCara (Eds.), *Cardiovascular psychophysiology*. Chicago: Aldine Publishing Co., 1974. Pp. 312–331.

OBRIST, P. A., HOWARD, J. L., LAWLER, J. E., GALOSY, R. A., MEYERS, K. A., AND GAEBELEIN, C. J. The cardiac–somatic interaction. In P. A. Obrist, A. H. Black, J. Brener, and L. V. DiCara (Eds.), *Cardiovascular psychophysiology*. Chicago: Aldine Publishing Co., 1974. Pp. 136–162.

PROUTY, L. R., AND HARDY, J. D. Temperature determinations. In F. M. Uber (Ed.), *Biophysical research methods*. New York: Interscience, 1950. Pp. 131–173.

PSHONIK, A. T. *The cerebral cortex and receptive function of the organism*. Moscow: Sov. Nauka, 1952.

RASKIN, D. C. Semantic conditioning and generalization of autonomic responses. *Journal of Experimental Psychology*, 1969, *79*, 69–76.

RESCORLA, R. A. Pavlovian conditioning and its proper control procedures. *Psychological Review*, 1967, *74*, 71–80.

RICHARDS, D. W. Circulatory effects of hyperventilation and hypoventilation. In W. F. Hamilton and P. Dow (Eds.) *Handbook of Physiology, Sec. 2: Circulation, Vol. 3*. Washington: American Physiological Society, 1965. Pp. 1887–1898.

ROBERTS, A. H., KEWMAN, D. G., AND MACDONALD, H. Voluntary control of skin temperature: Unilateral changes using hypnosis and feedback. *Journal of Abnormal Psychology*, 1973, *82*, 163–168.

ROBERTS, A. H., SCHULER, J., BACON, J., ZIMMERMAN, R. L., AND PATTERSON, R. Individual differences and autonomic control: Absorption, hypnotic susceptibility, and the unilateral control of skin temperature. *Journal of Abnormal Psychology*, 1975, *84*, 273–279.

ROBINSON, S. Physiology of muscular exercise. In V. B. Mountcastle (Ed.) *Medical physiology*, Vol. 1. St. Louis: Mosby, 1968, Pp. 520–552.

RODDIE, R. A. Effect of arm position on circulation through the fingers. *Journal of Applied Physiology*, 1955, *8*, 67–72.

ROESSLER, R. L., AND BROGDEN, W. J. Conditioned differentiation of vasoconstriction to subvocal stimuli. *American Journal of Psychology*, 1943, *56*, 78–86.

ROGOV, A. A. *Vascular conditional and unconditional reflexes in man*. Moscow–Leningrad: Izd. Akad. Nauk SSSR, 1951.

ROTHMAN, S. *Physiology and biochemistry of the skin*. Chicago: Chicago University Press, 1954.

SHARPEY-SCHAFER, E. P. Effect of respiratory acts on circulation. In W. F. Hamilton and

P. Dow (Eds.), *Handbook of Physiology, Sec. 2: Circulation, Vol. 3.* Washington: American Physiological Society, 1965. Pp. 1875-1886.

SHEAN, G. D. Vasomotor conditioning and awareness. *Psychophysiology*, 1968, 5, 22-30.

SHEAN, G. E., AND STRANGE, P. W. Effects of varied respiration rate and volume upon finger pulse volume. *Psychophysiology*, 1971, 8, 401-405.

SHMAVONIAN, B. M. Methodological study of vasomotor conditioning in human subjects. *Journal of Comparative and Physiological Psychology*, 1959, 52, 315-321.

SKINNER, B. F. *The behavior of organisms.* New York: Appleton, 1938.

SNYDER, C., AND NOBLE, M. Operant conditioning of vasoconstriction. Paper presented at the meeting of the Midwestern Psychological Association, Chicago, April 1965.

SNYDER, C., AND NOBLE, M. E. Operant conditioning of vasoconstriction. Paper presented at the meeting of the Psychonomic Society, St. Louis, October 1966.

SNYDER, C., AND NOBLE, M. Operant conditioning of vasoconstriction. *Journal of Experimental Psychology*, 1968, 77, 263-268.

SPIELBERGER, C. D., AND DeNIKE, L. D. Descriptive behaviorism versus cognitive theory in verbal operant conditioning. *Psychological Review*, 1966, 73, 306-326.

STEPTOE, A., MATHEWS, A., AND JOHNSTON, D. The learned control of differential temperature in the human earlobes: Preliminary study. *Biological Psychology*, 1974, 1, 237-242.

STERN, R. M., AND ANSCHEL, C. Deep inspirations as stimuli for responses of the autonomic nervous system. *Psychophysiology*, 1968, 5, 132-141.

STERN, R. M., AND PAVLOSKI, R. D. Operant conditioning of vasoconstriction: A verification. *Journal of Experimental Psychology*, 1974, 102, 330-332.

STOLTZ, S. B. Vasomotor responses in human subjects: Conditioning and pseudoconditioning. *Psychonomic Science*, 1965, 2, 181-182.

SURWIT, R. S., SHAPIRO, D., AND FELD, J. F. Digital temperature autoregulation and associated cardiovascular changes. *Psychophysiology*, 1976, 13, 242-248.

TAUB, E. Self-regulation of human tissue temperature. In G. E. Schwartz and J. Beatty (Eds.), *Biofeedback: Theory and research.* New York: Academic Press, 1977.

TAUB, E., AND EMURIAN, C. E. Autoregulation of skin temperature using a variable intensity light. Paper presented at Biofeedback Research Society Meeting, Boston, 1972.

TAUB, E., AND EMURIAN, C. S. Feedback-aided self-regulation of skin temperature with a single feedback locus, I: Acquisition and reversal training. *Biofeedback and Self-Regulation*, 1976, 1, 147-167.

TEICHNER, W. H., BEALS, J., AND GIAMBALVO, V. Conditioned vasomotor response: Thermoregulatory effects. *Psychophysiology*, 1973, 10, 238-243.

TEICHNER, W. H., AND LEVINE, J. M. Digital vasomotor conditioning and body heat regulation. *Psychophysiology*, 1968, 5, 67-76.

THAUER, R. Circulatory adjustments to climatic requirements. In W. F. Hamilton and P. Dow (Eds.), *Handbook of Physiology, Sec. 2: Circulation, Vol. 3.* Washington: American Physiological Society, 1965, Pp. 1921-1966.

WEINMAN, J. Photoplethysmography. In P. H. Venables and I. Martin (Eds.), *A manual of psychophysiological methods.* New York: Wiley, 1967. Pp. 185-217.

WINER, B. J. *Statistical principles in experimental design*, 2d ed. New York: McGraw-Hill, 1971.

9   *On the Nature of Alpha Feedback Training*

Martin T. Orne and Stuart K. Wilson

I. Introduction

A new kind of interaction between man and his body, *biofeedback*, elicited enthusiastic interest in many sectors of the scientific community in the late 1960s. A number of investigators had shown that automatic electronic sensing and feedback of a wide variety of usually unconscious physiological functions allowed individuals to directly influence internal processes that had previously been considered beyond volitional control. These included galvanic skin response (Crider, Shapiro, and Tursky, 1966), heart rate (Engel and Chism, 1967; Engel and Hansen, 1966), blood pressure (Shapiro, Tursky, Gershon, and Stern, 1969), evoked cortical potentials (Fox and Rudell, 1968; Rosenfeld, Rudell, and Fox, 1969), and EEG (Hart, 1968; Kamiya, 1969; Mulholland, 1968). Perhaps most impressive was the elegant demonstration by Miller and DiCara (1967) that curarized animals could acquire instrumental control over visceral and glandular responses.

EEG brain alpha wave feedback had particularly struck the imagination of researchers and public alike. Alpha waves—the large sinusoidal 8–13 cycle per second EEG activity—had been linked by earlier studies (Lindsley, 1952; Stennett, 1957) to intermediate levels of arousal. The alpha rhythm was felt to be most prominent when the individual was neither drowsy nor hyperalert. Within this theoretical context, Kamiya (1969) demonstrated that individuals could control

Martin T. Orne and Stuart K. Wilson · Unit for Experimental Psychiatry, The Institute of Pennsylvania Hospital, and University of Pennsylvania, Philadelphia, Pennsylvania.
The research reported here was supported in part by the Advanced Research Projects Agency of the Department of Defense and was monitored by the Office of Naval Research under contract #N00014-70-C-0350 to the San Diego State College Foundation, by grant #MH 19156 from the National Institute of Mental Health, and by a grant from the Institute for Experimental Psychiatry.

alpha density through feedback and consequently maintain higher alpha levels. Further, this enhanced alpha density was associated with pleasant, relaxed feelings (Brown, 1970, 1971; Hart, 1968; Kamiya, 1969). These results thus suggested that alpha feedback was a method by which modern man might achieve direct control over the level of his neurophysiological arousal and, therefore, over his anxiety and dysphoria. The potential, not only for the troubled individual but for everyone, appeared unlimited and held out the promise of our advancing beyond the age of drugs into an age of direct, conscious control of many psychobiological processes.

In the discussion to follow, we seek to evaluate the disparate scientific observations that made this dream plausible. We also focus on the line of research carried out at the Unit for Experimental Psychiatry specifically intended to clarify those aspects of alpha feedback training, and of the alpha mechanism itself, that are crucial to the potential therapeutic application of alpha feedback training. Finally, we try to spell out to what extent these hopes now seem justified and the possible directions of future research.

II. Studies Suggesting Alpha Feedback Training May Influence Subjective Experience

Berger (1929) demonstrated in his initial studies that the predominant EEG rhythm in relaxed individuals sitting with their eyes closed in a darkened room is alpha. He found that when the individual becomes drowsy, alpha activity rapidly disappears, while a stimulus that causes the individual to be startled, surprised, anxious, or frightened blocks the presence of alpha, at least temporarily. Later, Jasper (1936) suggested, and Lindsley (1952) and Stennett (1957) tried to document, that the relationship between alpha density and activation or arousal (both physiological and subjective) may be described by an inverted U-shaped function. They felt that during high arousal, as in anxiety-tension, alpha density seemed reduced and that it approached minimal levels with extreme excitement or panic. Alpha density was at maximal levels during alert, but relaxed, nonfocused mind-wandering. It disappeared from the EEG record with the onset of sleep. Thus, maximal alpha density appeared to reflect an intermediate level of arousal, that level at which an individual is neither drowsy nor hyperalert but rather comfortably relaxed. If alpha feedback training could teach an anxious individual to produce high alpha density he might concomitantly reduce his level of arousal to relaxed alertness, with its associated subjective state of pleasant relaxation.

The issue to be resolved seemed to be whether it was possible to learn to control such neurophysiological functions directly.

The initial enthusiasm for alpha feedback training appeared particularly warranted because brain functioning, in contrast to heart rate or blood pressure, logically seems to be more closely connected with subjective experience. Further, while not dealing directly with alpha feedback, the studies of feedback control over other visceral states, such as blood pressure or galvanic skin response, provided substantial scientific support for the view that feedback might be used to gain control over otherwise automatic physiological processes. Some investigators, from purely teleological deduction, felt even then that nature could never afford to leave life-supporting homeostatic systems to the capriciousness of conscious intent. However, the original study of heart rate feedback with curarized rats had dramatically shown that an animal could be induced to slow its heart, even to the point of death (Miller and DiCara, 1967).

A. *Subjective Identification of Alpha Production*

In light of the hypothesized relationship between alpha and arousal, Kamiya's (1969) anecdotal report of early work showing that subjects could learn to recognize the presence of alpha in their EEG was of great conceptual importance in providing a logical link to suggest that direct biofeedback of alpha wave production might produce desired subjective experiences. While observing the clinical EEG of a number of subjects, Kamiya instructed them to indicate whether they were producing brain wave state A (alpha) or brain wave state B (non-alpha) each time a bell rang. He provided feedback by telling them whether their statements were correct. Over a period of several hours some subjects apparently learned how to correctly identify alpha 100% of the time. Further, in Kamiya's later experiments on training the subject to enhance or suppress alpha, spontaneous alpha density during rests between training trials was higher than before, apparently because these subjects preferred the high alpha state.

Kamiya (1969) felt that it was not possible to conclude from the available data that the presence or absence of alpha was associated with perceptible alterations in subjective experience, but he reported that the subjects appeared to have gained some control over their brain wave states. It was not clear to Kamiya how and to what extent alpha production itself was represented in conscious experience; nor was it clear whether in order to identify it, the person was associating

certain levels of arousal or other behaviors with the concomitant
changes in alpha production. He proposed that the data did suggest
that it was possible to learn both to control alpha and to produce
specific subjéctive states by attending to simple biofeedback signals
based on EEG activity.

Given the above observations, it seemed reasonable to interpret
Kamiya's (1969) finding as indicating that feeding back the presence or
absence of alpha would allow an individual to learn to produce
maximal levels of alpha density. This, in turn, would produce a level
of arousal between drowsiness and hyperalertness—a state of mind
(and body) that, furthermore, might produce the salutary effects
reported by meditators, who also seemed to have high-amplitude and
high-density alpha in their EEG (Anand, Chhina, and Singh, 1961;
Wenger and Bagchi, 1961).

B. Meditation and Alpha Waves

Another important theoretical support for the use of alpha feedback training emerged from an increasingly widespread interest in
Eastern religions in general and meditation in particular. Previous
studies of the physiological status of Far Eastern meditators during
normal waking and meditation produced apparently striking confirmation of the notion that alpha waves were directly related to relaxed
states of mind. Anand *et al.* (1961) and Wenger and Bagchi (1961)
studied the EEG of yogis and reported that their brain waves showed
a predominance of very-high-amplitude alpha waves. Further, the
kind of stimuli that normally caused subjects to block alpha failed to
block alpha production in meditating yogis, whose discipline trains
them to turn inward and ignore the outside world. Kasamatsu and
Hirai (1966) studied Zen masters, who, in their meditation, are trained
to remain open and seek to experience even mundane stimuli as
continually new and fresh. They also noted very-high-amplitude alpha
in these subjects. In contrast to yogis, however, these individuals not
only showed the usual alpha blocking response to novel stimuli but
continued to block alpha indefinitely, even to the same trivial stimulus. In other words, the meditating Zen masters failed to habituate.

These studies of Zen masters and yogis, considered together,
were of special interest, not only because they suggested that meditators in general tended to have large amounts of high-amplitude alpha,
but also because their EEG demonstrated alpha characteristics com-
mensurate with their mental discipline. The meditating yogis failed to
show alpha blocking in response to a stimulus, while the Zen masters

failed to show habituation. Thus, particular states of mind seemed reliably associated with easily measured neurophysiological processes.

III. The Basic Alpha Feedback Experiments

Taken together, the several lines of preliminary inquiry described above were felt to be potential evidence for the idea that alpha feedback might be developed into a major tool for the self-control of subjective experience. All that seemed necessary was the proper electronic equipment, adequate training methods, and properly motivated individuals. A number of studies that supported this general hypothesis soon appeared.

A. Some Encouraging Alpha Feedback Results

Kamiya (1969), following up his early experiments on the identification of alpha, used electronic circuitry to identify the presence or absence of alpha waves in the EEG. He arranged the equipment so that either a light or a tone would go on whenever alpha waves were present. The subject sat in a dimly lit room and attended to either a visual or an auditory feedback signal. He then was trained to produce or block alpha by instructions to keep the signal on or off, respectively. Kamiya, as well as Hart (1968) and Mulholland (1969) independently, showed that in such conditions subjects could exert volitional control over the presence or absence of alpha. Kamiya pointed out that this control was manifested most dramatically in the ability to reduce alpha but added that subjects seemed to prefer the alpha state. Further, they tended to describe the state in characteristic terms, such as *relaxed, calm,* and *pleasant.* Brown (1970) found similar reports of relaxation, total concentration on the feedback light with a loss of awareness of the surroundings, etc. Interestingly, although Mulholland's subjects also were able to increase alpha, they did not report many of the striking subjective changes found by Kamiya and others.

The subjective experiences apparently associated with alpha wave production were explored more carefully by several investigators but substantiated perhaps most intricately by Brown (1971). Using appropriate electronic circuitry, she illuminated different colored lights, depending on the type of EEG wave in the subject's record. For example, blue or red lights were used for alpha, red or green for beta, and green or blue for theta. The subjects were encouraged to play with the lights for an hour and try to associate specific feelings with each of them. Forty-five subjects received this kind of feedback.

For each subject, one of the two possible light colors was associated with one of the three EEG frequency bands identified above. The subjects were then asked to sort more than 100 mood-descriptor terms into the appropriate red, blue, green, or white bin, symbolizing the three colored lights and no particular color association, respectively. Brown (1971) compared their sorting with the sorting performed by 45 control subjects who had not undergone the three-light feedback and had not associated any colors with the experimental situation. She was able to show that the experience of linking an EEG state with a colored light significantly changed the mood terms sorted with that color. Descriptors significantly associated more frequently with alpha colors were *calm, peaceful, pleasant, at ease, neutral, illusion, dreamlike, mysterious,* and *uncertainty.* Beta wave production (low voltage or small waves of greater than 13 Hz) was associated with feelings of being angry, aggravated, irritated, impatient, unhappy, troubled, frustrated, touchy, shaky, and investigative, as well as with feeling a void inside.

Thus, a much more specific assessment of the associated subjective experiences again seemed to confirm Kamiya's (1969) original reports. It appeared, then, eminently reasonable to try to utilize alpha feedback training as a means of helping the individual learn to gain control over the extremes of arousal. The only further requirements seemed to be an appropriate learning context for the subject and the necessary learning schedules.

IV. ESSENTIAL REFINEMENTS OF ALPHA FEEDBACK METHODS

If the therapeutic applications of the above findings were to be justified, several issues of both practical and theoretical importance required attention. Perhaps the most readily apparent problem was the wide individual differences in alpha density found among subjects—an observation Berger (1930) made early in his research. Some subjects in a darkened room show almost continuous alpha, which may persist even in the presence of light, while others show none. In a dimly lit room, under novel circumstances, Kamiya (1969) observed that most subjects had relatively low levels of alpha, which gradually increased over the session. Individual differences in baseline alpha density and the rising levels of alpha density that occurred during sessions presented serious methodological problems for efforts to document the effectiveness of feedback enhancement of alpha density.

A. Control of Subject, Methodological, and Situational Factors

The solution to the problem of individual differences originally attempted by Kamiya (1969) was to equate individuals with widely differing levels of baseline alpha production by setting the electronic filter gains arbitrarily for each subject so that the alpha-on signal would be presented 50% of the time regardless of the actual amount of alpha shown on the EEG record. Working in an operant conditioning context, Kamiya could equate, between subjects, the amount of positive reinforcement—the subject's feeling of success—in the task. Unfortunately, this procedure tended to focus attention away from the individual's actual changes in alpha density and artificially created a situation in which changes in apparent alpha density were emphasized. Only in later work (Nowlis and Kamiya, 1970) was any attention paid to the interaction between the initial level of alpha density and the effects of training procedures.

Other means of equating extreme differences between subjects were also employed in the later Kamiya studies. For example, Nowlis and Kamiya (1970) provided feedback to subjects with their eyes closed but asked some subjects to keep their eyes open if their initial alpha density was high. The latter condition would depress the high resting alpha levels and thus bring the starting alpha density of these subjects to a level more similar to that of individuals with moderate alpha density.

In these early alpha feedback studies the assumption was made that alpha density somehow reflected a basic psychobiological process, and little attention was paid to whether the individual's eyes were open or closed or to whether the circumstances were novel or the subject was well habituated; nor was there much concern with whether the feedback modality was auditory or visual. The possible interactions among initial baseline alpha levels, the circumstances of recording, and subsequent changes in alpha density were not considered. However, these issues must be taken into account, and extensive baseline measures of alpha density levels must be obtained before the results of feedback training can be compared between laboratories.

B. Replication of Alpha Feedback Results with Refined Methodology

Our first study sought to replicate the findings reported by Kamiya (1969) and others mentioned above (Brown, 1971; Nowlis and

Kamiya, 1970) but hoped, by attention to methodological detail, to gain a clearer understanding of the process. To facilitate analysis, eyes-closed and eyes-open baselines were obtained at both the beginning and the end of the experiment. The learning trials consisted of 2-min periods interspersed with 1-min rest periods. In order to demarcate clearly the beginning of rest, the feedback signal was arranged to provide a green light for the presence of alpha and a red light for the absence of alpha. The light was turned off to signal the onset of the rest periods. Instead of arbitrarily setting the electronic equipment to register 50% alpha, we set the equipment to reflect the presence of alpha as defined by standard definitions for the hand scoring of EEG wave forms. To accomplish this goal, a special filter with extremely sharp cutoffs, providing almost immediate discrimination of alpha, was developed (Paskewitz, 1971).

In addition to recording EEG from monopolar frontal (F4) and occipital (O2) electrode placements referenced to the ipsilateral mastoid, the procedure, followed in virtually all the early studies, also involved the recording of eye movements, heart rate, and the electrodermal response. Continuous paper recordings were made on a Beckman dynograph, and the data were also recorded on magnetic tape. The feedback system used occipital EEG signals, with the specially developed hybrid filters having step-function cutoffs at 8 and 12 Hz. There was a further amplitude criterion of 15 or 20 μV, depending on the particular experiment. At the completion of each session, a postexperimental interview was carried out during which the subject was asked about both the strategies employed to increase alpha density and the nature of his experiences during the experiment.

The first study included an initial session devoted to classical conditioning, followed by two feedback sessions on successive days (Lynch, Paskewitz, and Orne, 1974; Paskewitz, Lynch, Orne, and Costello, 1970). The results demonstrated that individuals did indeed learn to increase alpha density across trials, as had been reported by others. Figure 1 shows the effect of alpha feedback on seconds per minute of alpha produced by 16 males. Using visual feedback, subjects quadrupled the amount of alpha emitted during their first feedback session. However, we noted that this apparently dramatic increase took place from a very low initial level of alpha density. Thus, they went from an average of 2 sec/min of alpha density to an average of 8 sec/min of alpha density during the ten 2-min trials interspersed with 1-min rest periods.

Previous experimenters (Kamiya, 1969; Mulholland, 1969) had shown that subjects could volitionally block alpha as well as increase it when given appropriate instructions. We were also able to confirm

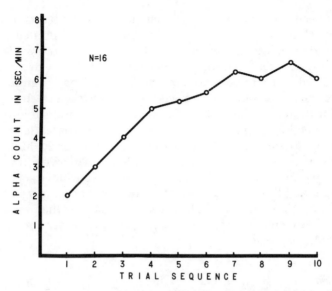

FIGURE 1. Seconds per minute of criterion EEG alpha produced during the first day of binary alpha wave feedback by visual display. Ten 2-min feedback trials are presented.

this finding in the same study. Thus, on the second day of feedback training, subjects had five feedback trials with instructions to augment alpha, followed by several trials during which they were alternately told to increase and decrease alpha density. Figure 2 certainly seems to document the claim that subjects can be taught to reduce, as well as to increase, alpha; however, careful examination indicates that something other than learning could explain this observation. On the very first trial during which subjects were told to "keep the red light on," alpha density dropped to a level nonsignificantly below the initial trial on Day 1, when feedback training with the visual display was started. Since subjects were producing almost no alpha under these circumstances, performance during subsequent "alpha-off" trials could not manifest any significant increase in alpha blocking from that seen during the first trial. It would, therefore, appear inappropriate to speak of subjects' learning to block alpha, since this is a skill that they seem to possess from the very beginning.

C. The Effects of Alpha Feedback on Subjective Experience

Care was taken in this study to solicit subjects for an experiment in conditioning rather than running self-selected individuals who wanted to be trained to increase alpha density. Only rarely did we encounter any subjective reports reminiscent of those described by

Kamiya (1969). In those occasional instances when subjects did report a kind of calmness or relaxation, it was invariably associated with the feedback trials, when the actual alpha density was, of course, far lower than during the rest periods in total darkness. While we were not prepared to dismiss the possibility that alpha feedback training might lead to systematic subjective effects, such effects were clearly not a simple function of alpha density. If this were the case, subjects would have reported being in an "alpha state" during the baseline periods of rest, when the actual alpha density was significantly higher than during feedback trials in the presence of light. We never encountered a subject giving such reports, and we therefore concluded, even at this early stage, that the subjective changes could not be simply a matter of the level of alpha density. However, it was felt that they might conceivably involve an increase in alpha density under circumstances that normally depress it.

D. Alpha Density during Light Feedback versus Resting in Darkness

The nature of the results of feedback training during the first study may be understood more clearly when placed in the context of

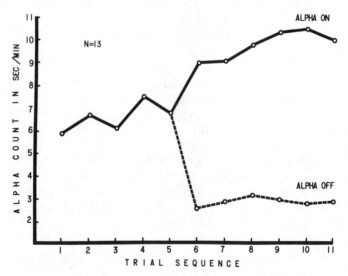

FIGURE 2.   Seconds per minute of criterion EEG alpha produced during the first day of binary feedback by light display. Five 2-min enhancement feedback trials were followed by 12 discrimination trials with alternating instructions to enhance and inhibit alpha production.

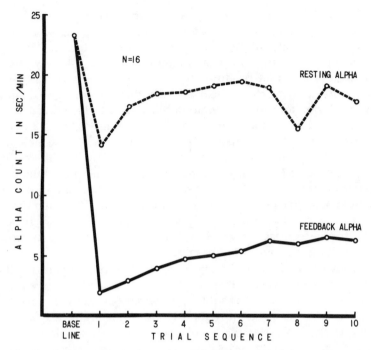

FIGURE 3. Seconds per minute of criterion EEG alpha produced during binary feedback with light display compared with baseline and rest period levels. The alpha feedback data are the same as those presented in Figure 1. Baselines and 1-min rest period alpha levels interspersed between 2-min feedback trials were obtained while the subject was in total darkness.

the alpha density during the initial eyes-open and eyes-closed baselines in total darkness as well as the alpha density during the rest periods. In these intervals, the feedback light was turned off and the feedback room again became totally dark. It is evident in Figure 3 that subjects in total darkness began with a spontaneously high baseline level of alpha density, which was promptly depressed by the visual feedback stimulus. However, during the rest period, when the room again was in total darkness, the alpha density returned to the much higher baseline levels.

V. The Significance of the Visuomotor System for Alpha Feedback Training

As Berger (1929) had already recognized, the presence of light is typically associated with a precipitous drop in alpha density. It seemed that the increase in alpha density associated with visual feedback, a circumstance that normally suppresses alpha, involved learning to avoid attending directly to the visual stimuli. Therefore, since the alpha density with visual feedback was of a far lower order of magnitude than that produced spontaneously in total darkness, it seemed more appropriate to speak of individuals' learning to disinhibit—in the Pavlovian sense—the alpha blocking effects associated with the presence of light, rather than to consider these data as a demonstration of learning to increase alpha.[1] Mulholland (1969) had independently shown that the process of habituation to the feedback stimulus is reflected by a gradual increase in the length of alpha bursts associated with it. Thus, the increase is also a product of adaptation to the feedback signal rather than of learning alone. This phenomenon explains in part why one typically sees a gradual increase in alpha density during feedback, regardless of the subject's success in producing alpha density greater than baseline levels.

In view of the dramatic effects associated with the visual feedback system, it seemed evident that if one hoped to find a true enhancement of alpha density, it would be necessary to carry out feedback training in the absence of light. Thus, we sought to determine whether individuals starting feedback training with alpha density already at a high baseline level could learn to increase alpha density to significantly higher levels. Accordingly, feedback signals were changed to tones, and all light was eliminated from the experimental room. The presence of alpha was signaled by a 75-dB tone presented at 360 Hz, and its absence was signaled by a 75-dB tone presented at 280

[1] We are seeking to make a distinction—which is a topic not commonly addressed in the learning literature—between the learning of a skill as opposed to the exercising of that skill under circumstances which normally inhibit it. Consider, for example, a student who is capable in mathematics but suffers from a test phobia which inhibits his test performance. If one were to operationalize learning to do mathematics simply by how well a student does on a test, one would confound the individual's true mathematical skill under optimal circumstances with the inhibition of that skill induced by the circumstance of taking a test. The most effective way to increase such an individual's performance would be through various procedures that would help disinhibit the anxiety effects associated with taking a test; in contrast, the student who cannot do mathematics will benefit most from encouragement, a good tutor, and lots of homework. Though in both instances one might observe improved test performance, it would be brought about by conceptually distinct processes: disinhibition in one case and learning in the other. There is little evidence to show that alpha feedback training leads to learning analogous to that of learning mathematics—despite feedback training, subjects rarely exceed their optimal alpha baseline level. Conversely, much apparent learning to increase alpha density seems to involve a process analogous to that of the student with the test phobia learning to effectively exercise a known skill during a test by disinhibiting his anxiety response to the situation.

Hz. The frequency difference was easily discriminated by the subject, and the tones were not experienced as noxious. In pilot studies, we determined that it made no intrinsic difference which tone was used to signal alpha and which was used to signal nonalpha.

A. Alpha Feedback in Total Darkness versus Dim Ambient Light

A study was conducted with nine subjects run in total darkness for six sessions, each separated by approximately one week (Paskewitz and Orne, 1973). Monopolar EEG recordings of the right occipital and the right frontal brain areas, each referenced to the right mastoid, were made. After an initial 3-min eyes-closed and a 3-min eyes-open baseline, an orientation period of 5 min was provided during which feedback was available, and the subject was encouraged to experiment with the tones to learn how his thoughts and behavior could affect them. The subject was then instructed to try to keep the high-pitched tone on and was given ten 2-min feedback trials interspersed with 1-min no-feedback rest periods. All feedback training was carried out in total darkness.[2]

Although during the first session subjects' initial high alpha activity was reduced markedly when they first opened their eyes in total darkness, they recovered much of this drop by the middle of the initial 5-min orientation period (Figure 4). These increases occurred within 2 or 3 min without instructions to augment alpha density. Whether they represent true learning or adaptation is unclear, but the rapidity of the increase was different from what was usually described as occurring with feedback training. Further, during the later sessions, this initial drop in alpha density during eyes-open baseline became

---

[2] At Dr. Kamiya's suggestion, two procedural changes were incorporated: (1) Subjects also received digital feedback indicating the amount of alpha they had produced during each of the 2-min periods by means of a digital display that indicated the number of seconds of alpha during the preceding 2 min and that was lit for 5 sec immediately at the conclusion of each 2-min trial before the 1-min rest period started. This feedback was deemed important to maintain motivation, since subjects could not really judge how well they were doing by listening to the tones. Further, the digital display provided information concerning even relatively small changes. Subjects were required to read the display out loud, thus providing feedback to the experimenter about their continuing alertness. (2) The frontal output was used as the basis of feedback. However, as in our previous studies, occipital alpha was also recorded, and the changes in occipital alpha, which were essentially parallel to those of the frontal alpha, were used as the basis for analysis.

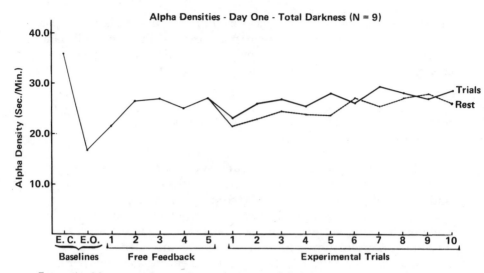

FIGURE 4. Mean seconds per minute of criterion EEG alpha produced on the first day of binary feedback by tones. The subjects were in total darkness during the auditory feedback as well as during baseline and rest periods. E. C.: eyes closed; E. O.: eyes open.

progressively less, presumably as subjects ceased to orient in a situation that was no longer novel.

The data suggested that subjects approached their maximal alpha density during the initial orientation period. The highest alpha density reached during any of the 10 alpha augmentation trials was only 7.2% more than that during this orientation period ($t = 1.81$, $p > 0.10$). Although in the group data the resting levels tended to be below trial levels, these differences were not significant.

When both trial and resting averages for all six sessions were examined with an analysis of variance, repeated-measures design, not one of the differences was significant (trials: $F = 0.19$, $p > 0.20$; rest: $F = 0.05$, $p > 0.20$). The largest difference between any two trial averages was only about 4 sec of alpha activity per minute. The trial average for the sixth session was not greater than the level of alpha density reached during the third minute of the orientation feedback period in the first session ($t = 0.35$, $p > 0.20$). Thus, within sessions or across sessions, no evidence indicative of learning to augment alpha density beyond the highest half-minute of alpha during the initial eyes-closed baseline period was noted in any of the subjects. Most important, subjects' initial eyes-closed baseline was not significantly exceeded at any time during the six days of training (Figure 5).

It appeared that by eliminating light from the feedback setting, one also eliminated any evidence of alpha augmentation during feedback training. These data, in conjunction with extensive pilot studies, led us to conclude that subjects do not appear to exceed their initial optimal baseline levels of alpha density with feedback training. Evidence of learning was present only if alpha density levels had somehow been depressed. To document this last point, it was necessary to clarify the relationship of these data to the effect of light on alpha density.

So that we could confirm the essential effect of the presence of light, the subjects who previously had failed to show any evidence of learning after six sessions spread over six days were asked to return for one additional day of feedback. Eight of the nine subjects were able to participate. Their EEG response in the identical experiment except for the presence of ambient light was far more similar to that of earlier subjects given light-signal feedback than it was to their own past performance during six sessions in total darkness (Figure 6). Recovery from the initial drop took place slowly, but their highest trial alpha density was 55.7% higher than their highest minute during the orientation period ($t = 3.04$, $p < 0.02$). The difference between trial and resting averages was significant ($t = 2.47$, $p < 0.05$). Tests between the results of the first session in total darkness and the subsequent session with dim ambient light indicated that the session with light for those same subjects was significantly different—both in reduced trial averages ($t = 9.11$, $p < 0.001$) and reduced resting averages ($t = 5.57$, $p < 0.001$)—from their performance in darkness.

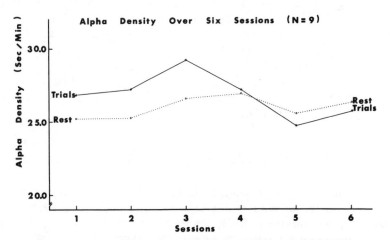

FIGURE 5.   Mean seconds per minute of criterion EEG alpha produced during each of six separate sessions of binary alpha wave feedback by tones. The subjects were in total darkness during the auditory feedback as well as during baseline and rest periods.

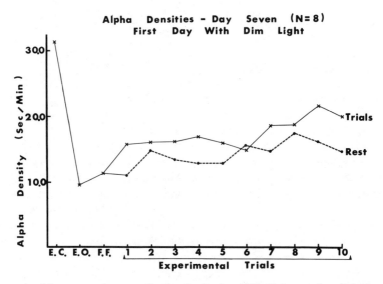

FIGURE 6. Mean seconds per minute of criterion EEG alpha produced during the seventh session of binary alpha wave feedback by tones. In this session, auditory feedback was presented while the subjects sat in a dimly lighted room. E. C.: eyes closed; E. O.: eyes open; F. F.: free feedback.

The importance of light, which had long been noted and again underlined in the earlier studies, was now clearly identified as being of major significance to any understanding of the alpha feedback experience. Further, the data supported the hypothesis that the apparent augmentation of alpha density during feedback occurred only when alpha density previously had been depressed by light. The increment in density shown during feedback seemed to involve the individual's gradually learning to ignore the stimuli that had been responsible for alpha suppression in the first place; that is, to cease orienting to visual stimulation.

B. "Looking" and Alpha Density

Mulholland (1969) previously suggested that alpha production was intimately related to visuomotor activity, specifically that of the triad of visual accommodation (convergence, pupillary constriction, and lens accommodation) rather than to visual stimulation, visual attention, or attention itself. He argued that only to the degree that attention is coupled with oculomotor control is it likely to be linked with alpha. This hypothesis regarding the connection between alpha production and the triad of accommodation was tested by Pollen and Trachtenberg (1972), who demonstrated that alpha blocking still occurred when the visual task was arranged so that feedback for accommodative effort was neither available nor required (accommodation was blocked with a cycloplegic agent, and lenses were provided to allow focused vision). Thus, although there are obvious limitations to the use of peripheral nerve blocks to examine central nervous system performance, this study suggested that the specific nature of the link between alpha and vision was still obscure. However, the general conclusions that could be reached included that, in some way, visual activity had a powerful influence on alpha density. Our data were also in agreement with this idea. Therefore, we sought to tease apart the relationship between visual attention and that of attention in general with regard to alpha density.

An unpublished study[3] compared attempting to see a barely perceptible visual stimulus with attempting to hear a barely perceptible auditory stimulus. Nine subjects participated in the experiment, which was conducted in a totally dark room. Baselines for eyes-closed and eyes-open alpha density were obtained. Counterbalanced sequences of an auditory and a visual attention task were then conducted as follows: The subject was told that sometime after a tone sounded a very dim light would be turned on. As soon as he perceived that the dim light was actually on, he was to press a button to let the experimenter know. The contingencies were arranged so that the very faint and difficult-to-identify light was turned on some 45 sec after the signal. A closely analogous task involved the identification of the presence of an auditory stimulus that was barely above threshold. This task, although equally difficult for the subject, had a significantly different impact on alpha density.

As Figure 7 shows, alpha density dropped precipitously—approaching zero in several subjects—as soon as the signal was given to search for the light and well before the stimulus was actually present. Once the light was identified, alpha density tended to increase again. In some cases, the light was not actually identified by the subjects, but the effort of trying to locate it was nonetheless sufficient to depress alpha density. Thus, even in total darkness, the attempt to see an object served to depress alpha density. Visual search produced alpha levels that were significantly below those during the auditory task (*t*s

[3] Paskewitz and Orne, 1973.

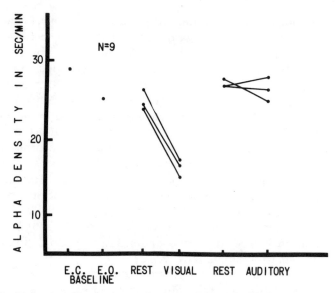

Figure 7. Mean seconds per minute of criterion EEG alpha produced during visual and auditory searches. The subjects sat in total darkness during both tasks. E. C.: eyes closed; E. O.: eyes open; Visual: visual search period; Auditory: auditory search period.

for the three trials, 3.08, 2.40, and 3.45; $p < 0.01$) and rests (ts for the three trials, 4.43, 2.60, and 3.08; $p < 0.01$). Alpha density during auditory search was not significantly below resting levels of alpha density (ts for the three trials, 1.23, 0.18, and 1.16; $p > 0.10$). Clearly, in contrast to visual search, the auditory search task caused very little drop in alpha density.

It is apparent that the attempt to see, even in the total absence of visual stimuli, is sufficient to produce alpha blocking. Thus, these findings replicated the visual-attention effects on alpha density reported by Adrian and Matthews (1934), supported by Durup and Fessard (1935), and suggested as part of the definition of alpha by Storm van Leeuwen and committee (1966). However, it would appear that the actual relationship of alpha rhythm to visual activity, brain activity, and subjective state is considerably less clear than one might expect 40 years after those simple and elegant studies that first demonstrated the connection between alpha density and the visuomotor system. Certainly, our work within the feedback setting did confirm and expand upon some of the original observations of the alpha rhythm's basic characteristics.

The primary finding was that the visuomotor system is of overriding importance in the suppression of, and in subsequent learning to enhance, alpha production in the typical feedback session. This connection between visual processes and alpha density is particularly direct for parieto-occipital alpha but, although still present to a considerable degree, is less so for temporal, central, and frontal areas of the brain. The importance of these regional differences in alpha density and alpha dynamics for alpha enhancement effects has not been fully clarified. However, early published reports (Brown, 1970; Kamiya, 1969; Nowlis and Kamiya, 1970) of the subjective effects of alpha increases did not direct attention to lateralized or regional differences in brain function. The enhancement of alpha and the subjective effects were demonstrated with occipital alpha recording but were assumed, or implied, to be whole-brain phenomena based on a change in overall psychophysiological state.

With the above data available, it seemed apparent that the effects of alpha feedback training should be reconceptualized as an experience that teaches the subject to augment alpha under circumstances that ordinarily reduce the amount of alpha in the EEG (Paskewitz *et al.*, 1970). The visuomotor system seems to be the overriding factor determining alpha levels in those circumstances in which the person can see visual patterns or, in a totally dark room, attempt to see them. Further, alpha enhancement under conditions that include the subject's eyes being open in a dimly lighted room seems to require different learning strategies, such as avoiding looking at anything directly. In addition, it may have different subjective effects when compared with alpha increases that might occur in a subject sitting with closed eyes in a totally dark room (Plotkin, 1976b; Travis, Kondo, and Knott, 1975).

Of considerable importance to the utilization of alpha feedback in a totally dark room is whether, under such conditions, a subject can increase his alpha density over an optimum eyes-closed resting baseline level. This question remains the center of current controversy. The recent papers by Hardt and Kamiya (1976) on the affirmative side and Plotkin (1976a) on the negative side adequately review the conflicting evidence. It would seem that it may be possible, as Hardt and Kamiya have pointed out, that different kinds of alpha recording and different feedback techniques, as well as longer periods of training than those described here, would allow subjects to demonstrate significant increases in alpha. However, we would agree with Plotkin that the burden of proof remains with those who make the claim. A convincing demonstration of such alpha changes has not yet been forthcoming.

Given that previous feedback enhancement of alpha wave density appeared to result from the lifting of alpha suppression mechanisms, such as those connected with light, the exploration of other potential sources of alpha inhibition seemed the most important area for further research. As we noted above, in the absence of light the suppression of alpha density that seemed to occur in the routine feedback setting could be seen only during the first session, when the subject opened his eyes in the total darkness. Once this relatively brief blocking effect is overcome—a process that occurs spontaneously during the first 2–3 min of the free-play period—the subject's alpha level again approximates that of the initial baseline, and no further augmentation can be seen during training. It seemed appropriate, therefore, to recognize that it might be necessary to reconceptualize the nature of the mechanisms underlying alpha density changes in the alert subject.

VI. ALPHA AND AROUSAL/ACTIVATION

The findings on levels of alpha density during visuomotor activity had begun to clarify some of the issues surrounding alpha blocking in the feedback context. At the same time, the basic link between alpha density and arousal began to appear to be much more complex than earlier workers had assumed. The initial experimentation, as reported above, had implicated the visuomotor system much more than arousal in alpha density changes, but no controlled manipulation of activation/ arousal had been carried out. Therefore, the most appropriate next step seemed to be to explore directly the key hypothesis justifying the use of alpha feedback in the clinical setting: that alpha density is linked to subjective and physiological arousal by an inverted U-shaped function.

In brief, both Lindsley (1952) and Stennett (1957) hypothesized that alpha density is related to activation or arousal by an inverted U-shaped function. That is, alpha density was felt to be at a maximum during alert, but relaxed, nonfocused mind-wandering, while dropping to zero with the onset of sleep. During physiological and subjective arousal, as in anxiety-tension, alpha density seemed reduced and approached minimal levels during periods of extreme excitement or panic. These assertions, based on laboratory-manipulated changes in arousal, appeared to receive further support from clinical research (Cohn, 1946; Costa, Cox, and Katzman, 1965; Jasper, 1936; Lemere, 1936; Ulett and Gleser, 1952; Ulett, Gleser, Winokur, and Lawler, 1953) on neurotic and schizophrenic patients with constant high arousal. Therefore, we began our exploration of the relationship of alpha density to levels of arousal with the assumption that the hypothesized relationships were essentially confirmed. However, it was apparent that visuomotor activity had to be controlled if we were to obtain uncontaminated observations on alpha-arousal interactions.

Since the previous data suggested that visuomotor activity in an alert subject under lighted conditions overwhelmed the effects on alpha density of any other behavior, the additional alpha blocking from activation/arousal might be difficult to discern under those circumstances. It was expected that a highly anxious person in a lighted room would block alpha more from his visuomotor activity than from the effects of fear itself. However, it was assumed that only learning to inhibit the fear effect would produce the dramatic subjective change relevant to controlling emotional turmoil in response to stress. For this reason, the presence of ambient light was eliminated from further experiments, and the hypothesized arousal mechanisms that might be responsible for reducing alpha density below optimal levels became the focus of attention.

A. High Levels of Arousal—Fear

We were left to confirm the assumption that since activation/arousal leads to decrements in alpha density, as did visuomotor activity, feedback training might permit the subject to disregard the alpha blocking effects of anxiety, just as it did those of light. It seemed entirely plausible that an anxious or aroused individual with reduced alpha in a totally dark room might learn to increase alpha density with feedback training and thereby learn to inhibit the mechanisms responsible for the physiological and psychological concomitants of anxiety.

Therefore, a study was specifically designed to: (1) establish during Day 1 the relaxed individual's optimal initial baseline; (2) create anxiety or fear in the subject over returning to the laboratory for a second session so that baseline alpha density for his second session presumably would be depressed; (3) show, then, how alpha feedback training can serve to increase alpha density even in total darkness, if it had initially been depressed by this situational anxiety; and (4) create a situation in which the subject would periodically be placed in jeopardy of being shocked (which would, presumably, again depress the level of alpha density) and in which an increase in alpha density would reduce or eliminate the likelihood of being shocked. In other words, the paradigm would approximate the all-too-common life situation in which the anxiety response is counterproductive and must somehow be controlled.

In an experiment by Orne and Paskewitz (1974), subjects first came to the laboratory to participate in a simple alpha feedback training experience. Every effort was exerted to make the subject comfortable and relaxed. A number of baselines were obtained, and feedback was given in the presence and the absence of ambient light. At the conclusion of this initial session, those subjects who had greater than 25% alpha were given the option of returning for a second session. It was explained that although it was very important for them to return, they were under no pressure to do so since the subsequent sessions involved receiving mildly uncomfortable to quite painful electric shocks to the calf of the leg. Thus, the experimenter refrained from actually reassuring the potential volunteers, although he made it clear that no injury would result. Of the 22 eligible subjects, 10 agreed to continue.

During the second session, two large silver electrodes and a ground were attached over the right gastrocnemius muscle, after the routine sensory electrodes had been positioned for recording EEG, EOG, GSR, and heart rate. The subject was informed about the nature of the silver shock electrodes but was given no instructions regarding when shocks might occur, since it was felt that any ambiguity about the shock would maximize anxiety. The experimenter left the room, the lights were turned out, and the entire session was conducted in total darkness.

Eyes-closed and eyes-open baselines as well as four routine 5-min feedback trials were given to the subject before shock instructions occurred. It was then explained that during the next part of the experiment he would, from time to time, receive electric shocks. "Jeopardy" periods (those times when he was in danger of being shocked) would be signaled by a third tone, clearly distinct from the alpha and no-alpha tones. This third tone would be on only when he was not producing alpha. Simply by turning on alpha, he could turn off the jeopardy tone and prevent his being shocked. It was emphasized that the only time he could be shocked would be while the jeopardy tone was on. Therefore, the more alpha he could produce, the less the likelihood of his being shocked.

Following these shock instructions, the subjects were given five 5-min feedback trials. Each of these trials was divided into 10 contiguous half-minute segments, 5 of which were jeopardy segments during which the third (or shock warning) tone was always present simultaneously with the no-alpha tone. During the other 5 segments, only the usual alpha or no-alpha tones were presented.

The shock contingencies were, in fact, arranged so that subjects received one to two shocks during each 5-min feedback segment.

Shock intensity was varied during the experiment, with only one or two being sufficiently intense to feel painful (since the purpose of the shock was to create apprehension rather than to inflict discomfort). These same procedures were repeated during a third visit to the laboratory.

The findings did not confirm the predictions of the theory. The initial alpha baselines during the second session were just as high as those in the first session, when no shock threat was present. During the first four feedback trials, alpha density was sustained at baseline levels (see Figure 8). The lack of alpha blocking following the shock instructions was most striking, in view of previous reports that fear causes drops in alpha density (Stennett, 1957). Alpha density did drop slightly, but transiently, during the first two jeopardy periods themselves. However, by the third jeopardy feedback period, alpha density levels were no different than those during nonshock feedback trials. The data from the third session showed alpha density differences between jeopardy and nonjeopardy periods only during the first jeopardy feedback trial. The group mean alpha density was equivalent to baseline levels during the rest of the trials. Thus, neither the anticipation of receiving electric shock nor the signal of the imminent

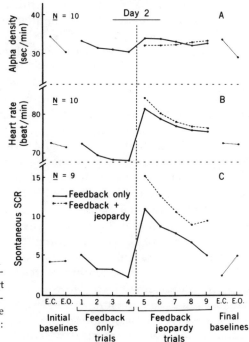

FIGURE 8. Mean seconds per minute of criterion EEG alpha, heart rate, and spontaneous skin conductance responses (SSCR) for the first day of shock (Day 2). E. C.: eyes closed; E. O.: eyes open.

onset of shock served to reduce the subjects' production of alpha density levels comparable to those found during resting baselines in the dark.

In an interpretation of these data, the first possibility to be considered was that the shock manipulation was not successful in making the subjects anxious. However, postexperimental inquiries clearly substantiated predictions that subjects would be anxious. Furthermore, during the experiment itself, visual observation (an infrared video system, included as a safety precaution, had permitted unobtrusive observation in the total darkness) revealed that the facial expression and demeanor of the subjects clearly suggested that they were anxious. Finally, other physiological data, notably heart rate and electrodermal responses, substantiated the subjects' reports and our behavioral observations. For example, as can be seen in Figure 8, when shock instructions were given, an instantaneous and dramatic increase in heart rate of well over 10 beats per minute took place (t = 2.98, p < 0.01). Pertinently, heart rate was significantly higher during jeopardy periods than during nonjeopardy periods (t = 2.05, p < 0.05), and when shock trials were over, heart rate returned to baseline levels. A second measure of activation, the number of spontaneous skin conductance responses (SSCRs), showed a closely analogous sequence of arousal. Data from the third session showed alpha, heart rate, and SSCR patterns very similar to those of the second and, therefore, replicated the findings.

Thus, neither the apprehension about the shock session in general, which might have been reflected in a drop in the second session's initial baseline densities, nor even the acute fear of being shocked resulted in the anticipated sharp drop in alpha density. The expected relationship between high levels of activation and reduced alpha density did not materialize. The data clearly indicated the lack of a necessary relationship between alpha density and the apprehension, anxiety, fear, or arousal levels of the subjects in this experiment. The discrepancy between these observations and previous reports (Lindsley, 1952; Stennett, 1957) of a link between alpha density, on the one hand, and subjective state and physiological arousal, on the other, clearly suggested that the old hypothesis required further exploration.

Insofar as the above results might reflect on the possible effects of alpha feedback training, they must be considered tentative because of the lack of yoked noncontingent feedback controls and the use of selected volunteer subjects. However, these findings call into question the assumed relationship between subjective anxiety–tension and alpha density, the basic notion upon which the rationale for the use of alpha biofeedback to reduce the effects of stress was founded. The study suggests that the simplistic assumption that alpha density always reflects a specific level of physiological activation/arousal does not hold, at least following and/or during alpha feedback training. Although these data, since they were collected during alpha enhancement feedback, cannot directly demonstrate the inadequacy of the inverted U-shape hypothesis describing the relationship between alpha density and arousal, they call into question the continued, unconsidered use of this conceptualization of the relationship of subjective and objective arousal with EEG alpha wave generation.

It is possible that the older literature (Lindsley, 1952; Stennett, 1957) suggesting a connection between high levels of arousal and decreased alpha density reflects a fortuitous combination of situation-specific factors and mediating influences that are not yet understood. Several phenomena were not adequately considered or controlled in previous studies. For example, the effects of novelty on the interaction between alpha density and arousal appear to be of considerable importance, particularly during the first visit to the laboratory. Johnson and Ulett (1959) found an inverse relationship between alpha density and Taylor Manifest Anxiety in 44 males during the first baseline recording session. However, they noted that this relationship was not present during the second and third visits to the laboratory. Johnson and Ulett recognized that they were not dealing with a simple relationship between optimal tonic level of alpha activity and anxiety but, rather, with a correlation that followed from differential response to a new and subjectively important experimental context. This point has been independently documented by Evans (1972) with regard to attempts to relate hypnotic responsivity to a subject's baseline alpha density. Most previous EEG studies of patients or of laboratory manipulation of fear have been carried out with subjects during their first experience with EEG recording. Thus, the interactions among the effects of novelty and fear with cortical activation cannot be separated without further controlled experimentation that takes these underlying factors into account.

The failure in earlier work to distinguish between studies performed with subjects having their eyes open in the presence of some ambient light versus those with subjects with their eyes closed or in the total absence of light produced even more confusion. The presence or absence of light not only interacts with habituation to the environmental situation but also plays a major role itself, with or without alpha feedback. Thus, attempts to relate current data to previous studies are frequently frustrated by the absence of standardized recording conditions in work performed before the effects of these phenomena were clearly recognized.

Early studies (Adrian and Matthews, 1934; Berger, 1929; Thiesen, 1943), which reported the alpha blocking effects of anxiety and arousal, typically used stimuli that were both novel and anxiety arousing. Further, little concern was given to concurrent visual activity. However, it now seems plausible to consider that any drop in alpha density that previous studies ascribed to arousal might actually have been the result of orienting to novelty or the visual activity provoked by the same stimulus responsible for emotional arousal.

Finally, Surwillo (1965) criticized Stennett's (1957) frequently cited study of the inverted U-shaped function as the result of an erroneous analysis of the data. Surwillo used the relationship between alpha amplitude and heart rate in his subjects to show that a single individual rarely demonstrates the inverted-U function. He found that his data, as well as Stennett's, produced such a curve only if subjects who increased alpha with increasing arousal were juxtaposed with those who decreased alpha with increasing arousal. The combination of the two limbs thus formed then created the inverted-U shape. However, this juxtaposition was possible only if the relative level of activation among the subjects was ignored. Thus, some of the key data ostensibly supporting the hypothesis have themselves been questioned.

It appeared possible, then, that our failure to find significant changes in alpha density with high arousal might be in agreement with Stennett's (1957) data as interpreted by Surwillo (1965), while still serving to discredit the inverted U-shaped function hypothesis. It was clear that it was necessary to reexamine carefully the nature of the high arousal end of the curve. However, the data for the low end seemed much less likely to be confounded by the above problems. For example, subjects falling asleep would have their eyes closed and would thus be exposed to the same low visual stimulation rates. Indeed, as will be demonstrated, our data seemed to confirm the older literature (Lindsley, 1960; Stennett, 1957) on the relationship between drowsiness and low alpha density.

B. Low Levels of Arousal—Drowsiness

Initially, practical concerns over obtaining valid baseline alpha densities against which to compare feedback results led us to examine some of the circumstances under which measures of alpha density were or were not characteristic of the individual. The initial 3-min eyes-closed and final 2-min eyes-closed baselines of subjects coming to the laboratory for a variety of feedback sessions were evaluated

(Paskewitz and Orne, 1972). The 24 subjects were primarily males who had participated in at least three laboratory feedback sessions.

The average intercorrelation (Pearson) between the mean alpha density for the six periods (two baselines during each of three visits) was 0.76, with individual coefficients ranging from 0.67 to 0.95. In spite of the generally high correlations, some baselines were highly atypical and failed to reflect the subject's usual alpha density. Baselines with reductions in alpha density of greater than 50% during 30-sec intervals were examined more closely in a subset of 9 subjects for whom eye movement data were available. Of 22 atypical baselines, 15 were accompanied by slow eye movements, a characteristic precursor of the onset of sleep (see Table 1).

Thus, a study of the reliability of baseline EEG alpha measures also clearly documented the now well-established relationship between the onset of drowsiness, which merges into Stage 1 sleep, and a corresponding decrease in alpha density. It is tempting to accept these data as documenting the relationship between low arousal and the absence of alpha. Here too, however, caution is needed. The drop in alpha density may not be a function of low arousal at all; rather it may be an incidental manifestation of the active processes associated with sleep onset.

For example, if one examines nighttime sleep records, there are periods when individuals show a great deal of arousal. Notably, REM is associated not only with the rapid eye movements that give the sleep stage its name but also with other manifestations suggesting heightened arousal, such as penile erection and marked variation in heart rate. Nonetheless, during these periods there is a disproportion-

TABLE 1

Number of Episodes of Slow Eye Movements Compared with Number of Periods of Atypically Low Alpha Density in 1-Min Samples from the Baseline Recordings of Nine Subjects

		Does Baseline Contain Atypically Low Minute?		
		Yes	No	
Are slow eye movements	Yes	15	5	**20**
present?	No	7	27	**34**
		22	**32**	**54**

$$\chi^2 = 13.27, p < 0.001^a$$

[a] The χ^2 values are based on data from 9 of 24 subjects. The authors recognize the compromise of the assumptions of the χ^2 statistic in that different subjects may be disproportionately represented. It seems reasonable to consider each depressed baseline as an independent event, however, even though it may occur more frequently in one subject than another.

ately small increase in alpha, especially when one considers the amount of mentation associated with dreaming as well as the auto-nomic arousal.

A similar paradoxical relationship between alpha density and arousal indices is suggested by the periods of GSR storms during Stage 4 sleep (Burch, 1965). This fascinating phenomenon does not seem to be accompanied by large changes in other physiological parameters, such as heart rate and respiration, but again, we are unaware of any evidence suggesting that alpha density normally increases during such periods.

Thus, activation within sleep appears to demonstrate a major separation of what seems to be a relatively unified physiological arousal in the waking individual. No considerable emergence of increased alpha density during normal sleep has been documented, yet arousal from these EEG sleep stages may be followed by reports of vivid dreaming experiences. We see, then, an apparent clear separa-tion of processes signaling increased subjective and physiological activation from cortical alpha production. The absence of evidence demonstrating a continued link between brain-stem activation, the cortex, and subjective experience strongly suggests that the decrease in alpha density seen as an individual approaches sleep may reflect an active disengagement of alpha-wave–producing mechanisms from the cortex, rather than a low level of general brain arousal. The specific concomitants of the connection between general activation/arousal and cortical arousal indices such as alpha wave production has yet to be determined.

At this juncture, it may be concluded that a number of subjec-tively and objectively different mechanisms might have one final common effect: a reduction in alpha production. As demonstrated by the preceding experiments, both attempting to see an object and drowsiness have alpha blocking effects. While high arousal appeared, in previous experiments, to result in reduced alpha density, it is not clear at this point whether this was an independent effect, secondary to increased eye movements, or the effect of unspecified mechanisms. However, given the several apparently fundamentally different types of alpha blocking, it would follow that different skills might be necessary to learn to augment alpha density, depending on the nature of the primary stimulus that is depressing alpha activity. With this new perspective, it becomes relatively meaningless to speak of alpha feedback training in a generic sense. We have to understand what influences have served to depress alpha density below the person's optimum levels in each specific feedback circumstance.

The problem of specificity of response in biofeedback has also been explored by Schwartz (1972, 1974, 1975), particularly with regard to cardiovascular parameters. His group's further work on brain processes has led them to postulate that patterns of brain and peripheral physiological processes, rather than isolated parameters, may be more meaningfully linked to cognitive–affective experiences. Schwartz (1976a,b) suggested that emotions and conscious states must be seen as emergent properties of neural patterning—perhaps, for example, in interactions between the two hemispheres—rather than merely as functions of general neurophysiological activation. Although such a perspective adds to our ability to plan meaningful experiments, an understanding of the nature of phenomena such as lateralization of hemispheric activation depends on the central issue of the significance of alpha density for brain arousal or activation, as a whole or in regions. This significance is by no means clear at this point, and therefore, we shall not seek to comment further on this line of inquiry.

VII. IS DIRECT AWARENESS OF ALPHA WAVE PRODUCTION POSSIBLE?

Since a number of underlying relationships between alpha and subjective experience were now at least vaguely apparent, the conceptual importance of Kamiya's (1969) early study—reported anecdotally, to demonstrate that subjects could rapidly learn to discriminate between alpha and no-alpha periods in their own EEG—became even greater. The most direct approach to the potential link between subjective experience and alpha production seemed to lie in attempting to replicate, with more rigorous controls, the original Kamiya finding that subjects could learn to identify periods of alpha wave production. Very early in our pilot work, we had run one subject in 2 of his total of over 30 sessions while providing him with a manipulandum so that he could signal the presence or absence of alpha as he thought it occurred. Visual inspection seemed to support Kamiya's observations that a subject could learn to identify alpha periods, but a number of problems made it very difficult to quantify such data. Therefore, we did not at that time pursue the matter further. However, the findings summarized above had convinced us of the need to address systematically the basic question of whether alpha bursts were reliably accompanied by an identifiable alteration in subjective experience.

An appropriate procedure was devised (Orne, Evans, Wilson, and Paskewitz, 1975) to allow for a more rigorous test of Kamiya's (1969) hypothesis. Subjects were automatically signaled periodically with a tone and required to indicate, by pressing the appropriate one of two buttons, whether they believed that they had or had not just been generating alpha. If the subject answered correctly, the signal tone was replaced by another, somewhat higher tone. If the choice was incorrect, the tone merely terminated. Thus, this situation provided "feedback" regarding only the presence or absence of alpha each time the subject responded to the tone. It is evident that this approach fits the classical signal detection model. Such a paradigm makes it possible to separate the accuracy of correctly identifying the presence of alpha independently from the accuracy of correctly identifying the absence of alpha. Further, it permits the identification of guessing strategies.

Though conceptually the experiment seemed straightforward and potentially elegant in its approach to the problem, the execution proved to present a series of unexpected problems. For example, even though care was taken to choose subjects with moderate amounts of alpha in order that alpha and no-alpha events would be equally frequent, these subjects, although well acclimated to the laboratory, showed a considerable increase in alpha, without feedback, during the second session and an even greater rise in the third session. Because of this dramatic increase in alpha density, finding periods of non-alpha with a duration of even 1–3 sec was very difficult. Thus, inequalities in the time intervals between alpha and no-alpha events developed.

The results were examined from several different perspectives. First, a day-by-day chi-square analysis for each subject suggested that correct discrimination was being acquired over time, but a more careful analysis showed that a significant chi-square reflected, in large part, an increase in correct guesses during alpha events with a corresponding increase in incorrect guesses during no-alpha events. Thus, the results were apparently a function of response bias on the part of the subjects, who seemed to believe that their alpha density gradually increased across days.

Further assessment through a one-sample runs test and a signal detection analysis confirmed that response bias was the central factor in producing the results. Although the relatively small number of trials and the possible violation of some of the underlying assumptions of signal detection make the results of such an analysis less than ideally clear, it did show that there was a very low d' index of discriminability. The response bias criterion showed signs of a strong "alpha" response bias effect that was relatively consistent throughout the series, except for the seventh session, when two of the subjects reported feeling extremely drowsy.

Legewie (1975) and Pavloski, Cott, and Black (1975) also used this alpha/no-alpha discrimination procedure in experiments attempting to replicate Kamiya's (1969) original findings. Neither group was able to demonstrate that their subjects could actually discriminate between these two EEG states. When trial probabilities and confounding cues were controlled, the subjects could not determine at any one moment whether alpha or no-alpha was occurring in their EEG recording. In summary, these alpha state discrimination studies suggested that the apparent ability to discriminate between alpha and no-alpha events during the pilot studies was probably an artifact of the individual's strategy within the experiment. For example, our subjects tried to increase their incidence of alpha without instructions to do so and followed this attempt with the strong tendency to choose "alpha" more often than "no-alpha" for their decision.

While it would be all too easy to dismiss Kamiya's (1969) anecdotal findings in light of the above studies, we are not yet prepared to do so. The number of subjects examined for the ability to discriminate alpha and no-alpha conditions is small, and our automated procedures may be obscuring the issue as much as helping to clarify it. Thus, our failure to replicate the earlier Kamiya results may be as much a function of our approach as of the nature of alpha. However, while it is, of course, possible that it is necessary to train individuals with longer windows than those that were used in these studies, it would seem essential that more carefully controlled positive observations be obtained before we are justified in assuming that the simple presence of alpha has cortical representation.

The line of inquiry into alpha and its connections with subjective experience had thus demonstrated that: (1) subjects do not appear to learn to increase their alpha density above their resting baseline through feedback; (2) visuomotor activity is of prime importance in depressing optimal alpha density and in subsequently learning to enhance alpha; (3) high levels of alpha density can be present even during very high arousal and subjective fear during alpha feedback; (4) the absence of alpha during activation/arousal changes during sleep suggests that whatever relationship exists in the waking state between alpha density and arousal levels is not readily seen during sleep itself; and (5) subjects may not be able to discriminate directly between alpha and no-alpha events during waking states. In sum, the view that alpha production is closely related to subjective experiences, has specific cortical representation, and alone reflects level of activation/arousal cannot be justified with currently available data.

Given these observations, it seems that the entire basis justifying the potential benefits of alpha feedback training is lacking, and accordingly, one might well choose to dismiss this entire line of inquiry. However, throughout our efforts to understand alpha feedback, we have become increasingly aware of the need to understand the underlying processes, and we have been forced to reevaluate issues that were assumed to be resolved by previous work in order to reconcile the conflicting reports in the literature. Of several issues that arose, the single most important factor, which has been essentially ignored in the reported work to date, related to systematic individual differences in the dynamics of the alpha response. Such differences may provide further clarification of the nature of the conflicting findings reported above.

VIII. THE EFFECTS OF COGNITIVE ACTIVITY ON ALPHA DYNAMICS

The view that alpha blocking is always associated with concentrated mental activity was first hypothesized by Berger (1929) and was supported by Adrian and Matthews (1934). Several subsequent studies seemed to demonstrate a clear relationship between mental tasks themselves and the blocking of alpha activity in the EEG (Chapman, Armington, and Bragdon, 1962; Darrow, Vieth, and Wilson, 1957; Glanzer, Chapman, Clark, and Bragdon, 1964; Glass, 1964, 1967; Lorens and Darrow, 1962). We also found, in early studies, that combining the task of incrementing alpha through feedback with a cognitive task such as subtracting by sevens produced more alpha blocking.

Individual differences in the degree of blocking, depending on the person's proficiency at the task and his self-paced rate of performance, seemed to substantiate such an interpretation. For example, one subject, choosing to do an arithmetic task more quickly than he could readily manage, showed large amounts of blocking, while another, going more slowly than justified by his skill in arithmetic, showed little blocking. It appeared obvious that the task difficulty at any given time was determined not only by the task itself and the individual's proficiency in the task but also by the individual's rate of task performance (Paskewitz and Orne, 1972). However, several other studies (discussed below) also seemed to indicate that there are other individual differences that might mediate the different alpha blocking reactions between persons.

A. Previously Reported General Effects of Tasks on Alpha Density

Mundy-Castle (1957) found that both mental arithmetic and imagery could be carried on without necessarily leading to alpha blocking. He concluded from his studies that there was no one-to-one relationship between alpha blocking and visual activity or attention. Further, Chapman et al. (1962) noted that mental arithmetic reduced alpha in an eyes-closed but increased it in an eyes-open condition. Kreitman and Shaw (1965) observed, in a study of eight subjects, that alpha density increased in some individuals during most tasks. Legewie, Simonova, and Creutzfeldt (1969) replicated a previous finding (Creutzfeldt, Grünewald, Simonova, and Schmitz, 1969) that a number of experimental tasks performed during an eyes-open condition increased temporo-occipital alpha in seven of eight subjects, while decreasing it when their eyes were closed. Thus, this group of studies tended to concentrate on the interaction between direction of alpha change during a task and visuomotor effects.

In contrast, Pollen and Trachtenberg (1972) focused on the impact of task difficulty. By varying the demand on mental effort, they found that in an eyes-closed condition, no alpha blocking occurred during the easier parts of their progressively more difficult range of tasks. In those sections that demanded greater mental effort, alpha blocking was present and continued until the problem was solved. Their results thus suggested that alpha augmentation might be expected only during lower-level mental effort. Any differences in alpha attenuation between subjects over different tasks could then be attributed to individual differences in task-related skills or effort.

In sum, the literature has concentrated on the effects of light on alpha changes during a task or on experienced task difficulty. However, the effects of the novelty of the experimental setting and the tasks were not well controlled. Further, the meaning of the fact that some individuals, when performing a mental task with their eyes open, augmented alpha was not clarified.

B. Individual Differences in Alpha Response to a Task

In view of the possible individual differences inherent in previous data and their potential practical and theoretical import, the effect of cognitive tasks on alpha density was reexamined (Orne et al., 1975), with particular attention given to the control of novelty effects and to the elimination of light from the experimental setting. Subjects were run through the same baseline recordings and essentially similar tasks on three different days, both as a preliminary familiarization with procedures in order to control novelty and to permit selection of those who were to participate in a feedback study to extend over several days.

The three sessions were designed to record alpha density while the subject sat in a totally dark room. Conditions included were eyes-open and eyes-closed resting baselines, as well as carrying out a number of tasks requiring different levels of cognitive effort. Following the initial eyes-closed and eyes-open baselines, a number of 90-sec serial subtraction tasks using several different numbers, as well as descending subtraction, were interspersed with 1- and 2-min baselines. The subtraction tasks varied in difficulty from simply counting backward by ones to the most difficult descending subtraction task. For the latter, the subject began by subtracting 9 from a three-digit number, then 8 from the remainder, then 7 from that remainder, and so on until reaching 2, when he began again with 9, 8, 7, etc., until told to stop.

The tasks were followed by ones designed to elicit left- or right-hemisphere activation specifically, such as verbal and mathematical problems for the left and visualization of scenes and visuospatial problems for the right. Five problems of each of the two types were performed in a counterbalanced order, with intervening 20-sec rests separating them. Essentially similar, although slightly modified, tasks and baselines were carried out during all three sessions. Thus, it was possible to compare alpha changes between tasks after novelty had been eliminated. All EEG data were obtained from bilateral recordings of monopolar occipital EEG, with the right mastoid used as reference, and recorded on paper. Criterion alpha was measured by use of a 15-μV amplitude standard for the presence of alpha.

During the first session, there was a general tendency to block alpha while performing the tasks, although some subjects blocked alpha much more than others. However, when the data from the second session were examined, strikingly specific individual differences in alpha dynamics emerged. Among these subjects, all of whom were used to the experimental procedures and were dark-adapted, seven responded to subtraction by ones by incrementing their alpha density above their own baselines and four responded by blocking alpha. However, given the Pollen and Trachtenberg (1972) findings on task-difficulty effects, one would anticipate that all subjects would block alpha during the difficult descending subtraction.

Subjects were therefore divided on the basis of whether they increased or decreased alpha density while counting by ones, so that we could see if this dichotomy would differentiate them when they performed descending subtraction. Figure 9 shows the mean percentage of left-hemisphere alpha density of two groups: four alpha blockers (dotted lines) and seven alpha augmenters (solid lines). The individual was assigned to the augmenting or blocking group on the basis of his alpha density change from baseline during subtraction by ones in the second session. Subjects who blocked alpha while counting backward by ones also did so during descending subtraction. However, contrary to expectations, those who increased alpha density while performing the simple task increased it during the difficult one as well!

As Figure 9 demonstrates, the two kinds of alpha response to a task are not related to differences in resting alpha density either during the initial baseline or in the rests preceding the tasks. Since the two groups were defined by the direction of their alpha response during subtraction by ones, it is hardly surprising that their alpha density is significantly different during that task. However, the continued differences (Trial 1, $t = 1.82$, $p = 0.05$; Trial 2, $t = 3.09$, $p < 0.01$) in their alpha response to the much more demanding descending subtraction task were remarkable, particularly since these differences were not related to the individual's success or speed in counting backward during the descending subtraction task.

The consistency of an individual's alpha response to a task is further demonstrated by the continued significant differences between these two groups, separated by direction of alpha change with subtraction by ones on Day 2, during the descending subtraction task

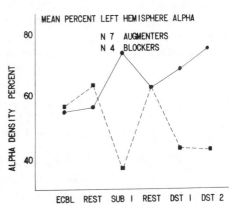

FIGURE 9.   ECBL: eyes-closed baseline; SUB 1: subtraction by ones (1's); DST 1 and 2: Descending Subtraction Tasks 1 and 2.

on Day 3. Again, the two groups showed their characteristic directions of response during the task, and their alpha densities were significantly different ($t = 3.02$, Trial 1; and 3.58, Trial 2; $p < 0.01$ for both). The Pearson correlations between Day 2 and Day 3 alpha density change scores during the descending subtraction tasks were 0.56, Trial 1, and 0.66, Trial 2 ($p < 0.05$). Pearson correlations of alpha density between tasks on the same day were uniformly above 0.66, regardless of the differences in the difficulty of the task. Thus, the individual differences in alpha dynamics appeared to be more important modifiers of alpha density response than task difficulty on the second and third days of the experiment.

The bimodality of these response characteristics, evident during the second and third days, was not present in the first day. On the contrary, a fairly uniform tendency to block alpha while performing a cognitive task was apparent. So that we could determine whether there were any individual differences reflected in Day 1 data, the number of subtraction tasks (total possible, five) during which an individual showed alpha augmentation was tabulated. Seven subjects identified as augmenters on Day 2 augmented alpha during a mean of 1.86 of the 5 subtraction tasks on Day 1, while six identified as blockers on Day 2 augmented during a mean of 0.33 tasks on Day 1 ($t = 2.69$, $p < 0.25$). (Two subjects who did not complete the third day are included in the Day 1 data.) Thus, an individual characteristic that was easily identified in Day 2 data was also present on Day 1 but not readily discernible because of the relatively uniform response to novelty.

These striking, reliable, and significant differences in the direction of alpha density changes during cognitive tasks, although observed by others in the past, have tended to be ignored because they were masked either by the presence of light or by novelty on the first day of testing. Therefore, they have been taken to represent random variation in alpha blocking. However, the persistent direction and amount of alpha change that occurred in our subjects across tasks and across days sugests that what may be manifest in these phenomena is a powerful and pervasive characteristic of the person's neurophysiological dynamics, rather than merely phasic changes whose nature is closely tied to his immediate mental effort or content. Thus, the same subjective experience and objective performance in some subjects may elicit considerable alpha blocking, in others alpha augmentation, and in still others little or no change in alpha density.

Clearly, such individual differences in response to cognitive tasks are not taken into account by current theories regarding alpha, activation, behavior, and subjective experience outside of the feedback context. Still, one might consider dismissing them as irrelevant to the general activation/arousal theory justifying the use of alpha feedback in a clinical setting. However, conceptually similar spontaneous changes in alpha density occurred during high activation/arousal in an alpha feedback experiment (Wilson, Orne, and Paskewitz, 1976). Some individuals blocked alpha during fear of electric shock and some showed no change, while others increased alpha; all these different responses occurred during periods of large increases in autonomic indices, such as heart rate and spontaneous skin conductance activity. Thus, these individual differences may be quite pertinent to an understanding of the conflicting reports in alpha feedback research.

Travis *et al.* (1975), for example, reported that only about 60% of their subjects felt the attempt to enhance their alpha density as a neutral or pleasant experience. This kind of variability in reports of positive subjective experience has been explained in a number of ways. For example, Walsh (1974) showed that subject expectations and demand characteristics of the experiment have a significant impact on whether the individual reports positive experiences. However, individual differences in alpha dynamics such as those reported here may help explicate the findings in a more basic and ultimately more useful manner. They may also clarify the controversy surrounding the potential of individuals to augent alpha density over baseline levels. Our data demonstrate that such increases are possible, at least in some persons. However, they have occurred in response to difficult cognitive tasks, or high activation/arousal, rather than during relaxation.

In sum, although there is little question that the nature of a cognitive task or an emotional experience has an impact on alpha dynamics, directing data analysis toward individual differences permits the identification of another important dimension in alpha phenomena. This dimension has previously been obscured by the effects of light or by orientation to novelty on the first day of participation in an experiment. Once these effects are controlled by the subject's being adapted both to darkness and to the circumstances of the experiment, individual differences in alpha dynamics become evident. It seems apparent that one cannot expect to apply alpha feedback to obtain predictable results unless these powerful systematic individual differences are better understood and taken into account. Otherwise, the results of alpha feedback can, at best, be no more than confusing and, at worst, detrimental to some of those whom we would hope to aid.

IX. OVERVIEW AND PROSPECTS

What may we then consider to be established conclusions regarding the relationship between alpha and subjective experience? *First,* contrary to our initial naive hopes, we cannot assume that high alpha density is uniformly accompanied by a moderate physiological arousal or subjective calm. It is now clear that a number of different mechanisms influence alpha density and interact to determine an individual's tonic levels and phasic changes in alpha. *Second,* visuomotor activity is of primary importance in determining alpha density and in the subject's learning to augment alpha in the presence of light. It would appear that feedback training carried out in light requires the development of different skills and may have very different subjective and objective results than that carried out in total darkness. *Third,* the widely accepted inverted U-shaped function hypothesized to relate alpha density to activation needs to be reevaluated. *Fourth,* while in early work we could not get people to exceed baseline alpha levels, it is now clear that some subjects do—in response to activation. *Fifth,* very important systematic individual differences in alpha dynamics must be taken into account in any further studies of the relationship between cortical electrical activity, subjective experience, and behavior, as well as in alpha feedback training research.

The disappointing overall results of alpha biofeedback training, compared with the initial hopes, have forced a reconceptualization of the necessary conditions for the clinical application of alpha feedback. Our results suggest that once novelty and visuomotor effects are eliminated, alpha augmentation may be the product of relaxation in one individual and of hyperarousal in another, while a third may show little relationship between subjective state and alpha density. Thus, regardless of the area of the brain from which recordings are taken, or the pattern of other autonomic parameters, uniform subjective experiences over a population of subjects are unlikely to emerge from a single direction of alpha change. Unless the individual differences are taken into account, it would seem foolhardy to expect that alpha feedback would lead to uniform effects once novelty and visuomotor factors are excluded.

In sum, the research that has followed the original reports of a reliable connection between alpha production and subjective experience has tended to negate and/or qualify the early results. However, three more recently defined areas of inquiry must be understood before the final chapter on the potential subjective effects of alpha enhancement through feedback training can be written. More careful examination of the relationship of specialized areas of the brain to behavior, as well as of the specific pattern of physiological reactions associated with particular emotional states, must be carried out. Perhaps most important to any future applications of EEG alpha feedback will be an in-depth exploration of individual differences in alpha dynamics. The potential new integration of basic neurophysiological and neuropsychological perspectives that may follow would then permit a more scientifically mature second approach to the use of this elusive method of interacting with man's neurophysiological self.

Acknowledgments

The line of research reported here would not have been possible without the close collaboration of David A. Paskewitz, who designed the equipment, ran the subjects, and supervised the analysis of all but the most recent studies. This later work was carried out in collaboration with Frederick J. Evans, Betsy E. Lawrence, Emily Carota Orne, and Anthony L. Van Campen. We would like to express our appreciation to them and also to William M. Waid for helpful comments and suggestions in the preparation of this manuscript and to Mae C. Weglarski and Lani L. Pyles for their technical and editorial assistance.

References

Adrian, E. D., and Matthews, B. H. C. The Berger rhythm: Potential changes from the occipital lobes in man. *Brain*, 1934, *57*, 355–385.

Anand, B. K., Chhina, G. S., and Singh, B. Some aspects of electroencephalographic studies in yogis. *Electroencephalography and Clinical Neurophysiology*, 1961, *13*, 452–456.

Berger, H. Über das Elektrenkephalogramm des Menschen, I. (On the electroencephalogram in man, I.) *Archiv für Psychiatrie und Nervenkrankheiten*, 1929, *87*, 527–570.

Berger, H. Über das Elektrenkephalogramm des Menschen, II. (On the electroencephalogram in man, II.) *Archiv für Psychiatrie und Nervenkrankheiten*, 1930, *40*, 160–179.

Brown, B. B. Recognition of aspects of consciousness through association with EEG alpha activity represented by a light signal. *Psychophysiology*, 1970, *6*, 442–452.

Brown, B. B. Awareness of EEG-subjective activity relationships detected within a closed feedback system. *Psychophysiology*, 1971, *7*, 451–464.

Burch, N. R. Data processing of psychophysiological recordings. In L. D. Proctor and W. R. Adez (Eds.), *Symposium on the analysis of central nervous system and cardiovascular data using computer methods*. Washington: National Aeronautics and Space Administration, 1965. Pp. 165–180.

Chapman, R. M., Armington, J. C., and Bragdon, H. R. A quantitative survey of kappa and alpha EEG activity. *Electroencephalography and Clinical Neurophysiology*, 1962, *14*, 858–868.

COHN, R. The influence of emotion on the human electroencephalogram. *Journal of Nervous and Mental Disease*, 1946, *104*, 351–357.

COSTA, L. D., COX, M., AND KATZMAN, R. Relationship between MMPI variables and percentage and amplitude of EEG alpha activity. *Journal of Consulting Psychology*, 1965, *29*, 90. (Abstract.)

CREUTZFELDT, O., GRÜNEWALD, G., SIMONOVA, O., AND SCHMITZ, H. Changes of the basic rhythms of the EEG during the performance of mental and visuomotor tasks. In C. R. Evans and T. B. Mulholland (Eds.), *Attention in neurophysiology*. New York: Appleton-Century-Crofts, 1969. Pp. 148–168.

CRIDER, A., SHAPIRO, D., AND TURSKY, B. Reinforcement of spontaneous electrodermal activity. *Journal of Comparative and Physiological Psychology*, 1966, *61*, 20–27.

DARROW, C. W., VIETH, R. N., AND WILSON, J. Electroencephalographic "blocking" and "adaptation." *Science*, 1957, *126*, 74–75.

DURUP, G., AND FESSARD, A. L'electrencephalogramme de l'homme: Observations psycho-physiologiques relatives à l'action des stimuli visuels et auditifs. (The electroencephalogram in man: Psychophysiological observations concerning the action of visual and auditory stimuli.) *L'Année Psychologique*, 1935, *36*, 1–32.

ENGEL, B. T., AND CHISM, R. A. Operant conditioning of heart rate speeding. *Psychophysiology*, 1967, *3*, 418–426.

ENGEL, B. T., AND HANSEN, S. P. Operant conditioning of heart rate slowing. *Psychophysiology*, 1966, *3*, 176–187.

EVANS, F. J. Hypnosis and sleep: Techniques for exploring cognitive activity during sleep. In E. Fromm and R. E. Shor (Eds.), *Hypnosis: Research developments and perspectives*. Chicago: Aldine-Atherton, 1972. Pp. 43–83.

FOX, S. S., AND RUDELL, A. P. Operant controlled neural event: Formal and systematic approach to electrical coding of behavior in brain. *Science*, 1968, *162*, 1299–1302.

GLANZER, M., CHAPMAN, R. M., CLARK, W. H., AND BRAGDON, H. R. Changes in two EEG rhythms during mental activity. *Journal of Experimental Psychology*, 1964, *68*, 273–283.

GLASS, A. Mental arithmetic and blocking of the occipital alpha rhythm. *Electroencephalography and Clinical Neurophysiology*, 1964, *16*, 595–603.

GLASS, A. Changes in the prevalence of alpha activity associated with the repetition, performance and magnitude of arithmetical calculations. *Psychologische Forschung*, 1967, *30*, 250–272.

HARDT, J. V., AND KAMIYA, J. Some comments on Plotkin's self-regulation of electroencephalographic alpha. *Journal of Experimental Psychology: General*, 1976, *105*, 100–108.

HART, J. T. Autocontrol of EEG alpha. *Psychophysiology*, 1968, *4*, 506. (Abstract.)

JASPER, H. H. Cortical excitatory state and variability in human brain rhythms. *Science*, 1936, *83*, 259–260.

JOHNSON, L. C., AND ULETT, G. A. Stability of EEG activity and manifest anxiety. *Journal of Comparative and Physiological Psychology*, 1959, *52*,284–288.

KAMIYA, J. Operant control of the EEG alpha rhythm and some of its reported effects on consciousness. In C. T. Tart (Ed.), *Altered states of consciousness: A book of readings*. New York: Wiley, 1969. Pp. 507–517.

KASAMATSU, A., AND HIRAI, T. An electroencephalographic study on the Zen meditation (Zazen). *Folia Psychiatrica et Neurologica Japonica*, 1966, *20*, 315–336.

KREITMAN, N., AND SHAW, J. C. Experimental enhancement of alpha activity. *Electroencephalography and Clinical Neurophysiology*, 1965, *18*, 147–155.

LEGEWIE, H. Subjective correlates of EEG feedback: Discrimination learning or superstition? In EEG alpha learning: State of the art. Symposium presented at the meeting of the Biofeedback Research Society, Monterey, Calif., February 1975.

LEGEWIE, H., SIMONOVA, O., AND CREUTZFELDT, O. D. EEG changes during performance of various tasks under open- and closed-eyed conditions. *Electroencephalography and Clinical Neurophysiology*, 1969, 27, 470–479.

LEMERE, F. The significance of individual differences in the Berger rhythm. *Brain*, 1936, 59, 366–375.

LINDSLEY, D. B. Psychological phenomena and the electroencephalogram. *Electroencephalography and Clinical Neurophysiology*, 1952, 4, 443–456.

LINDSLEY, D. B. Attention, consciousness, sleep and wakefulness. In J. Field, H. W. Magoun, and V. E. Hall (Eds.), *Handbook of physiology, Section 1, Neurophysiology III*. Washington: American Physiological Society, 1960. Pp. 1553–1593.

LORENS, S. A., JR., AND DARROW, C. W. Eye movements, EEG, GSR and EKG during mental multiplication. *Electroencephalography and Clinical Neurophysiology*, 1962, 14, 739–746.

LYNCH, J. J., PASKEWITZ, D. A., AND ORNE, M. T. Some factors in the feedback control of human alpha rhythm. *Psychosomatic Medicine*, 1974, 36, 399–410.

MILLER, N. E., AND DiCARA, L. V. Instrumental learning of heart rate changes in curarized rats: Shaping, and specificity to discriminate stimulus. *Journal of Comparative and Physiological Psychology*, 1967, 63, 12–19.

MULHOLLAND, T. Feedback electroencephalography. *Activitas Nervosa Superior*, 1968, 10, 410–438.

MULHOLLAND, T. B. The concept of attention and the electroencephalographic alpha rhythm. In C. R. Evans and T. B. Mulholland (Eds.), *Attention in neurophysiology*. New York: Appleton-Century-Crofts, 1969. Pp. 100–127.

MUNDY-CASTLE, A. C. The electroencephalogram and mental activity. *Electroencephalography and Clinical Neurophysiology*, 1957, 9, 643–655.

NOWLIS, D. P., AND KAMIYA, J. The control of electroencephalographic alpha rhythms through auditory feedback and the associated mental activity. *Psychophysiology*, 1970, 6, 476–484.

ORNE, M. T., EVANS, F. J., WILSON, S. K., AND PASKEWITZ, D. A. The potential effectiveness of autoregulation as a technique to increase performance under stress. Final summary report to the Advanced Research Projects Agency of the Department of Defense, monitored by the Office of Naval Research under contract N00014-70-C-0350 to the San Diego State College Foundation. Philadelphia: Unit for Experimental Psychiatry, July 1975.

ORNE, M. T., AND PASKEWITZ, D. A. Aversive situational effects on alpha feedback training. *Science*, 1974, 186, 458–460.

PASKEWITZ, D. A. A hybrid circuit to indicate the presence of alpha activity. *Psychophysiology*, 1971, 8, 107–112.

PASKEWITZ, D. A., LYNCH, J. J., ORNE, M. T., AND COSTELLO, J. The feedback control of alpha activity: Conditioning or disinhibition? *Psychophysiology*, 1970, 6, 637–638. (Abstract.)

PASKEWITZ, D. A., AND ORNE, M. T. On the reliability of baseline EEG alpha activity. Paper presented at the meeting of the Society for Psychophysiological Research, Boston, November 1972.

PASKEWITZ, D. A., AND ORNE, M. T. Visual effects on alpha feedback training. *Science*, 1973, 181, 360–363.

PAVLOSKI, R., COTT, A., AND BLACK, A. H. Discrimination and operant control of the occipital alpha rhythm. Paper presented at the meeting of the Eastern Psychological Association, New York, April 1975.

PLOTKIN, W. B. Appraising the ephemeral "alpha phenomenon": A reply to Hardt and Kamiya. *Journal of Experimental Psychology: General*, 1976a, 105, 109–121.

Plotkin, W. B. On the self-regulation of the occipital alpha rhythm: Control strategies, states of consciousness, and the role of physiological feedback. *Journal of Experimental Psychology: General*, 1976b, *105*, 66–99.

Pollen, D. A., and Trachtenberg, M. C. Some problems of occipital alpha block in man. *Brain Research*, 1972, *41*, 303–314.

Rosenfeld, J. P., Rudell, A. P., and Fox, S. S. Operant control of neural events in humans. *Science*, 1969, *165*, 821–823.

Schwartz, G. E. Voluntary control of human cardiovascular integration and differentiation through feedback and reward. *Science*, 1972, *175*, 90–93.

Schwartz, G. E. Toward a theory of voluntary control of response pattern in the cardiovascular system. In P. A. Obrist, A. H. Black, J. Brener, and L. V. DiCara (Eds.), *Cardiovascular psychophysiology*. Chicago: Aldine, 1974, Pp. 406–440.

Schwartz, G. E. Biofeedback, self-regulation, and the patterning of physiological processes. *American Scientist*, 1975, *63*, 314–324.

Schwartz, G. E. Biofeedback and physiological patterning in human emotion and consciousness. Paper presented at the NATO Symposium on Biofeedback and Behavior, Munich, Germany, July 1976a.

Schwartz, G. E. Self-regulation of response patterning: Implications for psychophysiological research and therapy. *Biofeedback and Self-Regulation*, 1976b, *1*, 7–30.

Shapiro, D., Tursky, B., Gershon, E., and Stern, M. Effects of feedback and reinforcement on the control of human systolic blood pressure. *Science*, 1969, *163*, 588–590.

Stennett, R. G. The relationship of alpha amplitude to the level of palmar conductance. *Electroencephalography and Clinical Neurophysiology*, 1957, *9*, 131–138.

Storm van Leeuwen, W. (Chm.), Bickford, R., Brazier, M. A. B., Cobb, W. A., Dondey, M., Gastaut, H., Gloor, P., Henry, C. E., Hess, R., Knott, J. R., Kugler, J., Lairy, G. C., Leob, C., Magnus, O., Oller Daurella, L., Petsche, H., Schwab, R., Walter, W. G., and Widen, L. Proposal for an EEG terminology by the Terminology Committee of the International Federation for Electroencephalography and Clinical Neurophysiology. *Electroencephalography and Clinical Neurophysiology*, 1966, *20*, 293–320.

Surwillo, W. W. The relation of amplitude of alpha rhythm to heart rate. *Psychophysiology*, 1965, *1*, 247–252.

Thiesen, J. W. Effects of certain forms of emotion on the normal electroencephalogram. *Archives of Psychology*, 1943, *40*, No. 285.

Travis, T. A., Kondo, C. Y., and Knott, J. R. Subjective aspects of alpha enhancement. *British Journal of Psychiatry*, 1975, *127*, 122–126.

Ulett, G. A., and Gleser, G. The effect of experimental stress upon the photically activated EEG. *Science*, 1952, *115*, 678–682.

Ulett, G. A., Gleser, G., Winokur, G., and Lawler, A. The EEG and reaction to photic stimulation as an index of anxiety-proneness. *Electroencephalography and Clinical Neurophysiology*, 1953, *5*, 23–32.

Walsh, D. H. Interactive effects of alpha feedback and instructional set on subjective state. *Psychophysiology*, 1974, *11*, 428–435.

Wenger, M. A., and Bagchi, B. K. Studies of autonomic functions in practitioners of yoga in India. *Behavioral Science*, 1961, *6*, 312–323.

Wilson, S. K., Orne, M. T., and Paskewitz, D. A. Individual differences in the interaction between alpha density and arousal. Paper presented at the meeting of the Society for Psychophysiological Research, San Diego, October 1976.

10 Passive Meditation: Subjective, Clinical, and Electrographic Comparison with Biofeedback

Charles F. Stroebel and Bernard C. Glueck

Early in this decade, a number of investigators began to study a variety of meditation-relaxation techniques that offered promise as alternatives to the increasingly widespread use, and abuse, of minor tranquilizers for alleviation of the discomfort and disability caused by stress-related disorders. At about this same time the concept of holistic medicine formally emerged, with an emphasis on individual self-responsibility in preventing and recovering from illness. Physicians, too, were developing an awareness of the limitations of scientific-technical medicine, which surgically or pharmacologically alters the body while ignoring the person, his personality, his memory, and important interpersonal issues. Animal studies confirmed this new awareness, correlating environmental stress with increases in mammary cancer, in hypertension, and even in the lymphocytic immune response to antigens. Further, consensus among anecdotal reports suggested that 50-70% of all complaints in general medical practice were stress-related, so that the symptom would not have occurred, or would have been less severe, in the absence of stress.

The potential of a nonpharmacological modality for dealing with stress thus had far-ranging implications, particularly if it were to operate at an earlier stage in the stress response mechanism than do chemicals. Minor tranquilizers and hypnotics are poor "soma" at best, only partially extinguishing the blaze once it has been kindled and at the same time frequently encouraging the user, through symptom

---

CHARLES F. STROEBEL AND BERNARD C. GLUECK · Research Department, Institute of Living, Hartford, Connecticut.

relief, to take on even more stress. The adaptation to new stress stimuli under this tranquilizer-dependent state, called *state-dependent learning*, is an important mechanism in tranquilizer tolerance and serves to enhance even further a person's proneness to perceive anxiety-stress stimuli when none really exist.

What is stress? Stress may be operationally defined as any perceived stimulus (extra- or intrapsychic) that elicits the normally adaptive, protective emergency fight-or-flight response. Cannon (1932) described the initial sympathetic nervous system activation of this response for immediate readiness to fight or flee, and Selye (1950) described the subsequent corticosteroid sequelae of chronic activation. Freud (1911), Miller (1948), and Rado (1969) differentiated the response into (1) real dangers to the body that require an emergency response (primary fear—an appropriate response) and (2) acquired or conditioned fears, called *anxiety*, where a previously neutral stimulus acquires the capacity, through classical conditioning, to elicit the genetically specified emergency response mechanism (anxiety, or secondary or acquired fear, which may be appropriate, called *signal anxiety*, or inappropriate, called *psychosomatic* or *neurotic anxiety*). Modern man, facing more frequent mental and less frequent physical conflict with an intricate system of symbolic representation (language) and an oftentimes rich fantasy life, begins to activate his emergency response system inappropriately with regard to time, place, and person. The "red alert" emergency response system for protection against real danger to the body is a protective genetic given; the "pink emergency," or even "white emergency" (imagined stress or threat), of acquired fear or anxiety is not. Chronic or inappropriate activation of the emergency response, termed *dysponesis* or "faulty effort" by Whatmore and Kohli (1974), is an unfortunate consequence of the pace of Western society and is a precipitating or exacerbating factor in the onset and/or expression of all forms of illness. Need it be inevitable?

Studies on state-dependent learning clearly suggest that even were an ideal "soma" (Huxley, 1932) to become available, man would reacquire the ability to sense stress in an increasingly perverted symbolic fashion, and inappropriately at that. It was from this basis that we began our studies on the concept of nonpharmacological intervention for the regulation of stress some seven years ago.

I. OVERVIEW OF THIS CHAPTER

This chapter presents a summary of studies we have conducted since 1970 into a variety of self-responsibility techniques that alter consciousness to create states that are incompatible with the fight-or-flight response to stress. Specific techniques investigated have included EEG alpha–theta enhancement biofeedback, EMG-thermal biofeedback, autogenic training, progressive relaxation, and three forms of passive meditation, including Carrington's derivative, clinically standardized meditation (CSM) (1977), Benson's derivative known as the *relaxation response* (Benson, Beary, and Carol, 1974), and the currently popular parent version, transcendental meditation (TM). In contrast to many idiosyncratic, esoteric, and ascetic yogic techniques, all of those studied seemed suited for incorporation into the life style of Western man. Our studies have varied in their formality and sequence but have in common central themes:

1. *Psychological.* Are there discernible differences in the effectiveness of these techniques with different personality styles, perceptual-orienting types, and diagnosed psychiatric conditions? Are there contraindications based on these issues? Does a technique encourage a fundamental change in orientation of a life style to stress, or does it function more like a tranquilizer, permitting the subject to encounter ever newer, more complex stress? Does the technique encourage long-term compliance?

2. *Physiological–physical.* Can the various techniques be differentiated physiologically? Striking here was the universality of reports for the different techniques of enhancement of the EEG alpha rhythm. Could direct training in enhancement of alpha rhythm *per se* provide an optimal strategy?

3. *Interaction–behavioral medicine.* The chapter concludes that an interaction of psychological and physiological factors is of crucial importance in unraveling the variance contained in the questions above.

II. Biofeedback

Prior to the introduction of the concept of biofeedback, Western scientists lacked a meaningful model for studying the voluntary self-regulation of visceroautonomic body functions achieved via hypnosis and/or Eastern meditation techniques. In fact, until recently, psychologists taught that it was impossible to condition the autonomic nervous system, smooth muscles, and glands by other than classical Pavlovian techniques. This assertion was in contrast to the very complex types of operant conditioning procedures employed in the behavioral laboratory, which enabled investigators to teach a wide range of mammals intricate skeletal muscle performance tasks. In 1960, Kimmel and Hill demonstrated the possibility of instrumental conditioning of the galvanic skin response (GSR). Since then, there have been reports of learned control of a wide range of autonomic nervous system responses, including the GSR (Shapiro, Crider, and Tursky, 1964; Fowler and Kimmel, 1962); heart rate (Engel and Chism, 1967; Engel and Hansen, 1966); blood pressure (DiCara and Miller, 1968); salivation (Delse and Feather, 1968); and the relaxation of striated muscle (Budzynski, Stoyva, and Adler, 1970).

Biofeedback provided a comparative scientific model for operational examination of altered states of consciousness and visceroautonomic self-regulation achieved by whatever means—yoga, hypnosis, or drugs. In contrast to our conscious awareness of the five senses, and the extensive kinesthetic-position feedback from the striate musculature, functional reporting at the conscious level from smooth muscles, glands, and the gamma efferent regulation of striate muscle tension is meager, except under conditions of malfunction. The major sensation with malfunction of the latter systems is the relatively crude sensation of pain, sometimes referred to a distant dermatome. In other words, we are relatively unaware of blood pressure, of gastrointestinal peristaltic activity, of cardiac mechanics, and of vasomotor regulation—the "involuntary" inner machinery of the body—except when significant malfunction occurs. While the adaptive regulation of inner machinery under conditions of normality indicates that relatively precise proprioception of its functioning does occur, this reporting is largely at an unconscious level, probably not ascending above the limbic system, and is not normally under "voluntary" control.

The basic psychophysiological principle of biofeedback is the provision of *parallel external proprioception* via an external biofeedback loop, so that an inner machinery function becomes observable at the conscious level. This proprioception is accomplished with suitable sensors (electrical, thermal, pressure, etc.), electronics, and audio, visual, or tactile feedback signals. Considerable experimental controversy currently exists as to how animals and man use this parallel external proprioception to gain voluntary control of the inner machinery function in question (e.g., operant conditioning, mediation, suggestion, placebo effect, etc.) (Stroebel and Glueck, 1973). However, voluntary control has now been demonstrated for many physiological systems under relatively passive learning conditions (i.e., voluntary control is difficult to demonstrate if the subject "tries too hard").

Procedures for self-regulation with biofeedback may be operationally specified, permitting laboratory scrutiny of relevant variables. For example, once a subject has acquired voluntary control over a visceral effector mechanism, it is possible to measure reaction times, as has been traditionally done with striate motor responses in psychology laboratories. Upon presentation of a stimulus, the subject is instructed to alter visceral functioning in a specific direction. The measured stimulus-response interval is the reaction time, as shown for seven variables in Table 1. These data suggest that parallel proprioception probably should not be instantaneous; instead, a time lag should be introduced into the extrinsic feedback circuit that is suitable for the function in question. This hypothesis has been tested in irritable colon patients, in whom the fastest learning of control of colonic motility occurred when biofeedback signals correlated with colonic activity lag by 6-9 sec. We surmise that the intrinsic proprioceptive report of colonic activity requires 6-9 sec to reach the unconscious brain via relatively slowly conducting general visceral afferent neurons.

In addition to its applicability in the treatment of a wide variety of psychosomatic conditions, biofeedback has provided psychophysiologists with an exciting new research strategy. Namely, biofeedback can be used to create a physiological steady state, that is, making some aspect of the physiological state a constant, permitting examination of the associated state of consciousness, both mentation and feelings. Normally, psychophysiologists must deal with a complicated mixture of additive and multiplicative factors, as shown in Figure 1. Psychophysiological variance may be divided into components assignable to physiology (P), behavior (B), and their interaction(I). In the analysis of a psychophysiological outcome, the effect of the last term (I) is crucial to an interpretation of the other two. For when the interaction is zero, the physiological and behavioral components are related to psychophysiological variance in a simple additive fashion, but when interaction is nonzero, vastly more complicated multiplicative relationships must be considered as well.

TABLE 1
Reaction Times for Voluntary Control of Seven Visceroautonomic Functions:
Pilot Study Data ($N = 5$)

Function	Median reaction time
EEG alpha blocking	0.3 sec
EEG alpha enhancement	0.75 sec
Heart rate change	1 sec
Hand warming	2 sec
Foot warming	3 sec
Electrodermal response	3 sec
Colonic motility change	6-9 sec

σ^2_{pp} Psychophysiological Variance	=	$\sigma^2_{physiology}$	+	$\sigma^2_{behavioral}$	+	$\sigma^2_p \times \sigma_b$ interaction	
Black Box Model	σ^2_{pp}	=	k^2	+	σ^2_b	+	$k \times \sigma_b$
Black Environment Model	σ^2_{pp}	=	σ^2_p	+	k^2	+	$\sigma_{p} \times k$

FIGURE 1. Schematic paradigm showing physiological, behavioral, and interactive components of psychophysiological (psychosomatic) variance. In the black box model, the physiological component is held constant. In the black environment model, the behavior component is held constant.

To take advantage of the simplicity of the additive relationship, neurophysiologists classically study the effects of drugs on nervous system functioning with immobilized (curarized or anesthetized) animal preparations with the environment held constant; this familiar black environment experiment holds interactive effects relatively constant. Similarly, pharmacologists study the effect of drugs on some aspect of physiological functioning in situations in which the environment is clearly limited, such as with isolated gut or isolated nerve preparations. Using comparable logic but a different strategy, experimental psychologists have studied the effects of drugs on the behavior of inbred animals with similar genetic constitutions, where p is relatively constant; this is the familiar black box experiment. In either the black box or the black environment experiments, the complexities of interpreting the multiplicative effects (exponential, logarithmic, rank reversal, or other) ascribable to interaction variance are minimized. Psychophysiologists, on the other hand, favor more realistic designs approximating real life in which both behavioral and physiological factors may vary; this situation is more like that faced by the clinician, who is confronted with a sick patient who needs help now, despite the presence of many complicating nonadditive factors.

Biofeedback, then, has enhanced the psychophysiologist's research armamentarium by permitting him to create a variety of relative physiological steady states in subjects under a variety of conditions. An analogy would be the mathematician's use of assymptotes and intercept crossings to analyze boundary properties of a mathematical function.

An example covering an area relative to this chapter may make this point clearer. Brown (1970) and Stroebel and Glueck (1973) created electroencephalographic (EEG) steady states by setting filters to provide biofeedback signals for three classically defined bands of EEG activity: theta, 4–7.5 Hz; alpha 8–12 Hz; and beta 20–35 Hz. Once a subject had achieved criterion levels of enhancement of activity in a given band, he was asked to describe his mental activity at the time (1) subjectively and (2) more objectively, using a variant of the Clyde Mood Scale (Clyde, 1963) adjective checklist. The results are tabulated in rank order along a spectrum of EEG activity in Figure 2.

Once an altered steady physiologic state has been achieved, psychological factors determine how the altered physiological state is subjectively interpreted. Orne (1962) has described some of these psychological factors as the "demand characteristics" of the situation, for example, the subject's expectations of a possible alteration in mood, or "high," from the experience, or implicit/explicit suggestions or cues provided by the experimenter (Stroebel and Glueck, 1973).

It is a distinct possibility that certain of the EEG states (theta and alpha) may make subjects especially prone to suggestion and/or uncritical of primary process thoughts, conceivably enhancing hypnotic phenomena and/or free association in psychoanalytic psychotherapy.

An alternative explanation for variations in subjects' mood reports correlated with a specific band of EEG activity would be the dissociation of EEG patterns and behavioral arousal that has been demon-

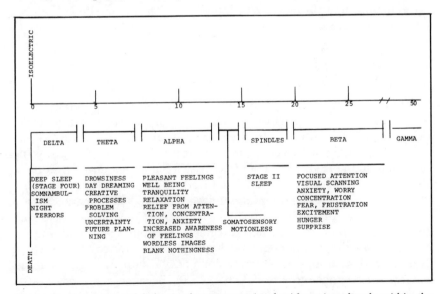

FIGURE 2. Emotions and behavioral states associated with various bands within the spectrum of EEG activity stabilized as steady states using EEG biofeedback.

strated pharmacologically and in sensory deprivation experiments (Bradley, 1958; Mathews, 1971; Zubek, 1969). For example, Lynch and Paskewitz (1971) have suggested that alpha biofeedback has certain similarities to sensory deprivation, including elimination of patterned external stimulation and unfocusing of attention. The important point is that all these many possible sources of variation may be manipulated systematically in the context of a relatively steady state achieved through biofeedback. This powerful new experimental procedure will very likely serve as the basis for many doctoral dissertations in years ahead, including the manipulation of other independent variables, such as drug states, illness states, etc.

Schwartz (1975) has extended this model, providing biofeedback for patterns of response for multiple variables. His work has emphasized that since variables such as blood pressure are multiply determined, some form of patterned biofeedback will probably be optimal in the treatment of conditions like essential (idiopathic) hypertension. This will very likely be the case for other psychosomatic illnesses as well.

As noted in Figure 2, most subjects report positive kinds of feelings—such as relaxed, floating, peaceful, very pleasant, and free from anxiety—as the main subjective awareness at the time that alpha frequencies are occurring. An occasional subject may report some feeling of discomfort from the detachment of dissociative feelings that arise at this time (Brown, 1970; Lynch and Paskewitz, 1971; Stroebel and Glueck, 1973).

III. PASSIVE MEDITATION

EEG patterns during passive meditation states also generally show an increase in the densities of alpha rhythms, particularly in the occipital areas, with a tendency toward a slowing of the alpha frequency, a gradual sweeping forward toward the frontal areas of the dominant alpha frequencies, and an occasional appearance of trains of theta waves, especially in the frontal leads (Banquet, 1973).

What might be termed the relaxed alpha state, marked by a predominance of alpha density in the EEG—whether achieved through EEG biofeedback, passive meditation, autogenic training, or naturally as the hypnogogic or hypnopompic transitions between waking and sleeping—is clearly incompatible with the fight-or-flight emergency response to stress (Selye, 1950). Because many psychiatric patients activate the emergency response system at inappropriate times and with inappropriate or misperceived stimuli, speculation has been widespread that training in self-recognition and voluntary control of the alpha state would be a useful adjunct in the treatment of emotional disorder. Would one alpha-state relaxation technique be preferable over others for patients with different psychiatric conditions?

In 1972, we began a study to answer this question, comparing progressive relaxation training, alpha EEG biofeedback, and a passive meditation technique as treatment adjuncts with a variety of psychiatric conditions in an inpatient setting where average length of stay is 5.5 months.

After investigating a number of meditation techniques, we decided specifically to evaluate transcendental meditation (TM) as our passive meditation procedure for the following reasons: the technique is standardized, with a large cadre of trained instructors available in most locales (hence, replication of the instruction and basic technique should pose no problems); the technique is simple, requiring 4–6 hr of verbal instruction and practice, and is entirely mental, not requiring physical exercise, special diets, or other ascetic demands; and published studies (Wallace, 1970a,b) had already documented physiological changes consistent with the relaxation response. Very briefly, TM is a mantra-type passive-relaxation technique that was introduced to the Western world in its present form by Maharishi Mahesh Yogi. The technique is quite simple, consisting of sitting comfortably, with eyes closed, for 20 min twice a day and thinking to oneself a Sanscrit sound, a mantra, that has been given to the meditator by a teacher of the technique.[1]

In the summer of 1971, we ran extensive psychophysiological studies on a number of subjects who were TM meditators of from four to six years' experience. Several of these individuals has been through the more intensive training process involved in becoming teachers of TM. These were all individuals under the age of 30, and all were males. Without exception, they showed significant amounts of spontaneous alpha on the EEG and showed considerable ability to control alpha density, being able to turn alpha on and off on request without the assistance of a biofeedback signal. In addition, two of the subjects who had been meditating longer periods of time showed frequent epochs of slower wave production in the theta range, with occasional delta density uncorrelated with eye movements. A number of the physiological changes described by Wallace (1970a,b)—for example, slowing of the heart rate, slowing of respiration, and an increase in the galvanic skin resistance (GSR)—were replicated in our studies,

[1] For a more detailed description, see Robins and Fisher (1972) or Forem (1973).

with the most consistent finding being a universal increase in the GSR in all subjects (up to 30% increase over baseline), although we never saw the extreme changes described by Wallace in his original studies (up to 400%).

The subjective reports of these meditators were generally positive, the meditational state being described as a special kind of free-floating attentional state that is essentially nonverbal and nonconceptual in nature, a state of restful alertness. All of these skilled meditators reported a marked reduction in their levels of anxiety and tension subsequent to starting regular daily meditation.

As a result of these findings, we began a series of experiments designed to test this hypothesis, namely, that if we could train volunteer subjects to produce increased alpha densities in their EEGs, we would help them toward a less tense and anxious general level of adaptation. The subjects were all volunteers, mainly college students and other young adults. The ability of these subjects to produce spontaneous alpha, particularly from the occipital areas, simply by sitting relaxed and closing the eyes varied considerably. It seemed to be related to the amount of psychopathology present in an individual as described on a self-report, the Minnesota Multiphasic Personality Inventory (MMPI) and on evaluation by two psychiatrist-observers during the course of the study.

In general, the higher the level of psychopathology, the greater the difficulty experienced by the subject in producing spontaneous alpha rhythms during eyes-closed control sessions. This same general pattern followed through during the biofeedback conditioning, with those subjects who produced the greatest amount of spontaneous alpha seeming to show a more rapid development of good control in turning alpha on or off on demand, frequently achieving maximum performance by the 10th training session. In contrast, three of the subjects who had the greatest amount of psychopathology experienced great difficulty in controlling their alpha frequencies and never really approached consistent performance over the entire 20-hour-long training trial.

The subjective reports of the alpha subjects during the alpha-on condition were generally feelings of well-being. However, a few of the subjects reported some discomfort, especially a feeling of lightheadedness or dizziness immediately after the sessions, which persisted for an hour or two.

A third approach to providing the increased general relaxation of the alpha state is the methods originally described as autogenic training by Schultz and Luthe (1959) and more recently formalized by Luthe (1965) and progressive relaxation by Jacobson (1929) and Wolpe and Lazarus (1966). Similar claims of reductions in the general levels of anxiety and tension have been made for this approach, which consists in gradually attempting to relax the voluntary musculature in a progressive fashion, starting with the toes and feet and sweeping upward to involve the whole body.

In the summer of 1972, we designed a research project to test the relative efficacy of these three types of general relaxation techniques in psychiatric inpatients at a private psychiatric hospital. Our reasons for utilizing three comparison groups were based upon the obvious impossibility of designing a blind study utilizing intervention techniques that demanded specific behavior activity obvious to everyone. A second important limitation was our inability to use the kind of strict controls of other treatment variables that would be preferred in a tight research design, since this would involve withholding other known effective treatment techniques in order to test the efficacy of these three unknown intervention modalities.

Patients were evaluated before beginning the study on the following psychophysiological measures: EEG recordings from eight channels—the right and left frontal, parietal, temporal, and occipital areas[2]; respiration, as recorded by a nasal thermistor; eye movements from bilateral leads over the external canthus; EKG from right and left wrist leads; and silver-silver chloride electrodes and isotonic saline paste for measurement of skin conductance between the middle finger and the wrist of the subject's right hand.

Measures of the patient's behavioral state and level of psychopathology were obtained by: a self-report, the MMPI, standardized descriptors of behavior obtained by the research psychiatrist and research staff utilizing the Minnesota Hartford Personality Assay (MHPA), and the automated daily nursing notes in use at the hospital, which give daily quantified measures of levels of acceptable behavior, anxiety, depression, antisocial behavior, disorganization, etc., as observed by nursing personnel on the patient's unit. These evaluations were repeated at intervals during the 16 weeks of the study.

In an attempt to equalize the amount of individual and group attention being given to the patients in the project, determined primarily by the amount of time spent by the TM instructors with the patients learning to meditate, we expected patients in all three groups to spend up to 20 min twice a day (which is the usual routine for the

---

[2] Electrode placements correspond to a modified International 10-20 Numeric system with leads placed over the frontal pole, the anterior temporal lobe, the posterior temporal lobe, the occipital pole, the motor area, and the parietal lobe of each hemisphere, plus a vertex lead. Reference electrodes for monopolar recordings are placed on the left and right ear lobe. A ground electrode is placed over the left mastoid bone.

meditators) practicing their technique and also to meet weekly as a group, since this was also part of the plan for the meditators.

Two groups of six patients each were started in the Wolpe-Lazarus version of progressive relaxation training to produce general relaxation. For the first 2–3 weeks, the novelty of the activity held their attention. However, it was rapidly apparent that they were not experiencing much in the way of a positive kind of subjective experience from the relaxation attempts and began to find the relaxation exercises quite boring. As a result, by their fourth week in the project, all of these patients had asked to stop, with some asking to switch to one of the other two experimental groups.

Most patients assigned to the EEG alpha biofeedback training were able to learn to control alpha density after 15 training sessions. They had considerable difficulty, however, in applying this training when they were not getting the biofeedback signals. This difficulty appeared to be related to an inadequate set of cues that would indicate to them when they were in the alpha state. For a number of patients in the alpha biofeedback group, the attempts to produce alpha resulted in an increase in tension and anxiety, because of the uncertainty about the results, and did little to promote the relaxation and tranquility that were the primary goals of the technique. We therefore terminated the alpha EEG biofeedback phase of the project after 26 patients had been through this type of biofeedback training.

Recently, other investigators, especially Green (1974), have reported that patients can learn effective control of alpha EEG and theta EEG densities if the biofeedback training is continued for a period of up to four months. Further investigation of this possibility certainly is necessary, but an argument against it would be the impracticality of this approach, which might require one hour a day of subject time five days a week for a period of four months, for a relatively small number of patients, over this long period of time. In contrast, learning passive meditation is a relatively simple matter that can be done quite easily and that requires no special equipment of any sort to learn.

The third experimental group consisted of patients who were taught to meditate using the TM technique. We decided to use a somewhat different procedure with our psychiatric patients from that followed in the usual course of instruction to the general public. Since, on occasion, individuals do experience considerable distress, both psychological and physical, during the early stages of meditation, usually stemming from a misunderstanding of the instructions or a misuse of the technique, we felt that our psychiatric patients might need a longer and more continuous follow-up period than is ordinarily given in order to learn to meditate properly. As a result, we established a policy of daily checking of the meditation process by the teacher during the first three weeks, meeting once a week as a group and individually on the other days. We believe that in most of our patients, this precautionary measure has minimized serious psychological or physiological upset that might have been a consequence of starting to meditate. One indication that this in fact has been the case is the relatively low attrition rate in the patients who have learned to meditate. Of the 261 patients who were taught TM in the hospital, 51 patients (19%) stopped meditating regularly—that is, at least once a day—during the first weeks after learning the technique. However, 35 of these patients did meditate occasionally and were quite cooperative in continuing with the data collection for the research project. Only 16 patients (6%) both stopped meditating entirely and refused further data collection in the project.

The loss of the two comparison groups—the alpha EEG biofeedback group and the relaxation training group—created a problem in the evaluation of the results obtained by the patients who were practicing TM, for the reasons discussed above. In an effort to provide a comparison group, we matched each patient in the experimental group with a "twin" in the general population of the hospital. This matching was done on the basis of sex, age within three years, and similarity of self-description on the MMPI, as indicated by a statistical analysis of the profile type. Some of the outcome data are based on a comparison between these two groups and the full hospital population. In addition, for the experimental group, their previous behaviors in the hospital, as indicated by the nursing-note factor scores and the medications utilized, provide a useful comparison of the patients' progress in the hospital before and after starting TM, permitting analysis by variable baseline crossover design (Blanchard and Young, 1974).

Clinical outcome data comparing TM patients and their matched controls receiving just the usual hospital treatment plan overwhelmingly favored the TM group by whatever measure has been evaluated (condition on discharge, MMPI admission–discharge difference scores, daily automated nursing-note evaluation of psychopathology, decrease in medication for insomnia, etc., with TM versus match group p values ranging from 0.05 to 0.001 using t tests and chi-square tests of significance, as appropriate) (Glueck and Stroebel, 1975).

What can be concluded from the clinical data of this study? First, passive meditation did not have an adverse effect on psychiatric inpatients, 40% of whom were diagnosed as schizophrenic. Second, a majority of patients subjectively reported that the calming effect of TM played a significant role in their recovery. Third, passive meditation was accepted more readily with longer compliance than training in progressive relaxation or EEG alpha rhythm enhancement.

However, we cannot conclude with certainty that passive meditation *per se* had any therapeutic value because of the difficulty in running controlled double-blind studies on patients with the current status of informed-consent regulations. The meditation patients were exposed to many demand characteristics that the matched group were not. For example, the meditation patients received considerable extra attention from charismatic instructors; they acquired a sense of importance from being members of an "elite" research group; and they had a sense of personal gain, receiving at no cost the TM training for which they would have paid outside the hospital. There was even some indication that the matched group felt shortchanged, as a goodly number requested that they be admitted to the research study, which was permitted only after their medical records had been accumulated for comparison purposes during a minimum of 16 weeks of hospitalization.

As data collection for the meditation study was nearing completion, two derivative passive meditation techniques very similar to TM emerged that will facilitate evaluation of the efficacy of TM *per se* but will require new studies. The first is the Benson relaxation response, which uses progressive relaxation, quiet breathing, and the mantra *one*. The second is Carrington's clinically standardized meditation, which permits the beginning meditator to experiment and self-select his own mantra from a list of 16 Sanskrit mantras. More recently, the public press has published a report revealing (accuracy unverified) that age to the nearest five years is the technique used for assigning one of 16 "secret" TM mantras. Additionally, ongoing research investigating the use of biofeedback for a variety of psychosomatic conditions has indicated that our original hypothesis—that EEG alpha enhancement would be the ideal comparison for the alpha state produced during passive meditation—was very likely an error.

Experience in our psychophysiology clinic, as well as in many other centers, strongly indicates that a combination of EMG frontal biofeedback (to lower the set point of the gamma efferent system of striate muscle tension) and thermal feedback (in which hand warming is accomplished by a lessening of vasoconstriction of smooth muscle in arteries) is an optimal strategy in enabling patients to produce a relaxed state correlated with enhanced alpha density. Further, with practice (4-6 months), the biofeedback state of reduced striate and smooth muscle tension can be achieved with a latency of several seconds, even with eyes open while the subject is carrying on fairly normal "Type A" behavior. This procedure is in marked contrast to passive meditation procedures, which require two 15-min quiet periods each day. We suspect that guilt over failing to adhere to this schedule is a major reason why people stop meditating.

This raises the issue of long-term compliance with self-responsibility relaxation–alpha state techniques. For general relaxation purposes, we have observed the following rank order of attrition rate with compliance from high to low at three-month follow-up: TM (80%) > Carrington's CSM, (60%) > Benson relaxation response (25%) > EMG–thermal biofeedback (10%). We are currently investigating the roles of personality style, perceptual orienting style, hypnotic suggestability, and the demand characteristics of each technique (very high for TM with its secrets and mystique, very low for biofeedback for general relaxation). In contrast, compliance is very high for EMG–thermal biofeedback applied to *specific* psychosomatic problems where symptom relief is self-reinforcing, as in reduction of headache pain; compliance is much lower for conditions with relatively "silent" symptoms, such as hypertension.

TABLE 2

Potential Applications of Biofeedback: General Stress Reduction and Specific Treatment Objectives

General	Specific

Objectives:
1. Relaxation
2. Lowering of tension
3. Creating states incompatible with emergency fight-or-flight response
EEG alpha biofeedback
EEG theta biofeedback
Frontalis EMG biofeedback
Nonbiofeedback modalities
  Passive meditation—TM
  Benson relaxation response
  Autogenic training
  Progressive relaxation
	Objective: To regulate or lower the activation of a target organ symptom
	Thermal (smooth muscle relaxation)
	  Classic migraine—vascular headache (rapid)
	  Common migraine—vascular headache (slow)
	  Raynaud's disease
	  Irritable colon syndrome
	  Essential hypertension
	  Angina pectoris
	Frontalis EMG
	  Tension—muscular contraction headache
	  Bruxism
	  TMJ syndrome
	Lumbar–sacral EMG
	  Muscular back pain
	EKG
	  Cardiac dysrhythmias
	GSR and thermal
	  Hypertension
	  Stress aspect of eczematous conditions

Based on compliance and the self-reinforcing aspect of specific symptom relief, we have differentiated potential applications of biofeedback into two categories: general stress reduction and specific treatment objectives, as shown in Table 2. Nonbiofeedback modalities with best compliance are probably the techniques of choice for general stress reduction unless a fundamental change in attitude toward preventive medicine occurs, for example, reducing insurance premiums for individuals who demonstrate continuing compliance with a self-responsibility relaxation technique.

IV. ELECTROGRAPHIC STUDIES

Each of the relaxation techniques we have studied produces augmentation of alpha density in subjects with significant alpha rhythm in the eyes-closed baseline condition. While subjects with minimal baseline alpha rhythm achieve very little EEG augmentation, they do report a comparable subjective "alpha state." We recognized that alpha density *per se* was probably only a portion of the physiological variance that was needed to clarify the possible psychophysiological differences among techniques. Our further, more sophisticated evaluation of meditators' EEG records revealed remarkable epochs of intrahemispheric alpha–theta synchrony for experienced subjects. This observation was subsequently confirmed by Banquet (1973) and Levine (1975) in their studies of intra- and interhemispheric EEG synchrony in experienced meditators.

Subsequently, we wrote machine and FORTRAN language programs for our PDP-12, PDP-15, and 15-graphics terminal configuration for analyzing monopolar and/or bipolar eight-channel EEGs[2] for isometric power spectra using the fast Fourier transform and associated measures of coherence and phase angle (for each cycle, 1–30 Hz) for any two placements, and also a measure of synchronicity expressed as a percentage of time that two electrode placements had a coherence greater than 0.80 (possible range is 0–+1.0) and a phase angle within ±20° for the subject's dominant alpha frequency.[3]

Figures 3 and 4 show the isometric power spectrum and coherence-phase angle graphics terminal displays for 1-min samples of an experienced meditator during meditation.

A study is in progress investigating these variables in subjects who are experienced in one of four relaxation techniques, as well as in a small sample of subjects experienced in all four: transcendental

[3] Documentation and calibration techniques for these programs are being published elsewhere or, alternately, may be obtained at reproduction cost from the authors.

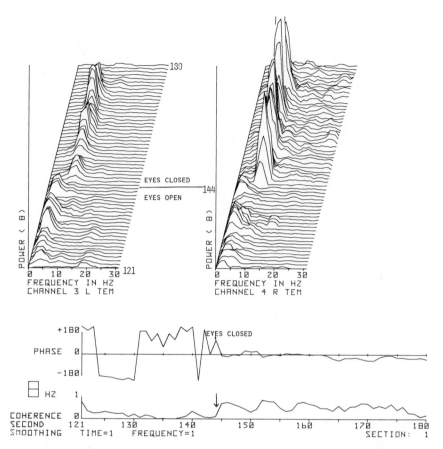

FIGURE 3. This is an isometric display of the power spectrum in an experienced meditator (four years). The two leads shown are from the left and right temporal regions and show 1 min of EEG data analyzed on a second-by-second basis. This is the 3rd minute of the recording and shows the change in the EEG patterns when the eyes are closed. The first 20 sec of the display show the slow frequencies seen with eyes open, probably reflecting eye muscle movement. Immediately after the closing of the eyes at the 140 sec point, the high amplitude alpha frequencies begin to dominate the record at about the 8-Hz frequency, although there is some higher-frequency activity, especially in the right temporal lead. The phase and coherence graphs show the lack of synchronization between the temporal areas during the eyes-open phase and the appearance of a considerable degree of synchronization shown by the movement of the coherence graph toward 1 and the phase angle toward 0 as soon as the eyes are closed.

meditation; the Carrington CSM; the Benson derivative relaxation response; and combined EMG–thermal biofeedback.

Figure 5 shows the interhemispheric synchrony in the upper panel and the intrahemispheric synchrony (dominant side only) in the lower panel for representative individuals experienced in TM (TM), in

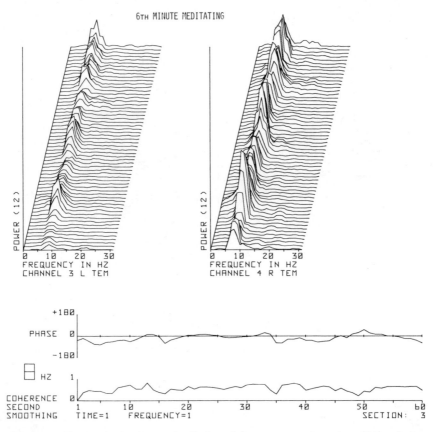

FIGURE 4.   This is another isometric display of the same experienced meditator during the 6th minute of meditation. The leads are from the two temporal areas and show the high degree of synchronization—as shown by the coherence graph approaching 1, and the phase angle graph approaching 0—that is seen in experienced meditators within the first few minutes of starting to meditate.

the relaxation response (RR), and in EMG–thermal biofeedback (BF) (no biofeedback present). Though sample sizes are still small, interesting differences in synchrony are emerging. The percentage of time that the synchrony measure was above criterion was obtained from a 20-min sample of each technique with each subject sitting with eyes closed in a comfortable chair under dim ambient light. Both TM and RR subjects have demonstrated significant interhemispheric synchrony between the temporal placements, while BF subjects have demonstrated virtually none. Compared to TM and BF conditions, RR subjects have had virtually no occipital synchrony. In contrast to TM and RR subjects, the BF subjects have demonstrated a relatively greater amount of intrahemispheric synchrony than have the meditating conditions. While none of the three techniques can be differentiated on the basis of enhancement of the dominant alpha frequency, these data suggest that significant differences do exist for measures of alpha synchrony (high coherence and low phase angle). Studies now under way with the Carrington technique, in which the beginning meditator self-selects the mantra most pleasing to him, may illuminate the issue of mantra uniqueness, which is a central claim of the TM

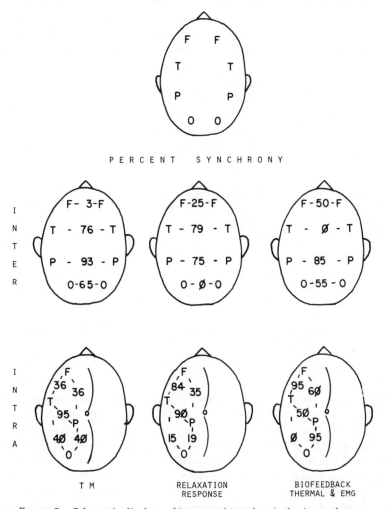

FIGURE 5.   Schematic displays of inter- and intrahemispheric synchrony.

organization. Will certain mantras produce greater degrees of synchrony than others? By age to the nearest five years? Can multiple pattern biofeedback of synchrony *per se* be used to replicate exactly the synchrony patterns that develop with the meditation modalities? (Fehmi, 1975.)

Pending outcome of these studies, we have several speculative hypotheses for interpreting the synchrony observations that are schematically illustrated in Figure 5:

1. *The mantra as a boring habituation stimulus.* This hypothesis suggests that the language-logic functions of the dominant left temporal cortex predominate mental activity under conditions of beta rhythm activation (desynchronization) with a tendency toward symbolic activation of the emergency response; that normalization of visceroautonomic homeostasis, regulated by the normally unconscious right temporal cortex-limbic system, predominates under conditions of alpha-theta synchronous activity; that "Type A" persons feel so much time pressure from depending on left cortical beta activation that they are in a state of relative deprivation of right cortical alpha activation; and that the mantra is a boring stimulus leading to habituation of beta activation and augmentation of alpha-theta synchrony.

2. *The mantra as a critical driver of synchronization.* If the mantra is a key factor in achieving the kinds of psychophysiological changes observed, it may represent an input stimulus to the central nervous system, most likely the limbic circuitry. We have been informed that analysis of the resonance frequencies of a number of mantras gives a value of 6-7 Hz, which is in the high theta EEG range and also approximates the optimal processing of the basic language unit, the phoneme, by the auditory system. (Lenneberg, 1967). Our current speculation is as follows. Since the mantra is a series of sounds, the formation of the thought mantra—for example, *oom,* which is a common, well-known mantra—probably takes place, according to most neurophysiologists, in the ideational speech area in the temporal lobe. Penfield and Roberts (1959) have mapped three areas involved in the ideational elaboration of speech: a large area in the posterior temporal lobe, an area in the posterior-inferior parietal region, and a small area in the posterior part of the third frontal convolution anterior to the motor-voice control area. Penfield and Roberts have claimed that the second two areas can both be destroyed and speech will return, so that the posterior temporal speech area is the fundamental locus for the formation of words. They have stated that the ideational mechanism of speech is organized for function in one hemisphere only, usually the dominant hemisphere. Therefore, when one thinks a

mantra, a significant stimulus is introduced in the temporal lobe and probably directly into the series of cell clusters and fiber tracts that have come to be known as the limbic system. Since limbic system activity is fairly well accepted today as the origin of much emotionally based behavior, and since an increasing excitation in the limbic system through a series of feedback stimulatory mechanisms has been postulated to explain disturbed behavior (Monroe, 1970), we are theorizing that introducing a driving mechanism with a dominant frequency of 6-7 Hz may act, with considerable rapidity, to dampen the limbic system activity and produce a relative quiescence in this critical subcortical area.

Since there are extensive connections running from the thalamic structures to the cortex, quieting the limbic system activity might allow for the inhibition of cortical activation, with the disappearance of the usual range of frequencies and amplitudes ordinarily seen coming from the cortex, and with the imposition of the basic resting or idling rhythms as shown by the appearance of very dense, high-amplitude, alpha wave production.

Similarly, since the autonomic nervous system is controlled to a considerable extent by stimuli arising in the midbrain, the rapid changes observed in the peripheral autonomic nervous system—such as the GSR changes and the change in respiratory rate, heart rate, etc.—could be explained by the quieting of the limbic system activity.

Presumably, in sleep, limbic system activity diminishes, mediated perhaps by the reticular activating system. One of the theories about the appearance of dreams, especially about the ideational content in dreams, has to do with an increasing access to the nondominant hemisphere, where repressed memories are presumably stored. The weakening of the repression barrier that occurs in sleep and in other altered states of consciousness, such as free association during the process of psychoanalytic therapy, *may* be produced in a relatively simple fashion during TM meditation. This phenomenon would offer an explanation of a phenomenon that has been reported by a number of investigators and that we have seen repeatedly in our patients. During meditation, thoughts and ideas may appear that are ordinarily repressed, such as intense hostile–aggressive drives, murderous impulses, and, occasionally, libidinal ideation. An impressive aspect of this phenomenon is that during the meditation, the intense emotional affect that would ordinarily accompany this ideation—for example, when obtained by free association—seems to be markedly reduced or almost absent.

Our speculation is that during passive meditation, the usual affective outflow from limbic structures is diminished, with enhanced

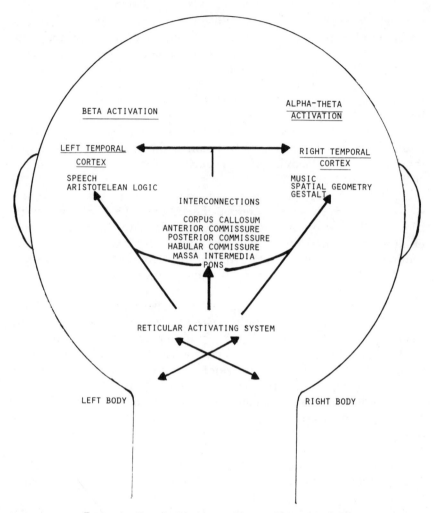

FIGURE 6.   Functional aspects of hemispheric specificity.

transmission of signals between the hemispheres via the corpus callosum or other commissures as shown schematically in Figure 6.

V. OVERVIEW OF CLINICAL INDICATIONS

As a result of approximately six years of experience with a variety of biofeedback procedures and teaching TM to psychiatric in- and outpatients, we feel that for general relaxation and creating a state incompatible with the emergency response, meditation is preferable to biofeedback. However, in patients with a specific psychosomatic symptom—that is, hyperactivation of an end organ supplied by the autonomic nervous system—a specific biofeedback treatment modality may be superior. Patients with a psychosomatic symptom may find a combination of passive meditation and specific biofeedback suitable.

Most members of Western society could benefit from learning a relaxation response that is incompatible with inappropriate fight-or-flight activation. The procedures seem to be particularly efficacious in individuals suffering from chronic anxiety, since with either biofeedback or meditation, the individual is given a relatively automatic stepwise process for relieving anxiety instead of being admonished to "just relax" (Otis, 1974). Biofeedback may have a virtue in that while he is hooked up to the feedback apparatus, the subject can experiment with various kinds of mental content—for example, boss, wife, children, work—to determine what kinds of stimuli activate his somatic reactions.

The generalized relaxation state that TM produces seems to affect most immediately and dramatically those psychiatric patients showing considerable amounts of overt anxiety, manifested by symptoms such as hand tremors, perspiration of hands and feet, "a knot in the pit of the stomach," or, in the present jargon, being "uptight." These individuals often are relieved of anxiety symptoms after the first meditation. Typically, the symptoms return after an interval of one-half hour to several hours, but during the next three to four weeks symptoms gradually subside. Thus, if the patient meditates properly twice a day for 20 min each time, by the end of an eight-week period, most of the overt anxiety symptoms disappear.

Another index of change is seen in the rapidly decreased requirement for night sedation, as chronic insomnia is replaced by a normal restful seven to eight hours of sleep. The need for various antianxiety psychotropic agents also seems to decrease. Patients with marked anxiety symptoms also seem to be more consistent in continuing meditation once they leave the hospital and return to the community.

Patients with more clear-cut overt psychotic symptoms, especially of the schizophrenic variety, also seem to be able to learn to meditate quite easily and show a somewhat slower, but nevertheless impressive, shift in the levels of anxiety, if this shift can be inferred from a decrease in overt psychotic symptoms. However, patients who are suffering from serious depressive symptoms, while able to learn the meditation technique fairly readily, seem to have considerable difficulty in being able to meditate comfortably and successfully twice a day without a great deal of encouragement and support. Of course, this difficulty is no different from these patients' impaired ability to perform any daily tasks because of the impact of the depression. Meditation does not seem to have the same immediate and obvious impact in depression that it does in the anxiety states mentioned above. In fact, four of the patients who were terminated early in the authors' research project were stopped because they received electro-convulsive therapy. All four were able to resume meditating success-fully after the series of ECTs, but the memory loss occasioned by the treatments required a relearning of the meditation technique.

The single most difficult group within the hospital setting appears to be patients under age 21. These patients, most of whom have been heavy users of various drugs, seem to show the least response to the initial meditation experience. To quote one of them, "There's nothing to this compared to the turn-on I get with my drugs." However, those who meditate regularly begin to admit, albeit grudgingly, after a period of eight to nine weeks that they sense changes. These changes seem to be in the general area of improved concentration, improved attention in high school class, and a general decrease in restless, impulsive activity that is part of their general clinical picture.

In contrast to the above, for patients who complain of specific psychosomatic symptoms—such as migraine headache, Raynaud's syndrome, and similar physiological manifestations of underlying chronic anxiety and tension—biofeedback interventions appear to be most effective. In general, the attempts to use TM to relieve psychoso-matic complaints—for example, migraine headaches or hypertension—have not been very effective (Benson, Beary, and Carol, 1974). Perhaps if TM is continued over a period of years, it will affect these stress-related conditions, but the life-threatening physiological changes that are associated with the psychosomatic illnesses do not permit this sort of slow, long-term intervention. The fairly immediate responses (within four to six weeks) achieved by biofeedback interventions provide the kind of prompt relief that these patients apparently require. Once this relief has been achieved, however, the addition of a generalized relaxation technique such as TM might be important for many of these patients, since most of them tend to resist strenuously any suggestion that their difficulties might have a psychological background and refuse any sort of psychiatric referral.

VI. SUMMARY

This chapter has reviewed some of our investigations into a variety of self-responsibility techniques that alter consciousness to create states that are incompatible with the fight-or-flight emergency response to stress. The remarkable range of physiological changes achieved through voluntary self-regulation techniques suggests that man need not be a pitiful victim of psychosomatic and other stress related illnesses.

It is true that once tissue pathology has occurred, whether through infection, trauma, poison, congenital defect, or tumor, external intervention by modern medicine to patch the defect is often impressive and largely beyond the subjective control of the patient. However, the vast majority of ills and the illness-onset situation itself (Shapiro, 1964) are clearly not beyond subjective control. These cannot be the private domain of the doctor–scientist but are a matter of the responsibility of each individual. Modern medicine does not sufficiently emphasize this need for individual responsibility. Acclimated as he is to be a recipient of rather than a participant in treatment, modern man may require personal demonstration through a structured period of self-learning to incorporate the concept of individual responsibility into his daily life-style in times of both health and illness. This learning may best be accomplished at an early age, with the teaching, for example, of the four Rs in the second grade: reading, 'riting, 'rithmetic, and *relaxation*.

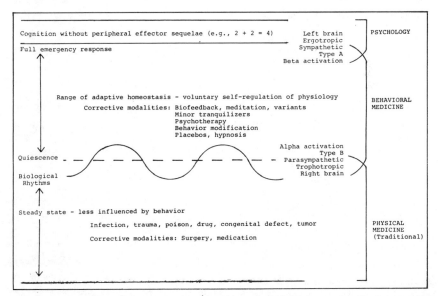

FIGURE 7. Relationships between traditional physical medicine and behavioral medicine.

By definition and tradition, the treatment of illness has been the focus of scientific medicine. The phenomenon of voluntary self-regulation requires that this definition be expanded to include the concept of *psychosomatic health* (Green, Green, Walters, Sargent, and Meyer, 1975). We need to recognize more widely that there is a large domain of our physiological functioning that is responsive to behavioral stimuli, is potentially adaptive, and is vulnerable to disregulation (Schwartz, 1977) as well as to voluntary self-reregulation. This behaviorally modifiable physiological domain is becoming designated as behavioral medicine, a formal recognition of the interaction of physiology and behavior shown in Table 1. Some relationships that have value in helping physicians oriented to traditional physical medicine to understand the concept of behavioral medicine are shown in Figure 7. In this age of organ transplants, we can conclude with certainty that behavioral medicine, using our evolving knowledge of variants of the self-regulation techniques we have discussed in this chapter, is a clearly superior alternative to increasing the use of tranquilizing medications or surgical intervention.

ACKNOWLEDGMENT

The support of the Fannie E. Rippel Foundation in creating the computer programs used in this study is gratefully acknowledged.

REFERENCES

BANQUET, J. P. Spectral analysis of the EEG in meditation. *Electroencephalography and Clinical Neurophysiology*, 1973, 35, 143–151.

BENSON, H., BEARY, J. F., AND CAROL, M. P. The relaxation response. *Psychiatry*, 1974, 37, 37–46.

BLANCHARD, E. B., AND YOUNG, L. D. Clinical applications of biofeedback training. A review of evidence. *Archives of General Psychiatry*, 1974, 30, 573–589.

BRADLEY, P. B. Central action of certain drugs in relation to the reticular formation of the brain. In H. H. Jasper (Ed.), *The reticular formation of the brain*. Boston: Little, Brown, 1958.

BROWN, B. B. Recognition of aspects of consciousness through association with EEG alpha activity represented by a light signal. *Psychophysiology*, 1970, 6, 442.

BUDZYNSKI, T., STOYVA, J., AND ADLER, C. Feedback induced muscle relaxation: Application to tension headache. *Journal of Behavioral and Experimental Psychiatry*, 1970, 1, 205.

CANNON, W. B. *The wisdom of the body*. New York: Norton, 1932.

CARRINGTON, P. *Freedom in meditation*. New York: Anchor Press–Doubleday, 1977.

CLYDE, D. J. The Clyde Mood Scale, Biometrics Laboratory, University of Miami, 1963.

DELSE, C., AND FEATHER, R. The effect of augmented sensory feedback on control of salivation. *Psychophysiology*, 1968, *5*, 15–21.

DiCARA, L., AND MILLER, N. Instrumental learning of systolic blood pressure responses by curarized rats: Dissociation of cardiac and vascular changes, *Psychosomatic Medicine*, 1968, *30*, 489–494.

ENGEL, B. T., AND CHISM, R. A. Operant conditioning of heart rate speeding. *Psychophysiology*, 1967, *3*, 418–428.

ENGEL, B. T., AND HANSEN, S. P. Operant conditioning of heart rate slowing. *Psychophysiology*, 1966, *3*, 563–567.

FEHMI, L. Abstract, *Proceedings of the Biofeedback Research Society*. Denver, Colo., 1975.

FOREM, J. *Transcendental meditation: Maharishi Mahesh Yogi and the science of creative intelligence*. New York: Dutton, 1973.

FOWLER, R., AND KIMMEL, H. Operant conditioning of GSR. *Journal of Experimental Psychology*, 1962, *63*, 536–567.

FREUD, S. (1911). Psycho-analytic Notes on an autobiographical account of a case of paranoia (dementia paranoides). In J. Strachey (Trans.), *Standard edition of the complete psychological works of Sigmund Freud*. London: Hogarth, 1958.

GLUECK, B. C., AND STROEBEL, C. F. Biofeedback and meditation in the treatment of psychiatric illnesses. *Comprehensive Psychiatry*, 1975, *16*, 303–321.

GREEN, E. E. Personal communication, 1974.

GREEN, E. E., GREEN, A. M., WALTERS, E. D., SARGENT, J. D., AND MEYER, R. G. Autogenetic biofeedback training. *Psychotherapy and Psychosomatics*, 1975, *25*, 88–98.

HUXLEY, A. *Brave new world*. New York: Harper-Row, 1932.

JACOBSON, E. *Progressive relaxation*. Chicago: University of Chicago Press, 1929.

KIMMEL, E., AND HILL, R. Operant conditioning of the GSR. *Psychological Reports*, 1960, *7*, 555–562.

LENNEBERG, E. H. *Biological foundation of language*. New York: Wiley, 1967.

LEVINE, P. H., HEBERT, J. R., HAYNES, C. T., AND STROBEL, U. *EEG coherence during the transcendental meditation technique*. Weggis, Switzerland: MERU Press, 1975.

LUTHE, W. *Autogenic training*. New York: Grune & Stratton, 1965.

LYNCH, J. J., AND PASKEWITZ, D. A. On the mechanisms of the feedback control of human brain wave activity. In *Biofeedback and self control*. Chicago: Aldine, 1971.

MATHEWS, A. M. Psychophysiological approaches to the investigation of desensitization and related procedures. *Psychological Bulletin*, 1971, *76*, 73.

MILLER, N. Studies of fear as an acquired drive. *Journal of Experimental Psychology*, 1948, *38*, 89–101.

MONROE, R. R. *Episodic behavioral disorders*. Cambridge, Mass.: Harvard University Press, 1970.

ORNE, M. T. On the social psychology of the psychological experiment: With particular reference to demand characteristics and their implications. *American Psychologist*, 1962, *17*, 776.

OTIS, L. If well integrated but anxious, try TM. *Psychology Today*, 1974, *7*, 45–46.

PENFIELD, W., AND ROBERTS, L. *Speech and brain mechanisms*. Princeton, N.J.: Princeton University Press, 1959.

RADO, S. *Adaptational psychodynamics: Motivation and control*. New York: Science House, 1969.

ROBINS, J., AND FISHER, D. *Tranquility without pills*. New York: Widen, 1972.

SCHULTZ, J. H., AND LUTHE, W. *Autogenic training*. New York: Grune & Stratton, 1959.

SCHWARTZ, G. E. Biofeedback, self-regulation and the patterning of physiologic process. *American Scientist*, 1975, *3*, 314–324.

SCHWARTZ, G. E. Psychosomatic disorders and biofeedback: A psychobiological model of disregulation. In J. Maser and M. E. P. Seligman (Eds.), *Psychopathology: Experimental Models*. San Francisco: Freeman, 1977.

SELYE, H. *The physiology and pathology of exposure to stress*. Montreal: Acta, 1950.

SHAPIRO, A. K. Factors contributing to the placebo effect: Their implications for psychotherapy. *American Journal of Psychotherapy*, 1964, *18*(Suppl. 1), 73-88.

SHAPIRO, D., CRIDER, A. B., AND TURSKY, B. Differentiation of an autonomic response through operant reinforcement. *Psychonomic Science*, 1964, *1*, 147-148.

STROEBEL, C. F., AND GLUECK, B. C. Biofeedback treatment in medicine and psychiatry: An ultimate placebo? *Seminars in Psychiatry*, 1973, *5*, 379-393.

WALLACE, R. K. Physiological effects of transcendental meditation. *Science*, 1970a, *167*, 1751-1754.

WALLACE, R. K. *Physiological effects of transcendental meditation: A proposed fourth state of consciousness*. Ph.D. thesis, Physiology Department, University of California at Los Angeles, 1970b. (Available from Maharishi International University Press, Fairfield, Iowa.)

WHATMORE, G. B., AND KOHLI, D. R. *The physiology and treatment of functional disorders*. New York: Grune & Stratton, 1974.

WOLPE, J., AND LAZARUS, A. A. *Behavior therapy technique, a guide to the treatment of neurosis*. Oxford: Pergamon Press, 1966.

ZUBEK, J. P. Physiology and biochemical effects. In *Sensory deprivation: Fifteen years of research*. New York: Appleton-Century, 1969.

Author Index

Subject Index